# medicine on trial

# medicine on trial

## Dannie Abse

Crown Publishers, Inc.
New York

**Editor** Jeremy Robson

**Designer** Roger Hyde

**Associate Designer** John Wood

**Art Assistant** Endre Boszin

**Picture Research** Lynette Trotter
Naomi Narod
Peter Fairfoul

**Text Research** Joanna Jellinek

Library of Congress Catalog Card Number: 68-57019

First published in the United States in 1969
by Crown Publishers Inc.

© 1967 Aldus Books Limited, London

Printed in Holland by N.V. Drukkerij Senefelder, Amsterdam

# Contents

## Introduction

Ask doctors from any part of the world why they chose to study medicine and the answers will be similar whatever their nationality: because, when young, they were idealistic; because the practice of medicine is an honorable vocation; because it would provide them with a decent standard of living; because there is a shortage of doctors in their country; because there is a tradition of doctors in their family. Not all these reasons will invariably figure, but few medical practitioners will exclude the idealistic one.

The youthful often indulge in rescue fantasies. In their daydreams, and in their night dreams as well, the beautiful and the good and the helpless are frequently saved from harm or death by a heroic protagonist who remarkably resembles the dreamer. Walter Mitty owns many faces, but one of the most popular of his disguises is Dr. Kildare or his counterpart. It is probably true that the urge to rescue the subjugated or the marooned stems, as the Freudians would have it, from our ambiguous desire to save our own mothers from the cruel embraces of the men they married. And it is just too terrible to contemplate why a person should choose to be a surgeon! No matter, whatever subjective factor plays a part in actuating a man to take up this or that career, it in no way argues against the value of the career: the medical profession is an honorable one and we are all honorable men.

I became a doctor not only for the reasons generally given, but also because I saw, when young, Edward G. Robinson in a film about the German bacteriologist Paul Ehrlich called *The Magic Bullet*. I came out of the Olympia Cinema in Cardiff, one Saturday afternoon at half past five, with my eyes shining. Before I had crossed St. Mary's Street, a metaphorical stethoscope in my pocket, I had saved an old lady from asphyxiating, administered first aid to a policeman shot by dockland gangsters, and operated on Adolf Hitler without success.

In due course I entered medical school and received there, like every other medical student in the world, an inadequate education. For almost two years I was taught the mysteries of anatomy and physiology. That I had to spend so many hours in the anatomy room, that students everywhere still have to learn in minute detail the anatomy of the human body (and embryology) seems ridiculous to me and to many other doctors. By the time students qualify most of them have forgotten all but the most important anatomical details. Their cloudy remembrance of the subject makes them no worse doctors, for the knowledge they acquired so obsessively and at such pains, and that they lost with such felicity, is quite useless for the most part in the general practice of medicine. Even those who, as postgraduates, specialize in surgery, have to relearn the subject.

There are those, I suppose, who believe that sooner or later medical students have to face up to the unpleasant realities of sickness and morbidity, and that the anatomy room, with its bodies and bits of bodies laid out on slabs in different stages of dissection, somehow serves as a useful introduction to a vocation where it is obligatory not to be oversensitive. Certainly the students soon become acclimatized to the sharp reek of formaldehyde that has "pickled" the dead bodies, and having hacked away with their silver-colored scalpels they become quickly immune to the grotesque scene of dismembered corpses.

I remember how, a few weeks after the commencement of our anatomy course, I observed one student, who earlier had been particularly fastidious, drop his lighted cigarette accidentally into the open cavity of a dead abdomen. Unthinkingly, he picked his cigarette end up, put it back in his mouth, and went on dissecting with no sense of disquiet or disgust. The medical student soon forgets that the body he is dissecting was once alive. It has become a model. Too often, during the clinical years, the live patient in the same way tends to become a "case." The attitudes absorbed in medical school cannot fail to find expression later when the doctor practices or when he, in turn, teaches a younger generation of medical students. So a tradition is established and only with difficulty modified.

10

My preclinical studies concluded and the examinations passed, I went on to Westminster Hospital, London, where for the first time I was confronted with patients, who repeated their case histories to me and to 12 other students with a quiet desperation. I now studied pathology, pharmacology, midwifery, gynecology, medicine, and surgery. I felt faint at my first operation, I quaked delivering my first baby, I felt a little nauseated at my first postmortem (I had known the patient, alive, in the ward, days earlier), and I winked at the nurses. I was given to understand by inference that medicine was a science—there were all the investigatory tests: the electrocardiograms, the encephalograms, the blood counts, the sedimentation rates, etc.— and I was encouraged to take "the scientific approach." If the Exception did not prove the Rule, then that merely demonstrated there was never such a thing as "never" in medicine. Most of my teachers, like doctors everywhere, had but rudimentary knowledge of human psychology, and the psychiatric wards were only utilized when everything else had failed.

Once a Mr. F. was brought into Casualty and he looked at us with dismal hopelessness. He complained that he was dead.

"Are you sure you're dead?" asked the doctor.

"Yes," said Mr. F.

"Do dead men bleed then?"

"Of course not, doctor."

With triumph the physician took a pin and grazed the skin of the patient, drawing blood. We all stood there quietly for a moment. Puzzled, Mr. F. said slowly, as he vacantly looked down at the little trickle of blood on his forearm: "It just goes to show, doesn't it doctor, that dead men do bleed?" The patient in this case, albeit with a great deal of reluctance on the physician's part, was eventually referred to the psychiatrist, for it seemed he was beyond the hope of real "science."

There were moments, I must confess, when I believed, after this or that small humiliation, or after finding myself in too much empathic correspondence with a suffering patient, that I had chosen the wrong career. I sympathized, then, with the composer Berlioz who, after studying medicine for a time, wrote: "Become a doctor! Study anatomy! Dissect! Witness horrible operations instead of throwing myself heart and soul into the glorious art of music! Forsake the empyrean for the dreary realities of earth! The immortal angels of poetry and love and their inspired songs for filthy hospitals, dreadful medical students, hideous corpses, the shrieks of patients, the groans and death-rattles of the dying. It seemed to be the utter reversal of the natural conditions of my life—horrible and impossible!"

Of course, there are many positive aspects of a medical education, and much, too, that is simply rewarding. Few medical students, however tough, have not experienced their moment of triumph after successfully delivering their first baby. Out of struggle, muscles tensed, shouts, palaver of blood, comes the child. All that has preceded it is forgotten: the voices that kept shouting, "Stop pushing"; the baby's head crowned; the sobbing of the mother; and even the parched face of the critical midwife in attendance. The cord has been cut, the sick-sweet smell of gas is over, and the mother invariably smiles that extraordinary, tender, satisfied smile when she hears, for the first time, the whimper of her own baby that sounds something like a seagull's cry. The rest seems superfluous, a curious trick even, the afterbirth, the blue-jellied cord descending. The student leaves the delivery room pleased. He feels his choice of vocation has been justified, was right after all. He is not displeased with his education. He does not, at this time, question it. He has seen those who have fallen out of "the splendid procession of life." He has seen patients recover. He has seen his teachers revered by others, and perhaps also he has thought with the pathologist A. E. Boycott: "I do not wonder that people die; that is easy enough. What I marvel at is that they go on living with bodies so maimed, disordered, and worn out." He has his final examinations to take.

Eventually I passed these examinations and was given the license I had so long worked for that allowed me to heal or inadvertently to kill. People called me "Doctor," and after a time I learned not to look over my shoulder when thus addressed. Soon I was journeying back to South Wales, having accepted an offer of a three-week locum tenens in my home town. By then I thought *The Magic Bullet* to be a rather corny movie; the old lady asphyxiating no doubt was rehearsing her act yet again in order to be saved by another youth with rescue fantasies; Cardiff policemen were inordinately fit, even if six inches smaller; and Hitler was dead and buried years before. But I returned, in 1950, to South Wales with a real stethoscope in my pocket and aware, as most doctors must be when they first practice, of my too obvious inadequacies.

The doctor who employed me showed me over his surgery while his wife packed the bags before they departed on their holidays. He kept telling me "Not to worry"—the favourite expression of all doctors and one I, there and then, privately swore not to use. The more he reassured me the more he exacerbated my own doubts in my proficiency. I was even more alarmed when he informed me that he generally dispensed medicines himself. "Here," he announced, opening the door of what seemed to be a pantry, "is my little dispensary." A row of large bottles containing different quantities of colored fluids stared at me. I had never dispensed medicines in my life: it had not been part of the hospital syllabus. True, I had passed an examination in pharmacology but few medical students failed this one-foot hurdle. The course consisted of very few lectures, and all I had to do, all the others had to do, was to learn a very small, thin textbook off by heart for examination purposes.

The whole emphasis of medical education was, and is, on diagnosis not on treatment. After all, it is only in recent years that specific drugs have been discovered that can deal with specific diseases. Since the training of a medical student is scientifically orientated, the timeworn prescriptions whose use was pragmatic or simply magical are, by and large, excluded from the curriculum. The therapeutic revolution in medicine that has taken place since the Second World War is still barely reflected in the medical student's education. The attitude that seems to inhere in medical teaching circles is that it takes a scientific detective to diagnose a syndrome of symptoms whereas the secondary question of treatment is sequentially arrived at simply by looking up the appropriate page in a book. In time, even the book can be dispensed with. The right hand side of the equation is known from experience.

"Not to worry," my employer said. "You will find labels on the different bottles."

Sure enough, the bottle of red medicine was marked, *For Nervous Complaints*; the bottle containing the white, flocculent mixture, *For Stomachs*. Even the doses were written out in such simple terms as a teaspoonful or tablespoonful three times a day. In the "pantry" no mystique of Latin obscurantism dominated. It was evident that this old, knowledgeable doctor had employed newly qualified men before, and knew their limitations. "This is white aspirin," he continued, "and this the pink aspirin for more sophisticated patients. You'll have to write out prescriptions for newer drugs, but up there you'll find plenty of samples you may want to try out." Soon he and his wife disappeared and after I had blankly weighed myself on the machine in the corner, I sat down at the desk idling through the advertisements from pharmaceutical firms. The time for my first evening surgery approached. Then the telephone on his desk rang clamorously, too loud. Before picking up the receiver I remembered the motto I had written on the flyleaf of some of my medical textbooks: *Nil Desperandum.*

It must not be thought that my experience, my feelings of inadequacy, were in any way idiosyncratic. My education had been typical, my lack of certainty natural. When, after a day or two, I saw innumerable patients whose symptoms were nebulous, though real— "This funny feeling I get here, doctor, often moves from place to place"—when they complained of pains in the back, sleeplessness, depression, headaches, indigestion, etc., I prescribed placebos, sedatives, or the pink or white aspirin. I soon discovered that diseases hardly ever presented themselves according to the textbook description and, in any case, for the most part the symptoms exhibited did not seem to derive from any known organic ailment. I began to feel I was earning my money for nothing. My advice was not based on the education I had received from medical school. "Yes," I was saying reassuringly, "not to worry." I felt a fraud.

Where were the subacute combined degeneration cases? Where the women suffering from thyrotoxicosis? Where the young man suffering from Hodgkin's disease? "Common things occur most commonly," they had taught me in hospital, meaning that certain signs and symptoms, say of an anemia, pointed to an iron deficiency rather than lead poisoning. If I prescribed an iron tonic it was without any rationale—for it was not for an anemia but for a complex of functional symptoms. Nor, on the whole, did my patients expect me to approach them too scientifically. When I requested an ex-miner to take off his shirt so that I could examine his chest with a stethoscope, his previous experience of doctors prompted him to say, surprised, "You're from 'Arley Street, are you?"

Of course, eventually I encountered patients with the definite illnesses that my medical education had prepared me for. I felt like a scientific doctor rather than an incompetent, bungling magician when I immunized children against diphtheria; treated people with asthmatic attacks or in heart failure; injected penicillin into those suffering from a febrile bacterial infection; gave morphia to incurable cancer cases; and had a young man admitted into hospital as an emergency case with an acute appendicitis. Too often, though, there were patients with organic symptoms whom I could do little for. There was no specific medicament that could cure them, but there were various drugs on the market that, the manufacturers claimed, might ameliorate their condition. More and more often I consulted the leaflets from these pharmaceutical firms. Perhaps I ought to try out this or that preparation?

The leaflets informed me that the product advertised had many advantages for a particular symptom or condition. They had an air of authority about them and, after all, they were sent out by pharmaceutical companies of high reputation. I had seen their advertisements in the authoritative and orthodox *British Medical Journal*, which surely would not print their copy if the product was valueless or dangerous? Perhaps not all newly qualified practitioners were as unworldly as I, yet surely many have been, and are continuing to be, persuaded by the text of such leaflets. And not only the newly qualified doctors either. On almost all of the advertisements the injunction "This product is almost free of undesirable side effects" can be read. Many firms even list the contraindication for prescribing the drug in question, which gives the rest of the copy a spurious authenticity. Again, one was persuaded by the knowledge that after the drug had been synthesized or extracted from natural sources it had not only been tested on laboratory animals but had also undergone, presumably, stringent clinical trials.

I had certain doubts. I recalled Alexander Pope's admonitory lines:

"Be not the first by whom the new are tried
    Nor yet the last to lay the old aside."

But Pope wrote in the 18th century when medicine, I knew, had its roots in folklore, ritual, magic, and superstition. Besides, to withhold a drug simply because it was new, because I had not gleaned enough information about it from scientific journals, might be under certain conditions morally indefensible. When a doctor is confronted by a suffering patient and he is not sure what to do, he is fair game for the propaganda of a leaflet, or a didactic article cleverly presented in the house magazine of a pharmaceutical company. On the other hand, it would be very wrong to propose that such leaflets are invariably misleading. On the contrary, often they are not, otherwise it would be easy to dismiss them always.

When I concluded my three weeks locum tenens in Cardiff I had learned several things. One was that whereas beforehand I *felt* I owned inadequate medical knowledge, now I *knew* that to be so. I thought then, though, that my inadequacy derived from the fact that I had not absorbed the medical education I had been offered. I did not question whether the education, apart from certain details, was itself inadequate. I thought that, with experience, my own in-adequacies would gradually dissolve. I still felt that 20th-century medicine was basically scientific and had no relation to the practice, say, of Alexander Pope's time. I had been conditioned to think in this way. W. H. Auden and Christopher Isherwood have satirized this con-ditioning of the medical student in their play *The Dog Beneath the Skin* where a chorus of students is obliged to say: "[I believe] in the physical causation of all phenomena, material or mental; and in the germ theory of disease. And in Hippocrates, the father of Medicine, Galen, Ambroise Paré, Liston of the enormous hands, Syme, Lister who discovered the use of antiseptics, Hunter and Sir Frederick Treves. . . ."

Where Auden and Ishwerwood are wrong is not in the implication of such a chorus but in thinking that medical students are taught the history of medicine—the vast majority would barely have heard of half the names they list! Because of their mechanistic and concentrated technological education, which allows them little leisure during their student years, doctors tend to be startlingly ignorant outside their subject. Nor is it easy for them to acquire broader knowledge immediately after they qualify, for they are too harassed and work over-long hours while they are juniors in the hospital hierarchy. Still, one might expect them at least to know where, let us say, hospitals originated. After all priests are aware of their tradition; painters know their art history; and even lawyers have to learn Roman law. Yet ask doctors to outline the historical origins of hospitals or other aspects of medical history and most of them would be at a loss.

Whether their general ignorance matters or not is debatable. Most would assume that the more widespread the knowledge and interests of a doctor the better equipped he would be to advise and help his patients. Yet the contrary may be true. When the writer Maxim Gorky suffered an illness and was advised to consult a medical man, Lenin is reported to have said: "Well whatever you do, don't go to a Communist doctor, for any man who has spent so much time on acquiring an historical and political perspective could only have done so at the expense of his medical education."

If medical students rarely question the basis of their education, still less do they query the practices of medicine as they observe them in the hospitals in which they are trained. They may grumble that Dr. X cannot teach or Mr. Y is a poor surgeon, but they are hardly likely to assess the virtue of medical orthodoxies. Individuals may be appalled at isolated happenings. I knew, for example, how unhappy a contemporary of mine was while "walking the children's ward." Despite the care and attention of the majority of nurses he felt it a mistake, from a medical point of view, that a young child or baby be separated from its mother. Simply, babies and infants have failed to thrive because of such enforced separation. Surely accommodation could be found in the hospitals for the mothers as well? There were, and are, many objections to such a reform. Doctors and nurses cannot, some of them say, continue with their work efficiently if parents interfere; or crisis conditions may arise and the very presence of the mother, who will naturally own a high emotional temperature, may affect the cold objectivity of the pediatrician. The same objections to relatives may apply in the medical and surgical wards. Often I have heard, in hospitals, the view expressed that "relations are a damned nuisance." And sometimes they are—asking questions when there are vital procedures to be carried out, interfering, or behaving hysterically, when all the medical attendants are doing their best and are hard pressed for time. Besides, when it comes to accommodation for mothers of infants, there are the physical practicalities to consider. There are just not enough beds for the patients, never mind for the relations. All the same, more and more authorities are stressing the psychological importance of allowing the mother to stay in the hospital with her sick child. The following letter, printed in *The Lancet* of December 18, 1965, from a mother to the National Association for the Welfare of Children in Hospital, London, is just one exhibit that argues potently, I think, for a reform that must come sooner or later:

"My little girl, Dawn, was admitted to hospital for a tonsils and adenoids operation when she was 3 years and 3 weeks old and she had never been anywhere without me, was very shy, and did not get on with strangers. I took Dawn to the hospital at 2.15 p.m. as arranged, was told to undress her and put her to bed. I was allowed to stay with her until 3 o'clock and told that I could return for the visiting hour 5 p.m. till 6 p.m. When I returned at 5 o'clock I was told by a little boy in the next bed that Dawn had cried after me ever since I had left her at 3 o'clock, her little face was quite puffed from crying when I left at 6 o'clock. I was told that I could not visit the next day because she was having the operation. . . .

"Wednesday, 17th. I telephoned at 12 noon and was told that Dawn had had the operation and was satisfactory. I asked if I could visit but was told not to do so after an operation but they said I could ring again at 6 p.m. if I wanted to. I again telephoned the hospital at 6 p.m. and was told that Dawn was bleeding heavily but not to worry and ring again at 8 p.m. This I did and was told that the surgeons had taken her back to the theatre to stop the bleeding and they said I could telephone at 9.30 p.m. This I did and was told that she had not come round yet but the bleeding had stopped and was told to ring at midnight. This I did and was told that Dawn was sleeping peacefully. They told me not to worry, to go home to sleep and telephone the hospital at 10.30 a.m. next morning. At this point I must point out that each time I rung up I begged to see my child but they said there was nothing to worry about and that I could not see her.

"Thursday, 18th, 10.30 a.m. I telephoned the hospital, spoke to the ward sister and was told that Dawn was a little improved and that I could visit at 4 o'clock. I arrived at the hospital at 3.50 p.m. and was asked to wait because the doctor was with Dawn. A few minutes later I was told that Dawn had collapsed but not to worry because the doctor was doing all possible. I asked if I could go to her but was told to wait. As I waited I prayed to God to help my little girl: a few minutes later the ward sister came and said that my dear Dawn had passed away at 4.15 p.m., so you see although I was there I couldn't go in to see her even though she was dying. They took me to see Dawn then but it was too late for my love to do its work because she had gone to rest.

"There had to be a post mortem on my little girl and they found that she had died from bilateral broncho-pneumonia. They said that she would have had pneumonia anyway but the doctor couldn't tell before the operation.

"Other mothers who had children in Dawn's ward were allowed to see their children because they hadn't had the operation and these mothers have told me that on the day of Dawn's operation she had been returned to the ward and was crying constantly for me and this, I believe, caused the bleeding.

"I do believe that my little girl died from pneumonia but I also think that if I had been with her it might have had a different ending because she wouldn't have needed to sob her heart out if I had been by her side, and if she hadn't cried she wouldn't have lost so much blood, and if she hadn't lost the blood then she would have had more strength to fight the pneumonia with.

"Who knows, perhaps if I had been with her, I still may not have saved her life but at least I could have given her comfort.

"This morning I have done the last thing I can do for my little girl, that is to attend her funeral. If this letter can help you in any way to get another youngster his mother's care after this operation I shall be pleased for you to use it, because after all a nurse's skill cannot mend a child's broken heart, only a mother can do this because there is nothing in the world like a mother's love when a child is ill and upset."

Reasonable criticisms of individual procedures in hospital management or in general practice are frequently made by patients and relatives, and sometimes their concrete illustrations are as poignant and persuasive as the letter above. Nor does the medical Establishment resent such focal criticism. After all, it does not undermine the basic tenets of orthodox medicine.

More radical critics, for their part, tend to overstate their case, praising medicasters and cranks, and too often only concede that there has been medical progress in our time in asides or in metaphorical footnotes. Writers like Bernard Shaw have taken the medical profession to task for not being scientific enough—"the rank and file of doctors are no more scientific than their tailors," he wrote characteristically— while others, like the British author Brian Inglis, complain that the medical profession nowadays is too rationalistic and does not take account of facts and mysteries that appear to be "unscientific."

As for the general public, it continues on the whole, I think, to show respect for the medical profession even in those Western societies that, year by year, show increasing disrespect—often justified—for establishments hitherto considered to be almost sacrosanct. True, an increasing minority consult fringe practitioners and there are always certain sophisticates who air hostile views about doctors and modern medicine; but the latter, anyway, seem to lose these attitudes when they, themselves, become sick and dependent. It is because of the general respect of the public that doctors, outside their surgeries, can sometimes use their titles to secure certain minor privileges for themselves. (Recently at Dublin airport I tried vainly to board a plane that was full, and informed the officials pompously that I had to be on it because I was a *doctor* and was expected in London within an hour. "Sure, I'm sorry," I was told, "but do you know that t'ree desperate priests have to be left behind also, sir?" To be classed with priests, even desperate ones, in religious Dublin, is to be honored indeed.)

Any thinking doctor, though, will sooner or later wonder whether the faith that most patients put in him as the representative of orthodox medicine is justified—and he will perhaps be prepared to counter the arguments of those who challenge the very concepts of the "science" that he practices. Not that this book is in any way intended as an apologia for orthodox medicine. Since those weeks when I completed my locum tenens in Cardiff I have become aware that the more I know, the more I read, and the more I experience, the more I journey into doubt and ignorance. There is no one view of modern medicine: it is both a success and a failure. So, in the following pages I have tried on the one hand to describe the dramatic achievements that have taken place in certain spheres of medicine during our time; but on the other I have also underlined—especially in the middle chapters—the failures as they have occurred and are occurring.

Thus, in the chapter "Drugs for the Sick Mind" attention is drawn to the plight of the mentally ill, and to the cheerless optimism of those psychiatrists—dangerous in my view—who rely on psycho-chemicals in healing them; in the chapter "The Human Guinea Pig" I have focused on those doctors who have engaged in "scientific research" under political pressures or have conducted experiments without due regard for patients under their care; in the latter chapter, too, as well as in those entitled "The Addicts" and "The Cost of Drugs," the suffering consequent on the misuse of drugs, the iatrogenic diseases, and the ethical responsibilities of those marketing and dispensing drugs are considered. Elsewhere the direct consequences of, and problems raised by, the failures and successes of modern medicine are discussed.

The use and misuse of drugs is central to such a discussion but is by no means the whole story. Today, unlike the Greeks, we do not hope that Aesculapius will appear in our dreams and reveal to us, through interpreting priests, what method of treatment we should follow to be cured. We do have psychiatrists, though, to unravel our night visions. Besides, much of modern medicine, even where it depends on mechanistic drugs to effect a cure, is quite unscientific. Disease often is a matter of abnormal function rather than damaged structure, and the etiology too frequently is unknown, the diagnosis a question mark, the treatment symptomatic, the prognosis uncertain. The wise physician, in his day-to-day confrontation with patients, could well take as his motto: Accustom thy tongue to say, "I know not."

# 1 The Very Small Enemy

To discuss without rancor the failure of modern medicine, the machinations and greed of the pharmaceutical industry, the obtuseness of the educational system that confronts the medical student, the too heavy reliance by the medical profession on drugs for both the sick mind and the sick body, the fallibility of individual physicians—all this can be a constructive exercise, providing the perspectives are not lost sight of. For the successes of modern medicine are just as real. The progress made lately has been rapid and remarkable.

Most spectacular has been the conquest of bacterial infection as a result of the discovery of antibiotics, which so many people now take for granted. We are apt to forget how different medical practice was before the Second World War. Not only were the wards of hospitals crammed with people suffering from acute infections such as pneumonia, meningitis, and septicemia, but the surgical wards too had their common quota of festering wounds—pus-discharging abscesses, weeping fistulas, and raw, angry carbuncles. One is reminded of Thersites's list of ailments in Shakespeare's *Troilus and Cressida*: "The rotten diseases of the south, the guts griping, ruptures, catarrhs, loads o' gravel i' the back, lethargies, cold palsies, raw eyes, dirt-rotten livers, wheezing lungs, bladders full of imposthume, sciaticas, limekilns

Molds from four different earth samples. Pure cultures from such molds are removed and grown separately before being tested for their antibiotic value.

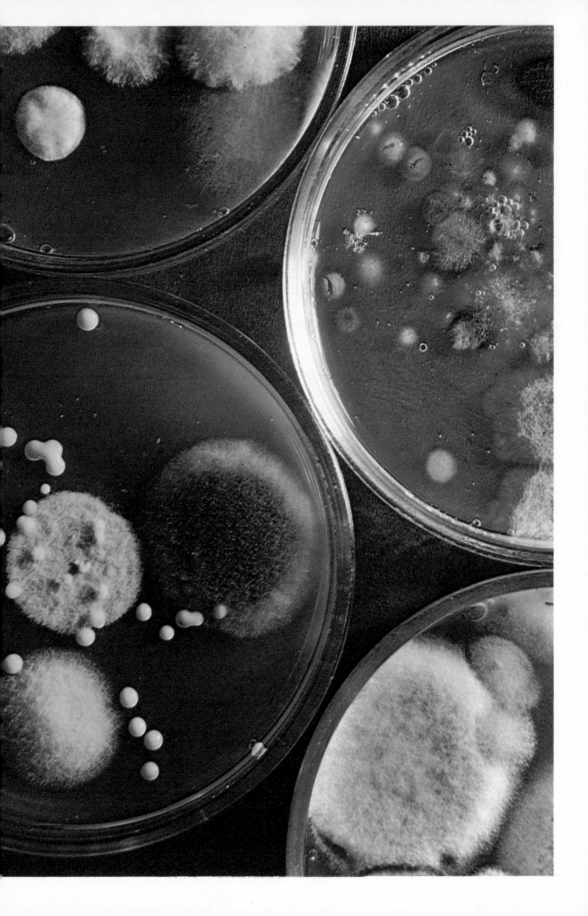

i' the palm, incurable bone-ache. . . ." The medical profession had evolved scientific nomenclature for such ailments but the remedies remained almost ineffective. Too many parents had to face the likelihood of losing at least one child from one or another infection. Too many vigorous adults succumbed to an infective process when their careers were only beginning.

Less than twenty-five years ago, the doctor with his black bag visiting a child with pneumonia could do little more than wait for "nature to take its course." His therapeutic position had progressed only minimally since the time of Hippocrates, the father of medicine (*c.* 400 B.C.), who advised for "peripneumonia," as the disease was then called (the term survived for 2000 years): "If the fever be acute, and if there be pains on either side, or in both, and if expiration be attended with pain, if cough be present, and the sputa expectorated be of a blood or livid colour, or likewise thin and frothy, or having any other character different from the common, in such a case the physician should proceed thus . . . the inner vein in the arm should be opened on the side affected and the blood abstracted according to the habit, age and colour of the patient, and the season of the year, and that largely and boldly if the pain be acute."

In the early 1930s the treatment of pneumonia commenced like a ritual with three grains of calomel to open the bowels. Every four hours an expectorant mixture was prescribed consisting of stomach irritants to encourage the discharge of phlegm and mucus. Every four hours digitalis (the dried leaf of the common foxglove) was given to strengthen the heart muscle. Chloral or bromides or barbiturates, along with brandy, were freely dispensed. So sedated, intoxicated, purged, and drugged, the patient lay in his hospital bed to await "the crisis." Meanwhile he was expected to drink as many as 15 pints of fluid every day "to flush the toxins out of the system." This, one must remember, was the therapeutic nightmare not of some distant past but of our own century.

In France "cupping"—the operation of drawing blood to or from the surface of the body by forming a partial vacuum over a certain spot—was still prevalent in some regions in 1945. Sixteen years earlier the British novelist George Orwell had been treated by this method in a gloomy Paris hospital, as he recounts in an essay, "How The Poor Die":

"I saw on a bed nearly opposite me a small, round-shouldered, sandy-haired man sitting half naked while a doctor and a student performed some strange operation on him. First the doctor produced from his black bag a dozen small glasses like wine glasses, then the student burned a match inside each glass to exhaust the air, then the glass was popped on to the man's back or chest and the vacuum drew up a huge yellow blister. Only after some moments did I realise what they were doing to him. It was something called cupping, a treatment which you can read about in old medical textbooks but which till then I had vaguely thought of as one of those things they do to horses. . . .

"I watched this barbarous remedy with detachment and even a certain amount of amusement. The next moment, however, the doctor and the student came across to my bed, hoisted me upright and without a word began applying the same set of glasses, which had not been sterilized in any way. A few feeble protests that I uttered got no more response than if I had been an animal. I was very much impressed by the impersonal way in which the two men started on me. I had never been in the public ward of a hospital before, and it was my first experience of doctors who handle you without speaking to you or, in a human sense, taking any notice of you. They only put on six glasses in my case, but after doing so they scarified the blisters and applied the glasses again. Each glass now drew about a dessert-spoonful of dark-coloured blood. As I lay down again, humiliated, disgusted and frightened by the thing that had been done to me, I reflected that now at least they would leave me alone. But no, not a bit of it. There was another treatment coming, the mustard poultice, seemingly a matter of routine like the hot bath. Two slatternly nurses had already got the poultice ready, and they lashed it round my chest as tight as a strait-jacket while some men who were wandering about the ward in shirt and trousers began to collect round my bed with half-sympathetic grins. I learned later that watching a patient have a mustard poultice was a favourite pastime in the ward. These things are normally applied for a quarter of an hour and certainly they are funny enough if you don't happen to be the person inside. For the first five minutes the pain is severe, but you believe you can bear it. During the second five minutes this belief evaporates, but the poultice is buckled at the back and you can't get it off. This is the period the onlookers enjoy most. During the last five minutes, I noted, a sort of numbness supervenes. After the poultice has been removed a waterproof pillow packed with ice was thrust beneath my head and I was left alone. I did not sleep, and to the best of my knowledge this was the only night of my life—I mean the only night spent in bed—in which I have not slept at all, not even a minute."

It is hard to understand why such primitive methods of treatment persisted so tenaciously until the advent of antibiotics—though in fairness it should be said that not all hospitals were as bad as the one Orwell described. Presumably doctors had to take some action when confronted with a suffering patient and *some* of the palliative

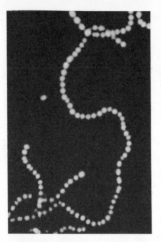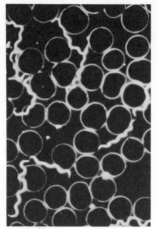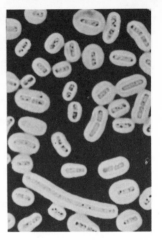

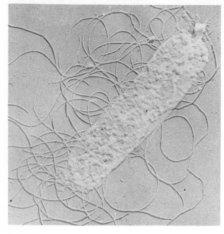

Most bacteria fall into one of three well-defined shapes—spherical (above left), screw-shaped (center), or rod-like (above right). Some bacteria are capable of moving, and do so by means of long, thin hairs known as "flagella" (left).

Right, cupping with bamboo sticks—an ancient cure for rheumatism practiced still in some parts of China.

measures they prescribed did make their patients feel more comfortable. Again, since many patients recovered (in spite of the doctors) the doctors concluded that their treatment had been partly responsible, and so were encouraged to repeat their prescriptions in the future. Such logic reminds one of the experimental biologist who, placing a grasshopper on his research table, shouted, "Jump." When the grasshopper jumped, the biologist measured the height of the jump. He repeated this exercise several times. Then the biologist cut off the legs of the grasshopper and once again shouted, "Jump." After the grasshopper failed to respond to such commands, the biologist concluded: "When a grasshopper has its legs amputated it loses its power of hearing."

However, even as George Orwell lay in the Paris hospital breathing in the sickly smell of its 19th-century atmosphere, the events that were to change radically the whole pattern of therapeutics had begun. For in the same year, 1929, the bacteriologist Alexander Fleming published a paper about penicillin in the *British Journal of Experimental*

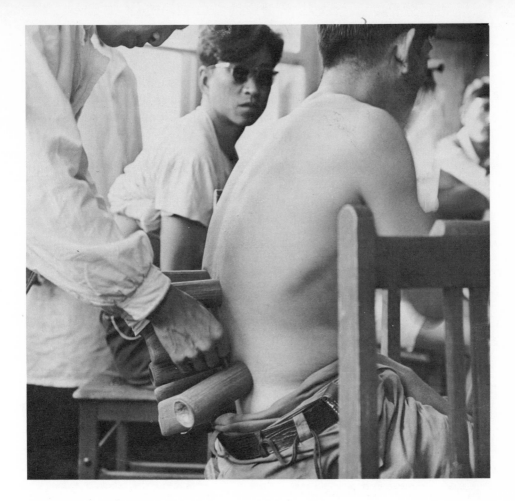

*Pathology.* The previous September, Professor Fleming had made a startling discovery while working in his laboratory at St. Mary's Hospital, London. He had inspected the glass culture plates on which he was growing staphylococci and noticed how one of the culture mediums had been contaminated.

This was not in itself an unusual occurrence. Thousands of bacteriological workers have been, and are, bothered by the growth of contaminating molds on their culture plates. This sort of contamination is regarded critically as a reflection on the technique of the bacteriologist. As a result such plates are discarded and the bacteriologist has to begin again. So, of course, Fleming was irritated when he observed the contamination. Obviously some spores (fungus) rather like that seen on old bread or stale cheese had blown into the laboratory. He was about to dispose of the culture plate when something made him hesitate and tilt the plate to catch the afternoon light from the window. He looked closer. He put the plate under a microscope. He saw the usual blur and then, as he focused the lenses, the distortion cleared to reveal how the growth of the staphylococcus colonies had partly dissolved. Why? What mold had alighted, spun onto the plate to kill off the bacteria? These were the questions Fleming asked himself. He did not throw the culture plate away.

Professor Fleming said later: "There are thousands of different moulds and there are thousands of different bacteria, and chance put that mould in the right spot at the right time. If my mind had not been in a reasonably perceptive state, I would not have paid any attention to it. I might have been in a bad temper say after a quarrel with my wife; I might have just become engaged and my mind might have been full of the young woman, or I might have been suffering from the after effects of too heavy a meal and been mentally too sluggish to notice it or do anything about it." Fleming was emphasizing the luck or chance involved in his discovery of penicillin—for the mold contaminating that culture plate sired the substance we now call penicillin. But chance was not the only factor. As Louis Pasteur had written years earlier: "In the field of observation, chance favours only the prepared mind." That remark perhaps defines both scientific and artistic inspiration. In any event, Fleming subcultured the mold, encouraged the "yellow magic" to grow profusely, and found that even a minute dilution of it could be strongly antagonistic, not only to the staphylococcal bacteria but to streptococci and other bacteria also—the germs that caused untold suffering and fever, killed man, woman, and child alike, and filled the beds of hospitals like the one George Orwell described.

Strangely, certain molds had been part of the armory of folk-medicine for centuries. In certain regions of Brazil, for example, the peasants believed in the magic value of field mold when applied to cuts and wounds. In the Ukraine, Greece, and Yugoslavia, too, peasants cured septic wounds and some infections with the growth on moldy bread, believing it to be more valuable than doctors' drugs.

In 1640, one apothecary of London, John Parkinson, had recommended, perhaps with clairvoyant insight: "The Mosse upon dead mens Sculles. Let me here also adjoyne, this kind of mosse somewhat like unto the mosse of trees, and groweth upon the bare scalpes of men and women that have lyen long, and are kept in Charnell houses in divers Countries, which hath not onely beene in former times much accounted of, because it is rare and hardly gotten, but in our times much more set by, to make the Unguentum Sympatheticum, which cureth wounds without locall application of salves, the composition whereof is put as a principall ingredient, but as Crollius hath it, it should be taken from the sculls of those that have beene hanged or executed for offences."

John Parkinson's remedy of penicillin mosses from "dead mens Sculles" was not taken up by other 17th-century apothecaries. In 1929, Fleming's yellow magic, it seemed, would also be ignored by the medical profession—though Fleming did receive encouragement from a former student of his, a Dr. C. G. Paine, who was practicing in Sheffield. Paine asked Fleming for some filtrate of the mold so that it could be tried out clinically.

Dr. Paine used the filtrate on four newborn babies suffering from gonococcal conjunctivitis—a condition that often resulted in permanent eye damage and blindness. The babies' lids were sticky with pus and the whites of their eyes were obscured. Two days later, in three of the four cases treated by Dr. Paine, the eyes cleared spectacularly. The filtrate had cured the conjunctivitis so that somewhere in the world today there are, presumably, three adults who can see because of Fleming's original mold and Dr. Paine's initiative, whereas others remain blind because the manufacture of large quantities of pure penicillin was not tackled for 10 long years. Fleming was a bacteriologist, not a biochemist. He had neither the laboratory equipment nor the training for concentrating penicillin. He needed chemists to reduce his mold to a stable salt that could be marketed and used generally; and for the time being this help was not forthcoming.

Meanwhile another "miracle" drug was on the point of being discovered, in western Germany. In 1933, Dr. Gerhard Domagk, who was employed by the Bayer Dye Works in Elberfeld, tested the effect of several dyes on mice that had been infected experimentally with lethal doses of streptococci. The medicinal value of dyes had already been demonstrated in 1907 by Paul Ehrlich, the German instigator of modern chemotherapy, who discovered that the dye trypan red was active against sleeping sickness. Ehrlich had gone on to treat other diseases by chemical injections and his experiments had culminated in the discovery of 606, Salvarsan, the "magic bullet" against syphilis (the six hundred and sixth arsenical compound he had tried out on this disease). Ehrlich's discovery had raised the hope that other drugs would, in time, be discovered that could be "aimed" at specific species of bacteria, killing them without harming the human host.

The mice Domagk infected with hemolytic streptococci generally died within a few days from septicemia; but he discovered that if he fed the mice with red dye, Prontosil, before infecting them, they survived the infection. It so happened that in February 1935 Domagk's own daughter, Hildegarde, developed a festering finger after she had handled a culture of streptococci in her father's laboratory. The infection grew worse, despite surgery, and soon she developed the general signs of blood poisoning: an irregular fever, rigors, etc.

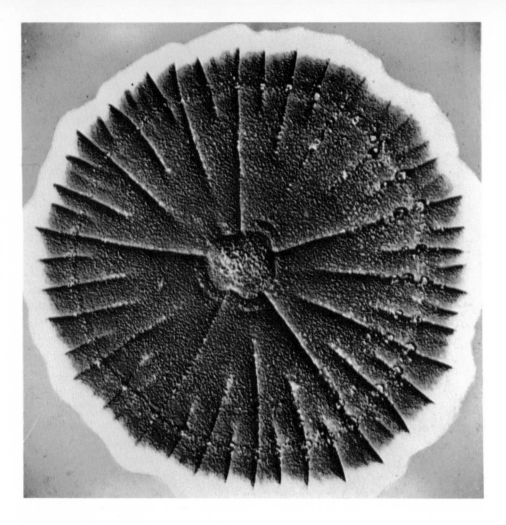

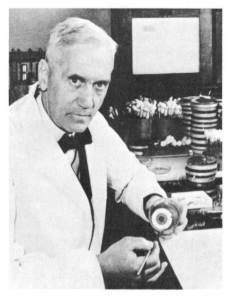

Above, the symmetrical colony of the *Penicillium chrysogenum* mold, a variant of the original penicillin mold discovered by Sir Alexander Fleming (left) in 1928. It is from this more fertile mold that most of the world's commercial penicillin is now being produced.

Above right, testing a variety of isolated antibiotic cultures for their efficacy against a specific disease organism. Plugs of the different cultures are placed on a plate of infected nutrient jelly, and left to incubate overnight. The clear circles around some of the plugs show where an antibiotic culture has proved strong enough to kill or inhibit the growth of the disease organism.

Right, an Indian girl before and after treatment with the antibiotic Aureomycin for trachoma—an eye disease that afflicts some 400 million people.

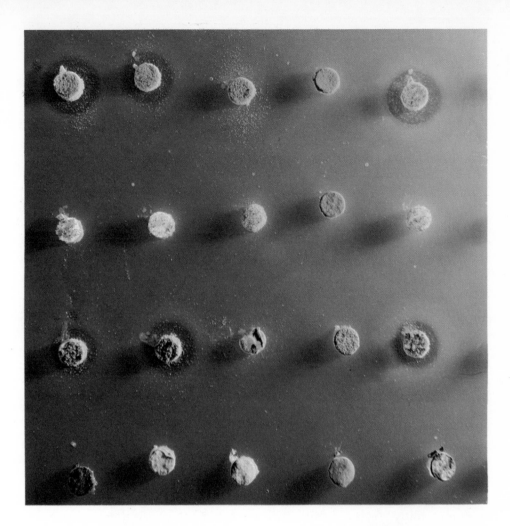

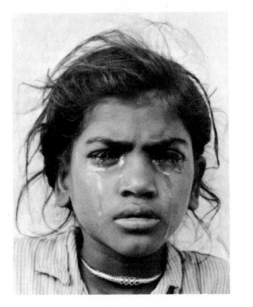

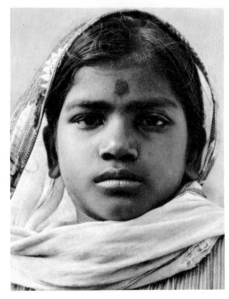

Domagk knew that if the septicemia was not curbed abscesses would develop in the pleura of her lungs, in the joints, in the pericardium (the membranous covering of the heart). What had happened to the mice would probably happen to his daughter: she would die. It was a desperate father who urged his febrile daughter to swallow a large dose of Prontosil. How deeply felt was his relief when he observed his child revive and finally recover completely.

Later in 1935 Domagk published a paper on the work he had done in his laboratory over the last two years. He called it emotionlessly, "On the behaviour of Prontosil towards Streptococci"—and soon there were to be worldwide repercussions. One small detail seems worth recounting here. As an honored guest, Gerhard Domagk was invited to London to give an address on Prontosil to the Royal Society of Medicine. One of those present, listening to his success story, was Alexander Fleming.

Prontosil was soon to be used in the treatment of puerperal fever. This illness—commonly known as childbed fever—was dreaded by mother, father, and doctor alike. For after the birth of a child the new mother was especially liable to contract an infection that, if uncontrolled, could develop into a peritonitis and septicemia. Too often medical attendants had to stand helplessly by while the young mother suffered prostration, delirium, and an increasing feebleness of the heart's action. Death of a young mother has always been a particularly poignant tragedy. In the 50 years preceding the discovery of Prontosil, some 100,000 young women in England and Wales died of puerperal fever, leaving behind them stunned husbands, wide-eyed children, and the new baby crying in its cot. In the late 1930s the number of maternal deaths in the United States from puerperal sepsis alone amounted to five in every 1000 births.

Dr. Leonard Colebrook described in the *British Medical Journal* how he first used Prontosil in 1935 at Queen Charlotte's Hospital, London: "It seemed clearly worth while to try the drug on some of our puerperal fever cases which we knew to be infected with haemolytic streptococci. At first we treated only the more severe cases, for which we had no promising therapy. The grave prognosis in such cases had become all too familiar to us. The death rate had ranged consistently between 20 and 30%.

"Almost at once, with the new drug, there was a surprising and most gratifying change. Signs of incipient peritonitis did not develop as we expected; positive blood cultures changed quickly to negative—I recall one woman in particular whose blood for the first three days of treatment grew over 3000 colonies of streptococci per c. cm., on the fourth day it grew none, and at the same time her temperature fell from 104 degrees F. (40° C.) to normal, and never rose again above 99 degrees F. (37.2° C.). This was something that we had never seen before in ten years' experience of the disease.

"The case mortality in the first series of 64 patients (all infected by haemolytic streptococci) was 4.7%. In the previous five years before prontosil it had ranged from 16.6 to 31.6% averaging about 25%. It seemed clear to most of us that in red prontosil we had at last got a drug which could change the course of a haemolytic streptococcal infection in human beings."

Soon after this triumph it was demonstrated at the Pasteur Institute in Paris that, in the body, Prontosil was broken down into a simpler constituent: p-aminobenzene sulfonamide. This constituent of Prontosil proved to be the active agent in curing the streptococcal infection. Moreover this sulfonamide had been discovered and known about since 1908 and not patented as Prontosil was. As a result, all kinds of sulfonamide preparations were now manufactured chemically and tried out in laboratories throughout the world. Few doctors realized in 1936 that with the discovery of the sulfonamides medical practice was to undergo a revolution. As Dr. Colebrook wrote: "We had no idea that within a couple of years the grim shadow cast by lobar pneumonia over the human race would be practically lifted and that cerebrospinal meningitis, gonorrhoea, many urinary infections, middle ear and mastoid disease, and a host of other infections would lend themselves to successful treatment by the new drugs. . . ."

Before the end of 1936 two American doctors, Perrin H. Long and Eleanor Bliss of Johns Hopkins University, Baltimore, reported that the sulfonamides had caused "quinsies to melt away, the advance of erysipelas to stop in its tracks, and running ears to dry up in a short time." Franklin D. Roosevelt's son was cured of a raging streptococcal infection by the new drug. Seventeen years later, in December 1943, another sulfonamide preparation, M & B 693, was given to Winston Churchill, then seriously ill with pneumonia in North Africa. Churchill, typically, said afterwards in a broadcast: "The intruders were repulsed." Countless other microbe intruders into less famous human bodies were repulsed between 1936 and 1943 by the sulfona-mide drugs. They continue to be so to this day.

Meanwhile renewed interest had been taken in Fleming's penicillin mold in Britain. An Australian, Howard Florey, and a brilliant refugee from Hitler's Germany, Ernst Chain—who had read Fleming's paper of 1929—now, 10 years later, began work on Fleming's original culture and eventually produced a brown, stable powder. By July 1, 1940, they were ready to test its therapeutic properties on 50 mice that had been given a lethal dose of streptococci and staphylococci. They injected their crude brown penicillin into 25 of the mice at three-hourly

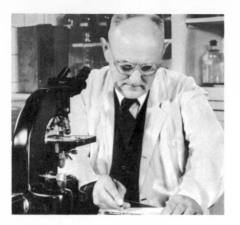

Left, Dr. Gerhard Domagk, discoverer of Prontosil, the first of the sulfonamides. Below, the effect of a sulfonamide on a pus-discharging streptococcus. In the right-hand picture, the streptococcal chain (shown left) has been attacked by the sulfonamide and inhibited.

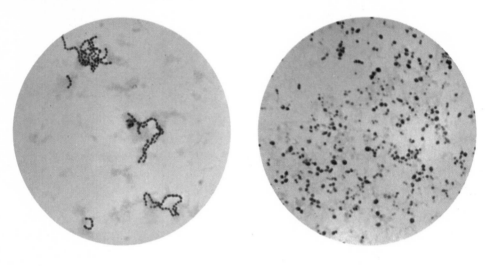

intervals. These survived, whereas the other 25 died within 16 hours. Though the salt manufactured by Chain and Florey was only 1 per cent penicillin and 99 per cent impurity, the chemical road to mass manufacture had begun. Fleming visited Florey and Chain at Oxford, where they were working. Afterwards he said rather wistfully: "They have turned out to be the successful chemists I should have liked to have had with me in 1929." He was now optimistic. He felt that his penicillin would soon be in competition with the sulfonamides. On November 15, 1940, he wrote to Florey: "I have been comparing the solid penicillin which I got from you with the sulphonamides, and it seems to be, weight for weight, a great deal more potent than the most powerful of them on the ordinary septic microbes. It only remains for your chemical colleagues to purify the active principle, and then synthesise it, and the sulphonamide will be completely beaten."

After much difficulty, the active penicillin principle was purified and manufactured in bulk. By 1943, Britain was producing 300 million units a month, the U.S.A. 1700 million units. By 1945, 26 thousand million units were being manufactured in Britain and 570 thousand million in the U.S.A. In 1956 the journal *Antibiotic Medicine and Clinical Therapy* could say: "Thanks to antibiotics, a million and a half lives [in the U.S.A.] were saved in the first fifteen years of the sulfon-amide and antibiotic era. These lives represent those persons who might have died if the percentage of mortality from certain infections had continued in the same proportion after 1937—when sulfonamides began to be used in the U.S.A.—as in former years. Of the lives saved from 1938 to 1952 inclusive, 1,000,000 would have died of pneumonia and influenza, 76,000 mothers would have died from puerperal fever, 136,000 of syphilis and 90,000 of appendicitis. . . ."

The antibiotic revolution had triumphed beyond Domagk's and Fleming's dreams. True, sulfonamides did sometimes cause side effects. Their crystals, on occasions, were deposited in the kidneys, damaging them. This complication was largely solved, however. But more worrying was the fact that the toxic action of the crystals on the bone marrow could lead to the dangerous blood condition of agranulo-cytosis. This meant they could be prescribed for only a limited number of days. The toxicity of penicillin too had to be considered. It was found that a small dose of penicillin injected into guinea pigs usually proved fatal in a few days, and when the dead guinea pigs were examined, necrotic and hemorrhagic lesions were to be found in many organs—in the liver, in the kidneys, in the adrenals, in the heart muscle. It was also found that penicillin is 100 to 1000 times more toxic for guinea pigs than for mice. Happily, penicillin's toxicity in man is comparable to that in mice. Penicillin and its main therapeutic derivatives, developed in very recent years, are virtually nontoxic in human beings.

It was fortunate that basal patents were not taken out for either penicillin or the sulfonamides. Thus they could be made by anyone. All the information regarding penicillin's production was published and when Florey visited America and other countries he demonstrated the methods of extraction he and his co-workers used at Oxford. The result has been that, because of competition, the price has remained low. The manufacturers receive less for the penicillin than they do for the package in which the antibiotic is marketed. The discoveries of the sulfonamides and penicillin—unlike some recent patented drugs—have been made available without the public having to pay extortionate sums to profiteering pharmaceutical companies.

However, the antibiotic revolution had only begun with the discovery of sulfonamides and penicillin. Many other disease-defeating antibiotics were soon produced, notably streptomycin (in 1943), chloramphenicol (in 1947), and the tetracyclines, Aureomycin and Terramycin (in 1948 and 1950 respectively). Streptomycin in particular has captured the public imagination since, unlike the sulfonamides and penicillin, it has been used to treat tuberculosis—along with para-aminosalicylic acid (PAS), which was discovered in 1946, and isonicotinic acid hydrozide (INAH), discovered in 1952.

Tuberculosis has been a scourge of man for thousands of years. Exhumed, prehistoric skeletons of hunchbacks show that it raged to wreck and twist and cripple its victims long before the era of recorded history. It is known that in the 14th century B.C. the priests of the Indo-Aryans treated the disease by chanting, "Oh Fever, with thy Brother Consumption, with thy Sister Cough, go to the people below." In ancient China, tuberculosis of the lungs was known as *lao-ting*. The Greeks suffered from the disease and they bore it, with better gifts, to Rome. The conquering Romans, in their turn, spread it throughout the countries of Europe.

In Britain, glandular tuberculosis (scrofula) was known for centuries as the "king's evil," and was treated by the royal touch.

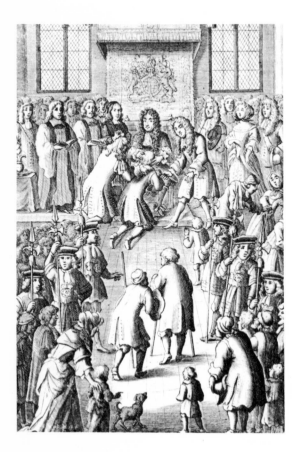

Left, Charles II of England administering the royal touch to a tubercular patient—a contemporary engraving from John Browne's *Adenochoiradelogia, or Kings-Evil Swellings* (1684). According to Browne, Charles II "actually touched, on an average, 4000 persons every year." Today, teams especially trained by the World Health Organization vaccinate whole communities against T.B. and give treatment where necessary. Right, members of a mobile WHO X-ray unit at work in a village of Basutoland.

Dr. Samuel Johnson, when a child, was one of the last to receive the royal touch—from Queen Anne, at the beginning of the 18th century. But the kings' divine right to rule did not bestow on them the divine gift to heal, for tuberculosis continued unchecked. The philosopher John Locke (1632–1704) recorded that in the London of his time one death in five resulted from tuberculosis.

It was not until 1882 that the tubercle bacillus was discovered by the German bacteriologist Robert Koch, who demonstrated that the various manifestations of tuberculosis—the bone malformations, scrofula, the lung disease, and so on—were all due to the same crafty, destructive germ. It is remarkable that in our time, after such a long and dramatic history, the disease tuberculosis should be virtually conquered by the discovery of streptomycin, PAS, and INAH.

Consider for a moment the roll call of the famous dead brought down by the tubercle germ and the great works that might have been created had a specific cure been available then. Here are a few names taken at random from the phthisic casualty lists of the younger

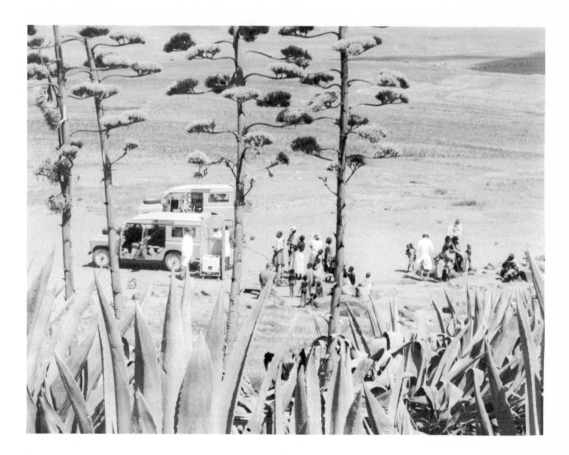

dead for whom streptomycin came too late: Charlotte and Emily Brontë, Edgar Allan Poe, Robert Louis Stevenson, Franz Kafka, D. H. Lawrence; Raphael, Watteau, Modigliani, Aubrey Beardsley; Mozart, Chopin, and Purcell. These knew the menace of the tubercle germ. They could have understood John Keats when he said, after coughing up blood: "I know the colour of that blood. It is arterial blood. I cannot be deceived in that colour; that drop of blood is my death warrant:—I must die."

Streptomycin was discovered by Professor Selman A. Waksman and co-workers Albert Schatz and Elizabeth Bugie, at Rutgers University, New Brunswick, in 1943. Waksman had for years been examining molds and soil cultures. He had been interested in the mysteries of the soil and the different varieties of microorganisms living in it ever since he studied agriculture at Rutgers in 1911. Later, this Russian-Jewish immigrant to the U.S.A. had become a research assistant in soil bacteriology at the New Jersey Agricultural Experimental Station. During his studies he noted how rarely he found disease-producing microbes in the soil, and wondered why this should be so. (The tubercle bacillus, for example, does not live for any length of time in the earth.) Waksman began to think that they did not thrive there because they were destroyed by other soil organisms. If this were so, then it was quite possible that these latter organisms could be used to combat disease in man.

The concept of the soil as a form of medicine has an age-old tradition. It is not only pet animals that eat soil from time to time instinctively. The widespread custom of earth-eating was partly religious but also partly medicinal. The ancient Egyptians recommended soil-eating as a therapy in their papyri. The Otomac Indians ate a fine, yellowish, greasy clay. The Peruvians believed a clay soil called "chacco" to be valuable in treating dysentery. The negroes on the coast of Guinea chose to eat a particular yellow soil. And it is written in *Ecclesiastes*: "The Lord hath created medicines out of the earth: and he that is wise will not abhor them."

It seems a far cry from such primitive wisdom to modern scientific exploration, but Waksman's examination of soil cultures led him, in 1940, to discover his first antibiotic, actinomycin. This substance, alas, proved too toxic for use on human beings; but Waksman felt that sooner or later he would find another, less toxic antibiotic. "I shall never forget," he wrote, "the bright morning of June 1st, 1943, when a small group of people met in one of the rooms at the Pennsylvania Hotel in New York to discuss possible approaches to the problem of the chemotherapy of tuberculosis. . . . The sulfa drugs, which had been available for a few years, were effective against many infectious diseases, but seemed to have little or no effect against tuberculosis. Penicillin, which had recently made its appearance and was beginning to find a place in the treatment of various infections produced largely by cocci and certain gram-positive bacteria, was likewise ineffective against tuberculosis. . . . What was to be done now? Could one suggest new approaches that seemed to be promising and should be investigated further? William C. White [of the National Tuberculosis Association] spoke about the possible isolation of digestive enzymes from earthworms. . . . I expressed sincere doubt whether such an approach through the study of the digestive mechanisms in an animal body would work at all, and even whether further investigations in this direction were justified. I said, 'After all, the bacteria causing tuberculosis are to be destroyed not in the test tube, but in the human body, and any enzyme system powerful enough to bring this about would certainly digest the human organs as well.' White was not very happy about my comments, and spoke up rather angrily: 'How do you propose to go about this problem?'

"My answer was simple: 'The antibiotics will do it. Just give us time. Sooner or later we are bound to find one or more chemical agents that will be able to bring this about. They will kill the bacterium not by digesting it, but by interfering with its metabolism and its growth, without injuring the host. After all this would be based upon the principle of chemotherapy, as enunciated by Paul Ehrlich. Let us hope that such antibiotics will be found, and that they will not be too toxic to the human body.' "

So Waksman's search continued and he and his team examined hundreds of thousands of soil cultures. In 1943 one of them, streptomycin, proved to have marked antibiotic activities, and was active in laboratory conditions against the bacterium tuberculosis.

At this time one man in every seven afflicted with tuberculosis died. The rest, though "cured," suffered from the residual effects of the tubercle germ. Would streptomycin prove clinically capable of combating "the white plague"? During the clinical trials Eve, a young daughter of one of Waksman's colleagues, contracted tuberculous meningitis. The doctors knew the case was hopeless. Under these circumstances they decided as a desperate measure to give Eve the as-yet-untried drug.

Daily, over a period of four months, she was given intraspinal injections of streptomycin. Some improvement occurred almost at once. Gradually, Eve's distressing symptoms cleared until, finally, it could be said that here was the first case of meningitis ever to have been cured with an antibiotic. The story of Eve reminds one of Domagk's daughter. In each case a child was cured. In each case this cure was but a prologue to a million others. In 1952 Waksman, like Domagk, like Fleming, Florey, and Chain before him, was awarded the Nobel prize for medicine.

Later when Waksman traveled round the world he was often confronted by children bearing him flowers. One such confrontation awaited him at the famous Hôpital Sâlpetrière, in Paris. In his book *The Conquest of Tuberculosis* Waksman recounts how two children, a boy five years old and a girl eight years old, were brought in to see him: "They were dressed in colorful provincial costumes and each carried a large bouquet of flowers. 'These children are Michel and Janet,' said the physician. 'They were brought to this hospital six months ago, from distant regions of France. They were almost in a state of coma upon arrival. We began at once to treat them with streptomycin. As you see, they have both made a complete recovery. All the tests for residual tuberculosis appear to be negative. We were going to send them home last week, but we heard that you were coming to Paris and we have kept them here so that you could see them yourself. Are they not pretty!' With these words he presented the children to me. The little girl curtsied. Both children kissed my hand, handed me the flowers, and I patted their lovely curly heads. As I leaned over them, I felt like crying."

Waksman was invited into the hospital courtyard to be photographed with the youngsters. "This was the first photograph," he wrote, "in which I posed with children saved by streptomycin. On leaving the hospital, with the flowers in my hand, I looked back to see the two little ones waving goodbye. This was enough compensation for all the sleepless nights and the endless days spent in the study of the lowly microbes of the soil."

But the use of streptomycin had its hazards. On occasions it led to worrying side effects and could cause an incurable deafness. Also worrying was the fact that, after a time, the tubercular germs seemed to resist its antibiotic effect. What happened was that one in every million or so tubercle germs mutated to become resistant to strepto-mycin. This one individual germ multiplied—though the others were overcome—to produce families, colonies, populations of streptomycin-defiant bacilli, so that after a time streptomycin was powerless. With the discovery of PAS in Sweden in 1946, however, the problem was solved: the two drugs could be given together so that the mutant germ resistant to one drug was overcome by the other. With the discovery of INAH in February 1952, a third permutation was available to defy other resistant strains of the tubercle bacillus. Today, then, two or three of these drugs are given in combination, and tuberculosis is no longer the dangerous disease it was such a short time ago.

Right, some of the thousands of soil samples from many parts of the world sent to a research laboratory in New York for examination. Below, bedouins help in the collection of soil samples from the Sahara desert.

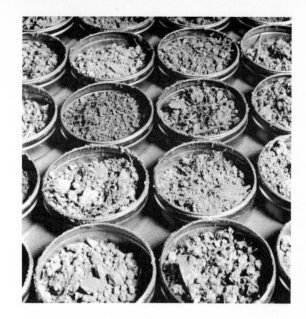

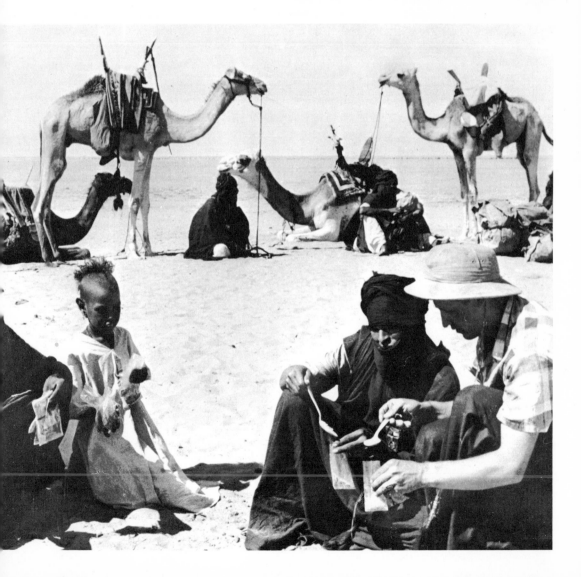

With the discovery of streptomycin the hunt for other antibiotics raced ahead. The pharmaceutical firm that could patent a new antibiotic seemed likely to make a fortune. The soil was now seen to contain antibiotic gold. In 1947 a soil sample collected from a mulched field near Caracas, Venezuela, yielded the powerful antibiotic chloramphenicol, while from the soil of Missouri and Indiana research workers eventually extracted the tetracyclines—Aureomycin and Terramycin. More antibiotics thus became available and more diseases—for example, typhoid fever—became susceptible to modern methods of treatment.

Of course there were abuses in the use of the new antibiotics. Often doctors, baffled by conflicting reports and pressurized by the propaganda of pharmaceutical firms, tended to prescribe antibiotics indiscriminately, sometimes even before a diagnosis had been made. Too frequently antibiotics have been unnecessarily prescribed for people suffering from benign and mild infections. Such a procedure is like dropping a hydrogen bomb to kill one man. Warfare—and the use of antibiotics is a kind of warfare—always brings its complications. Drug-resistant strains of bacteria appeared. Dangerous side effects occurred. Chloramphenicol, for example, was found to cause aplastic anemia from which people died. Thus its use has been restricted. Physicians no longer give it automatically for whooping cough, as they used to do; but when the disease itself is extremely dangerous—say, typhoid fever—then chloramphenicol will be prescribed. The danger of its complications has to be weighed against the peril of the disease from which the patient is suffering—especially when there is no alternative drug of value.

One of the consequences of the triumph of antibiotics has been the over-reliance on drugs by doctors and patients alike. With their use they have seen terrible symptoms melt away. The magic pill seems to have induced the idea that *all* pills—not just antibiotics—have magical properties. In 1963 the Department of Commerce in America estimated that public and private expenditure for prescribed and non-prescribed drugs totaled 4.2 billion dollars a year ($22 per capita). In 1965, it was estimated that in Great Britain 12,000,000,000 pills, capsules, and tablets were swallowed. In 1965, Britain's drug bill was over £120,000,000 (about $336,000,000); 9,000,000 tranquilizers were ingested, and some 2,000,000 antidepressive tablets. If Britain is spending £1000 ($2800) *every hour* on drugs, then this is not simply because the country is populated by hypochondriacs. Rather it is the result of the efficacy of antibiotics, which has given doctors a new faith in themselves and their patients a new faith in drugs generally.

The antibiotic revolution, then, has had far-reaching consequences. However, nothing irritates the general physician more than the fact that, while he has "magic bullets" against serious, bacterial infections, he is helpless to deal with something as simple as the common cold— a condition that leads to 35 per cent of all industrial absenteeism in the United States. It is hardly surprising, then, that "virus infection" is the most common diagnosis family doctors and pediatricians make today. But viruses do not only infect us with the common cold: different varieties are responsible for influenza, virus pneumonia, shingles, infective hepatitis, poliomyelitis, certain kinds of meningitis and encephalitis, rabies, and other diseases.

Viruses are composed chiefly of nucleoprotein and small amounts of lipide and carbohydrate; some scientists believe them to be the nearest known links between living and non-living matter. Certainly they are a much lower form of life than bacteria; and they are also much smaller. The largest single virus particle is about one twelve-millionth of an inch across whereas the smallest is twelve times smaller than that. So almost all viruses are beyond the range of an ordinary microscope. Only a powerful electron-microscope can reveal the vast majority of them. They exist as invisible organic dusts that can come alive and reproduce themselves at a fantastic rate when conditions such as temperature and acidity are right for them. These conditions are found in susceptible living cells of a particular host that may be either human, animal, insect, plant, or even a bacterium, depending on the viruses' idiosyncratic and particular proclivities. All human beings are inhabited by a multitude of these small parasites, many of which are harmless. Some, like the herpes virus, cause symptoms only during periods of fatigue and stress; then they can produce the well-known cold sores. In all, there are more than 1000 known varieties of viruses. Since 1960 it has been recognized that the *typical* common cold is generally a result of an infection by one particular family of viruses— the so-called rhinoviruses.

Those suffering from a common cold find no solace in knowing that in recent years a great deal has been learned about the properties of rhinoviruses. Nor are they reassured when told that virologists have discovered from clinical experiments that a *full-blown* cold is not particularly infectious. The highly infectious period, apparently, is during the maturation period before any cold symptoms are manifested. Nor will most people forgo their well-tried home remedies, even though the scientists tell them that their belief in the value of vitamins, whiskey, aspirin, etc., is a deluded one.

Sir Christopher Andrewes, in his book *The Common Cold* (1960), writes that during the 17 years of the existence of the Common Cold

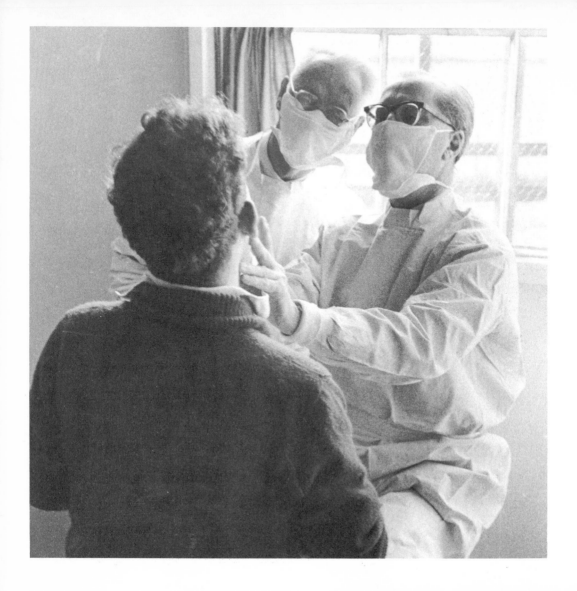

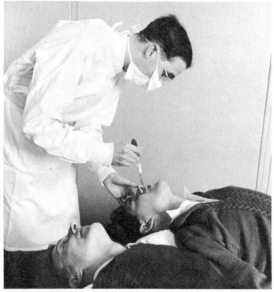

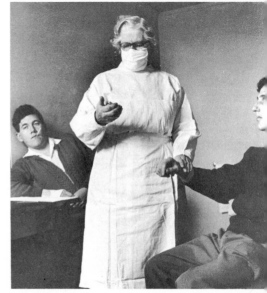

Unit at Salisbury, England—a center specifically set up for research into colds, and of which he was the scientific director—innumerable letters have been received. Many of the correspondents "knew" how to prevent or cure colds, and offered to disclose their secrets for cash. Some recommended sniffing pepper or cinnamon snuff; some local treatments such as washing the nose out with sodium bicarbonate, or water and salt, or potassium permanganate; some inhaling the vapor of ammonia, iodine, formalin, or eucalyptus. Other letters contained even more bizarre recommendations: "rubbing methylated spirits into a bald head, rubbing the body with vaseline . . . transient exposure to tear gas . . . wearing a gas mask for an hour, inhaling powdered, dry, liquorice leaves, working with lime . . . mental concentration especially on mathematics, growing a moustache right up to the nostrils, sweeping chimneys, standing on one's head under water, or wearing on the back between the kidneys a bag containing onions. . . ."

Though no drug effectively inhibits the cold virus, doctors can, through inoculations, protect people from a number of more virulent virus infections. These include smallpox, rabies, yellow fever, and poliomyelitis. Inoculation, at least in its crude form, was introduced into western Europe through the missionary zeal of the remarkable Lady Mary Wortley Montagu (1689–1762), the authoress who quarreled notoriously with the poet Alexander Pope. Lady Mary was the wife of the British ambassador in Constantinople. In Turkey she observed how the girls of the local harems had excellent complexions, unspoiled by pockmarks. These girls, like their predecessors in ancient China and Egypt, had been ingrafted. That is to say, infected material from smallpox pustules in mild cases had been scratched at one time on to their bodies. Subsequently they had suffered a mild attack of

The WHO supports intensive research into the common cold at a special unit established at Salisbury, England. Above left, doctors examine a new arrival at the center. Far left, volunteers are given nasal drops containing the particular virus under study. Left, a nurse checks the pulse and temperature of a volunteer as part of the daily medical routine.

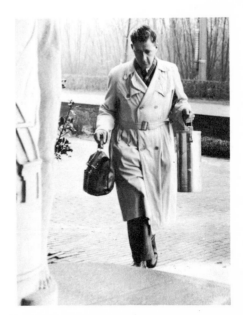

Right, in Leiden, Holland, throat washings—packed in dry ice—are brought to a national laboratory to be examined for influenza virus.

smallpox and this had left them with unblemished skins and an immunity to further smallpox infections, however severe. It was a risky procedure but Lady Mary, impressed with the results, inoculated her own young son. Back in London in 1718 she persuaded Princess Caroline to inoculate her daughter. The cautious princess wished first to see the results on condemned criminals and orphaned children. When these ingraftings proved successful she agreed to Lady Mary's promptings. And afterwards this method became a fashionable means of crude inoculation in western Europe, though the results were not always happy.

Some 80 years later, at the close of the 18th century, a more satisfactory method of inoculation against smallpox was discovered in Britain by Dr. Edward Jenner (1749–1823), a Gloucester physician. It had been common rustic knowledge for some time that milkmaids who had suffered a cowpox infection were immune to the more dangerous smallpox. Dr. Jenner acted upon this knowledge. In 1796 he scratched infective material from a cowpox pustule on to the arm of an eight-year-old boy named James Phipps. He was sure that the youngster would be immune to smallpox. To prove his thesis he tried, six weeks later, to infect the boy with material taken from a pustule of a smallpox patient. Since the boy did not contract smallpox, showing no symptoms, Jenner's theories were clinically corroborated. Despite opposition Edward Jenner's method of vaccination gained support and within a few years some 100,000 people throughout the world had been vaccinated—and for a time the death rate from smallpox was reduced. (Jenner did not at once realize that re-vaccination became necessary after some years.) In 1801, shortly after he became president of the United States, Thomas Jefferson is said to have vaccinated

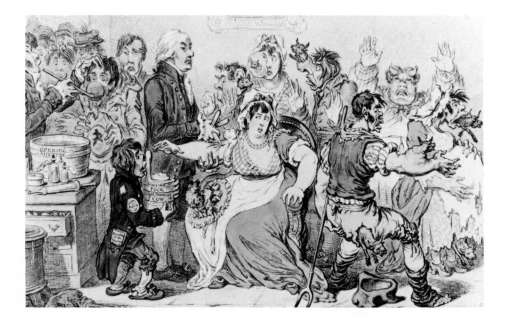

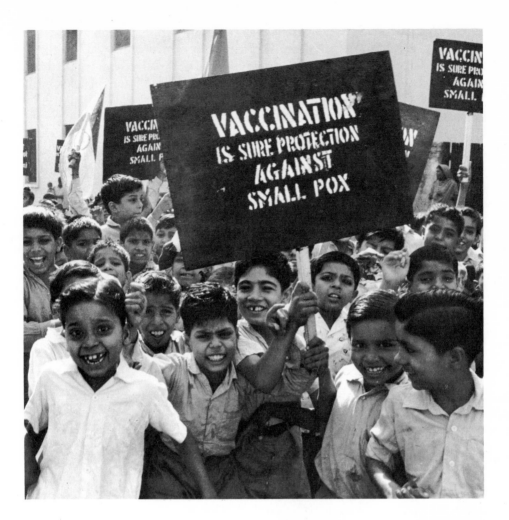

Left, *The Cow Pock—or—The Wonderful Effects of the New Inoculation*—the Gillray caricature of Edward Jenner published by the Anti-Vaccine Society in 1802. The value of inoculation is now generally recognized. In India, where two thirds of the world's smallpox cases occur, a massive vaccination program was launched in 1964 (above). By the beginning of 1965, more than 64 per cent of the population (some 279 million people) had been vaccinated. Right, an Afghan girl, victim of smallpox.

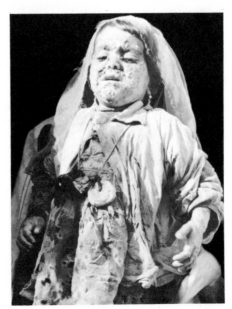

Indians personally. Jenner had said, "I will build a rock," and he continued his human experiments until the objective value of vaccination became incontrovertible. His methods, with only little modification, have withstood the test of time, and are used to this day. In Russia alone, where compulsory vaccination was introduced in 1919, it has been estimated that more than half a million lives have been saved as a result.

Vaccination has the rare hazard, it is true, of postvaccinial encephalitis (inflammation of the brain) and there has always been minority opposition to it. Men like George Bernard Shaw doubted the veracity of statistics that overwhelmingly proved the efficacy of vaccinia. "Even trained statisticians often fail to appreciate the extent to which statistics are vitiated by the unrecorded assumptions of their interpreters," he wrote in the Preface to his play *The Doctor's Dilemma* (1906). "Their attention is too much occupied with the cruder tricks of those who make a corrupt use of statistics for advertising purposes. There is, for example, the percentage dodge. In some hamlet, barely large enough to have a name, two people are attacked during a smallpox epidemic. One dies: the other recovers. One has vaccination marks: the other none. Immediately the vaccinists . . . publish the triumphant news that at such and such a place not a single person vaccinated died of smallpox whilst 100 per cent of the unvaccinated perished miserably. . . ." Those with the strong prejudices of a Bernard Shaw will always think of statisticians as liars when figures defeat their arguments; and, from the occasional complication resulting from vaccination, will find confirmation in their belief.

In 1947 5,000,000 New Yorkers were vaccinated against smallpox after the infection was introduced into the city from Mexico; 49 of these suffered from postvaccinial encephalitis and there were eight fatal cases. Such an event allows the antivaccinationists to raise their banners high. But Jenner did build a rock. Mass vaccination has not only saved innumerable lives but has prevented even more people from suffering ugly disfigurements such as those visited upon the immoral but once beautiful Madame de Merteuil, in Laclos's 18th-century novel *Les Liaisons Dangereuses*. Madame de Volanges writes to Madame de Rosemonde: "Madame de Merteuil's destiny seems at last, my dear and worthy friend, to have been fulfilled. It is such that her worst enemies are divided between the indignation she merits and the pity she inspires. I was quite right to say that it would perhaps be fortunate for her if she died of the smallpox. She has recovered, it is true, but horribly disfigured: more than anything by the loss of an eye. As you may imagine, I have not seen her again; but I am told she looks hideous. The Marquis de —, who never loses an opportunity to be spiteful, said yesterday in speaking of her, 'that the disease has turned her inside out, and that her soul is now visible on her face.' "

Almost a century passed after Jenner's discovery before the preparation of a second virus vaccine. On July 6, 1885, Louis Pasteur, a great admirer of Jenner, performed the first inoculation against rabies. A nine-year-old boy, Joseph Meister, had been bitten on the hands and legs by a rabid dog. The inoculation saved the boy's life. (When he grew up, Joseph Meister became a gatekeeper at the Pasteur Institute in Paris. He committed suicide in 1940, following the German invaders' attempts to open the crypt where Pasteur was buried.)

Rabies has infected animals and man ever since early Greek and Roman times. Nowadays the disease is associated in the public mind with mad dogs, but in previous centuries other animals were carriers of the rabies virus. In 1886 the deer in Richmond Park, just outside London, were found to be infected, while in more recent times vampire bats have been implicated in the transmission of the virus. During 1928 there was an epidemic of rabies among the cattle of Paraguay, after they had been bitten by vampire bats. The disease killed off 30 per cent of them. Indeed, it is probable that vampire bats throughout the entire eastern sector of South America are heavily infected with rabies, and human beings need to put wire screens on their houses as a protection at night. More recently it has been recognized that the ordinary insect-eating bats as well can, on occasions, transmit the disease.

Sixteen per cent of people bitten by rabid animals die. Pasteur's vaccine, if given soon enough, reduces the fatalities to one per cent. Rabies is a terrifying disease. Patients suffering from it complain of a dry throat and extreme thirst, but as soon as any water passes their lips the head is thrown backward, jerking, and reflex spasms make breathing difficult. The water is then ejected. It is because of this symptom that the disease has been called *hydrophobia* (fear of water). After three days, maniacal grimaces and paralyses manifest themselves, to be followed by convulsive seizures. Moreover, consciousness is retained almost until death.

It was this very nightmare aspect of rabies that induced Louis Pasteur to study the disease: he had never forgotten how, when he was a boy, a number of men in his village had been attacked by an infected wolf. Pasteur knew that the causative agents of rabies infected the brain and spinal cord. He took spinal cords from rabbits that had died from the infection and hung up the cords in dry, sterile air. He found that by this method he could attenuate the virulence of the rabies virus, and finally he prepared a vaccine by making an emulsion from these spinal cords. His vaccine proved effective in protecting dogs infected by rabies, as it was later to protect Joseph Meister and many other human beings. A commission set up in Britain in 1888 not only recognized the value of Pasteur's discovery but believed that it showed a way "to avert by inoculation . . . other diseases besides hydrophobia."

The first two vaccines to be discovered, then, were against virus infections. After Pasteur the development of immunization was essentially against diseases caused by bacteria. Bacteria were easy to grow on culture media in the laboratory; but early virus workers did not know then, as they do now, how to grow viruses on living tissues outside the body (culture tissues). They had to infect animals with viruses and such experimental work was clumsy and expensive. Yet without growing the viruses in large, controllable quantities it was virtually impossible to produce vaccines from attenuated strains. Hence the long delay in the discovery of the third major vaccine against a virus infection: yellow fever.

Yellow fever, or yellow jack, as it has been called, is a mosquito-transmitted infection endemic in certain tropical and subtropical areas, especially in South and Central America and Africa. A description of a yellow-fever epidemic that broke out during the Siege of Cartagena in 1740 is given by Tobias Smollett in *Roderick Random*, and shows how lethal the infection can be: " . . . the bilious fever amongst us . . . raged with such violence that three fourths of those whom it

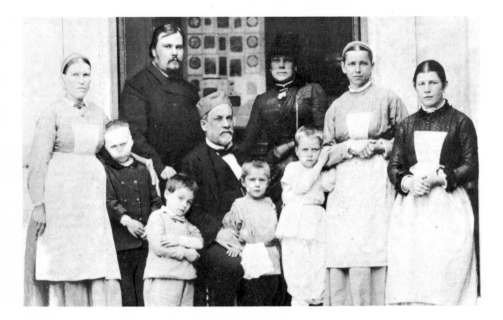

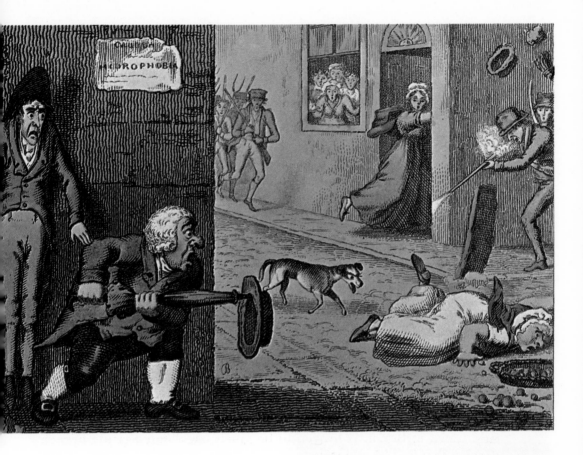

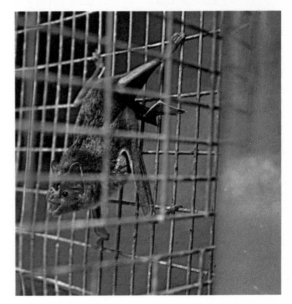

Left, Louis Pasteur with his nursing
staff and some of the first children he
inoculated successfully against rabies.
Above, the widespread fear of rabid dogs
and hydrophobia in 19th-century Britain
is caricatured in *Mad Dog,* an engraving
by T. C. Busby (1826). Today, rabies'
most dangerous carrier is the vampire bat
of Mexico and South America (right).

invaded died in a deplorable manner: the colour of their skin being, by the extreme putrefaction of the juices, changed into that of soot. . . ."

From time to time outbreaks of yellow fever have occurred in international ports such as Swansea in South Wales (1865), and New Orleans (1905). Roughly 15 per cent of cases are fatal, and many scientific investigators have contracted the disease. In 1927 two eminent bacteriologists and pioneers in the conquest of yellow fever, Adrian Stokes (an Englishman) and Hideyo Noguchi (a Japanese), who had been sent on separate missions to Africa by the Rockefeller Institute, died of the fever. Noguchi's last reported words were: "I don't understand."

Earlier that year, though, the first step in the discovery of a vaccine against yellow fever had been taken by Stokes when he found that rhesus monkeys could be infected with the virus. An American, Max Theiler, took the second step in 1928 when he injected small particles of an infected monkey's liver into the brain of a white mouse. Theiler also discovered that as the virus passed through the brains of more and more mice, the strain became increasingly virulent for mice but at the same time less virulent for monkeys. Eventually, in 1936, Theiler managed to produce an attenuated virus—after it had been passed through other tissues, including chick embryo. Now harmless to human beings this virus, which still brought forth antibodies against yellow fever, could be used as an immunizing agent. Theiler's vaccine —derived from the so-called 17D strain of yellow-fever virus—was field-tested in Brazil. It proved to be much safer than a crude French vaccine that had been developed from a strain grown by Theiler in the brains of mice.

All the same, 56 million people were vaccinated with the French vaccine between 1939 and 1953; and though frequent reactions resulted there were few fatalities. The World Health Organization reported that yellow fever, in humans, had almost vanished from those territories (Western Equatorial Africa) where this French vaccine had been used. Between 1940 and 1947 the Rockefeller Foundation produced 28,104,420 doses of Theiler's 17D vaccine and gave it to the American forces and to other agencies to be used in 33 different tropical countries. Today both vaccines are readily available.

The most recent vaccine to be developed is against poliomyelitis. This virus infection has never been associated with a high death rate and indeed most recover from it without any ill effects whatsoever. Nevertheless it is a disease particularly feared, for most people have read reports in newspapers of children crippled by polio, or perhaps have met adults who suffer some permanent disability as a

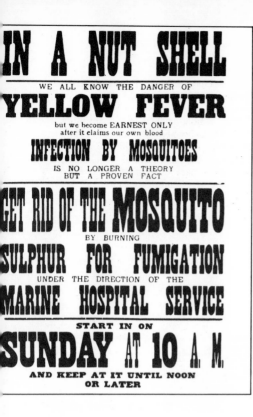

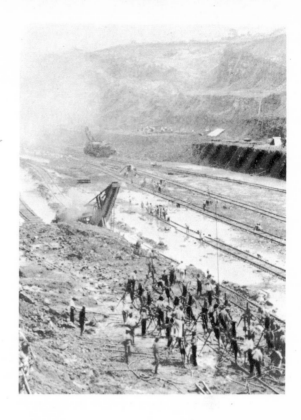

Above, one of the many posters issued in New Orleans during the yellow-fever epidemic of 1905. Above right, workers on the Panama Canal in 1913. Repeated outbreaks of yellow fever frustrated the French attempts to cut the Canal during the 19th century, and it was completed—by American engineers—only in 1914.

consequence of a virulent attack years before. Epidemics of poliomyelitis, moreover, seemed to be most prevalent in the advanced countries such as Sweden, New Zealand, and Australia. The U.S.A., in 1949, suffered its worst epidemic when 43,000 cases were reported. The cleaner and more hygienic a nation the more frequently it seemed to be visited by the poliomyelitis virus. This strange fact has been explained by Richard Fiennes in *Man, Nature and Diseases*:

"In epidemics of poliomyelitis, while the effects can be serious in a large proportion of the younger children, those under the age of three are rarely if ever affected. During the first three years of life, there is a 'safe' period when infection with the virus is harmless; it can, however, create immunity, so that a child who has been in contact with poliomyelitis during the first three years of life will not succumb to infection at a later age. In communities not dedicated to high standards of child welfare it is found that a large proportion of infants become infected during the safe period; indeed virtually the whole population

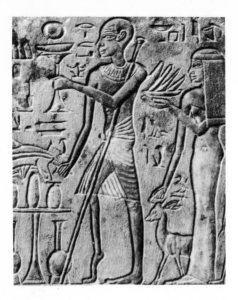

Left, an Egyptian stele of the 18th Dynasty (1567–1320 B.C.) shows a young man with a withered leg, a characteristic feature of poliomyelitis. In modern times polio has become most manifest in the more prosperous communities. Below, in Pittsburg, U.S.A., Dr. Jonas Salk helps during the mass inoculation trial of his then controversial polio vaccine.

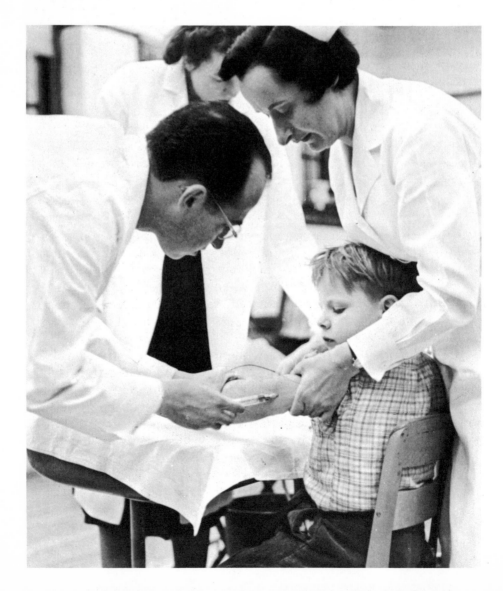

is immune by the age of three, so poliomyelitis never becomes a serious problem. In advanced communities, by contrast, the younger children are largely protected from the sources of infection, but become exposed at the time they are sent to school and begin to mix with other children. At this age, they are not only susceptible to infection but more liable to develop symptoms of paralysis. The reasons why this happens are related to the method of transmission. The virus is one of the 'entero-virus' group, whose members are natural inhabitants of the intestinal tract of animals and man. The polio virus only affects the human species, and transmission is therefore directly from one human to another. Some experts believe that infection is by so-called 'droplet' means; this is to say that the virus is carried on droplets of moisture in expired air. It is, however, more generally accepted that the virus is transferred from one host to another by means of inapparent con-tamination of the hands and fingers with excreta or stools; by this means the virus may be transferred to the food and passed from person to person."

During the 1930s, news of two new anti-polio vaccines had been welcomed with great jubilation. Both, later, were discovered to be useless and one was found to be positively dangerous in certain circumstances. As recently as 1953, gamma globulin, a constituent of human blood, was used for mass injections in 23 areas of the U.S.A. in a hopeless bid to beat the poliomyelitis epidemics. Such was the general fear of poliomyelitis that during their tour of Australia in 1953, Queen Elizabeth and the Duke of Edinburgh received this same, useless injection of gamma globulin.

But in 1949 an event of importance had occurred: scientific workers of Harvard Medical School cultivated the polio virus in monkey kidney cells. Dr. Jonas Salk took advantage of this new discovery, and selecting the different varieties of the virus, killed them with formal-dehyde. Eventually he managed to produce a vaccine of dead viruses that, when injected into animals, had no ill effect yet called forth poliomyelitis antibodies. In 1953 he was ready to test his vaccine on human beings—and such was his confidence that he chose his own three young children as "guinea pigs" for the experiment.

Convinced of the soundness of Dr. Salk's work the National Foundation for Infantile Paralysis, which had originally been spon-sored by President Roosevelt (himself a polio victim), arranged mass trials to test the new Salk vaccine. Altogether 1,830,000 children were given an injection of the vaccine and the results were convincing. The association arranged a huge press and television conference to announce the new wonder vaccine, and the press covered the event as massively as if it had been the ending of some major war. The American

Medical Association's Board of Trustees confirmed: "This vaccine is one of the greatest events in the history of medicine." It was intended that, during 1955, 13,000,000 American children should be vaccinated, and various commercial firms were contracted by the American government to manufacture the Salk vaccine. One of the firms was the Cutter Laboratories, and some of their vaccine was later found to contain live virus. As a result 79 people in Idaho alone contracted poliomyelitis and as news of new cases came in from other parts of the country the chiefs of Cutters were obliged to send the following telegram to chemists: URGENT NO FURTHER INJECTIONS CUTTER POLIO VACCINE TO BE MADE STOP IMMEDIATELY ADVISE YOUR PHYSICIANS STOP PLEASE RETURN UNUSED SUPPLIES.

The Cutter firm had supplied Idaho, parts of California, Nevada, New Mexico, Arizona, and Hawaii. The decision to stop the Cutter vaccine injections was too late. Two hundred children suffered from paralysis, and 11 of them died. Subsequently no such catastrophic accidents occurred and by May 1959 more than 150,000,000 children and young people in 90 countries owed their protection against paralytic polio to the Salk vaccine.

Other workers, like the American Dr. Albert Sabin, believed in the efficacy of a live attenuated vaccine, and this was seen to have advantages finally, for it could be given in sweets or on sugar which children obviously preferred to injections. Dr. Sabin persuaded the Soviet Union to use his live vaccine and massive trials were carried out there, which proved to be a success. By 1960 over 80,000,000 people had been given the Sabin oral vaccine and this along with the Salk injections has markedly reduced the incidence of poliomyelitis. In New Zealand, for example, where 80 per cent of the population were immunized during 1962 and 1963, not one case of poliomyelitis has been reported. Sabin, like Salk, could righteously quote Emerson: "The reward of a thing well done is to have done it."

No doubt, in the future, other vaccines will be discovered to protect us against this or that infection. Yet while the old adage "prevention is better than cure" is valid as a generalization, it is unlikely to cheer those who are unhappily, and perhaps tragically, suffering from a virus disease. They will continue to hope for the discovery of specific drugs that can act against viruses as antibodies can against specific bacteria. The progress of modern medicine does not depend on a succession of empirical accidents. Rather, successes follow on the discovery of pathological processes. Fortunately, with every year that passes, more and more is revealed about the nature of viruses and how the body summons forth its defenses against them. It has been known for a long time that vaccines for smallpox and poliomyelitis, for example, conscript into the blood the specific antibodies of these illnesses and so give protection against them. So it was natural to presume that antibodies played an important role in the recovery of a patient suffering from any virus infection. That fact, it is now realized, does not explain everything about the process whereby the body overcomes viruses. For since antibodies combine with viruses outside the cells, how can antibodies attack those viruses that spread directly inside the cells? Recent research has shown how, under the stimulus of virus infection, the cells themselves respond by producing an anti-viral substance. This substance has been called *interferon*.

If interferon plays such an important part in overcoming a virus infection—be it poliomyelitis, or influenza, or the common cold— perhaps this substance can be used as a means of attacking viral infections. This question engages the attention of research workers at this moment in time. Other investigators are not so much looking for a drug to overcome viruses directly, but are searching out ways and means whereby the body cells can be stimulated to increase their own natural output of interferon and so conquer the invading viruses with greater ease and rapidity.

What seems likely is that in the next decade or two there will be a further major advance in the battle against infection, and this advance will involve the virus diseases. Such progress will have as far-reaching social consequences as the discovery of the antibiotics, and much human misery will be averted or at least deferred. Already, the control of infectious diseases has so progressed that its very reality would have seemed to an earlier generation an optimistic and pretty dream. George Orwell, whose description of a primitive French hospital was quoted at the beginning of this chapter, wrote later, when sick and dying of tuberculosis, of the nightmare world he imagined could exist by 1984. At least the progress against infection, and all that that entails, is one, forlorn, concrete sign, in a world divided and often at war, that the wit of man is not directed exclusively on destructive purposes.

# 2  Against the Grim Horseman

Before the Battle of the Plains of Abraham at Quebec in 1759 General James Wolfe is reported to have said: "I would rather have written Gray's *Elegy in a Country Churchyard* than have the glory of conquering Quebec." I imagine many people, however honored they may be in their own field, must have thought, at least in their more messianic moods, "I would rather have been awarded the Nobel Prize for Medicine." In recent years that honor has frequently been gained by those who have discovered drugs to combat infection. Thus Gerhard Domagk in 1939, Alexander Fleming, Ernst Boris Chain, and Howard Walter Florey in 1945, and Selman Abraham Waksman in 1952. But there have been other winners of this high award, and the gradual evolution of medicine toward being a science, along with much avoidance of misery and death, has been a sequel to their achievements.

In 1923, Frederick Grant Banting (Canada) and John James Richard Macleod (Scotland) were awarded the Nobel Prize "*For their discovery of insulin*"; in 1929 it was the turn of Christiaan Eijkman (Holland) "*For his discovery of the antineuritic vitamin*" and of Frederick Gowland Hopkins (Britain) "*For his discovery of the growth-stimulating vitamins*"; in 1934 the prize was awarded to George H. Whipple (U.S.A.), George Richards Minot (U.S.A.), and William P. Murphy

American tennis star Ham Richardson— a diabetic—in play during the Wimbledon Tennis Championships, 1965. Until the discovery of insulin, diabetes was feared as a crippling and often fatal disease.

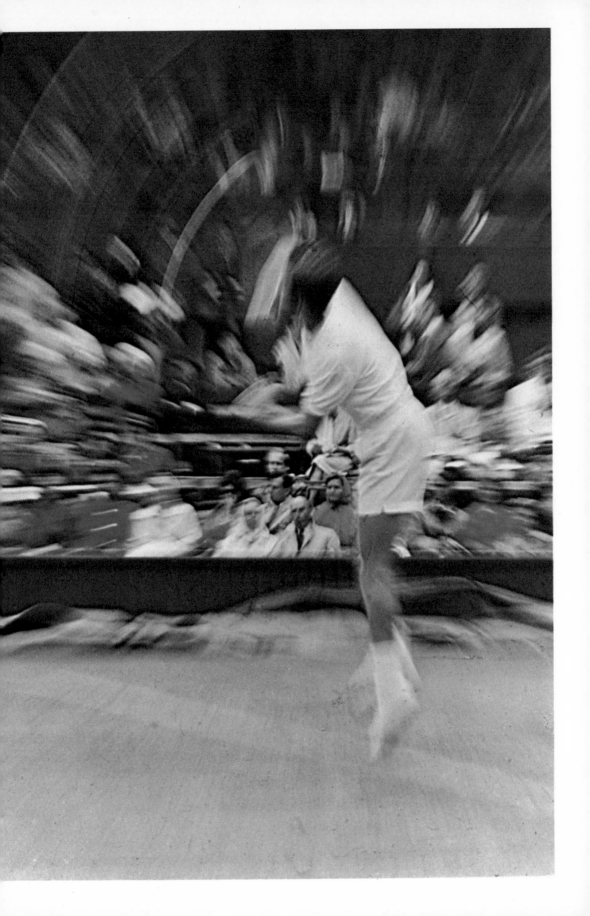

(U.S.A.) *"For their discoveries concerning liver therapy against anaemias"*; in 1937 to Albert von Szent-Györgyi (Hungary) *"For his discoveries in connection with the biological combustion processes, with especial reference to vitamin C and the catalysis of fumaric acid"*; in 1943 to Henrik Dam (Denmark) *"For his discovery of vitamin K"* and the American Edward A. Doisy *"For his discovery of the chemical nature of vitamin K"*; in 1947 to Bernardo Alberto Houssay (Argentina) *"For his discovery of the part played by the hormone of the anterior pituitary lobe in the metabolism of sugar"* and to Carl and Gerty Cori (Czechoslovakia) *"For their discovery of how glycogen is catalytically converted"*; in 1950 to Edward Calvin Kendall (U.S.A.), Philip Showalter Hench (U.S.A.), and Tadeusz Reichstein (Poland) *"For their discoveries concerning the suprarenal cortex hormones, their structure and biological effects."*

I have called out this selected register of names to indicate where in particular, in our time, formidable medical progress has been made, apart from that against infection. There have been other notable medical Nobel Prize winners, but these multiple citations are all concerned directly or indirectly with hormones and vitamins. Conditions such as diabetes and pernicious anemia still cannot be cured; but as a result of this progress those suffering from such illnesses are now neither reduced to chronic invalidism nor condemned to death, as so recently was the case, which is both cheering and spectacular. If I have drawn attention to the nationalities—or at least to the country of origin—of these Nobel Prize winners, it is simply to underline the fact that the alleviation of suffering has resulted from international contributions, and that science—it needs saying over and over—like disease itself, knows no man-made frontiers.

How important such progress in medicine has been can perhaps be fathomed from the fact that in advanced countries today millions of people—more than three people in every 1000—suffer from diabetes but are still able to lead almost normal lives simply because they are taking insulin. Without it these same people would be subject to the tragic complications of diabetes, such as blindness and gangrene, and would soon be dying or dead.

Diabetes mellitus has been known to exist for thousands of years. The first accurate description of the disease was by Aretaeus of Cappadocia (now Central Turkey) during the second century A.D. He recounted how diabetes was "a melting down of the flesh and limbs into urine," and described other symptoms of the disease. "The patient is short-lived," he noted, ". . . for the melting is rapid, the death speedy. Moreover, life is disgusting and painful; thirst unquenchable; excessive drinking which however is disproportionate to the large quantity of urine . . . passed."

Later the Romans observed that bees were attracted to the sweet urine voided by diabetics, and in the fifth century A.D. an Indian, Susrata, observed directly that the taste of diabetic urine was sweet. It was not until the 18th century, however, that a British doctor from Yorkshire, Matthew Dobson, demonstrated chemically that diabetic urine has a sweet taste because it is loaded with sugar.

During my early days as a medical student at Westminster Hospital, I and 12 others were asked by the consultant how we would diagnose diabetes from a urine sample. "By finding sugar in it, Sir," I replied. And how would we discover whether or not there was sugar in such a sample? No one replied. A nurse was requested to fetch a sample of urine, and then the consultant dipped a finger into it before apparently tasting his finger with the tip of his tongue. The sample was passed around. Each student dipped his finger into it. Each one foolishly licked his finger. "Now," said the consultant, grinning, "you have learnt the first principle of medical diagnosis. I mean the power of observation." We were all baffled. "You see," he said, "I dipped my middle finger into the urine but *I* licked my index finger!" Indeed, it is not necessary, nowadays, to taste urine in order to detect whether it is loaded with sugar, nor for that matter to wait hopefully for the bees of summer to buzz through the window. A simple chemical test exists.

But why, in diabetes, is so much sugar present in the urine? The answering of this question leads one indirectly to the cause of diabetes and to the story of the discovery of insulin. In 1889, Oskar Minkowski, assistant to the professor of medicine at Strasbourg University, discovered that when the pancreas, the sweetbread lying behind the stomach in the loop of the duodenum, was removed from a dog, the animal's urine contained 5 per cent sugar the next day. The removal of the pancreas led, in short, to diabetes. Minkowski carried out further experiments and these confirmed that the activity of the pancreas was in some way related to the production of diabetes, but he went no further in trying to elucidate this relationship.

The pancreas produces two types of "juice." It secretes digestive fluids that pass through a duct into the duodenum and help to break down the food that has been emptied from the stomach. But the pancreas is also an endocrine organ—that is to say it secretes a chemical substance, a hormone, directly into the blood. This second substance derives from particular cells in the pancreas, the so-called islets of Langerhans. It was a young American pathologist, Eugene Lindsay Opie of Johns Hopkins University, Baltimore, who first noted that the islets of Langerhans underwent degeneration in diabetes. This he discovered when examining sections from the pancreas of dead diabetic patients under the microscope. In 1916 the British physiologist Sir

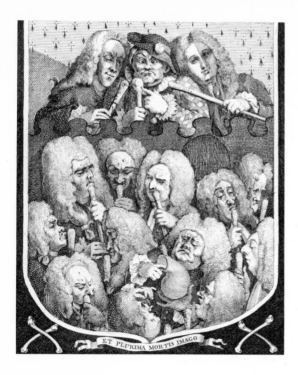

Distinguished contemporary physicians are represented in Hogarth's *The Arms of the Honourable Company of Undertakers* (1736). The two in the foreground are inspecting urine in a flask, and one is about to taste it, for sugar, on his finger.

Edward Sharpey-Schafer put two and two together and suggested that diabetes resulted from a lack of a hormone secreted by these islets of Langerhans. Sir Edward called this hypothetical hormone "insulin." It was only a matter of time, now, before scientific investigators would substantiate that such a hormone actually existed and go on to extract it from the pancreatic Langerhans cells.

To make such an extract, however, was not easy. Whole pancreatic extracts were of no use because the digestive juices in them destroyed the active principle (insulin) of the Langerhans cells. In 1921 a Canadian, Frederick Banting, read a scientific paper on "The Relation of the Islets of Langerhans to Diabetes" by Dr. Moses Barron of Minneapolis. Dr. Barron recounted how earlier experimenters had tied off the pancreatic ducts in rabbits. As a result the pancreas had degenerated but the islets of Langerhans had remained intact—and, importantly, as a consequence the rabbit had not suffered from glycosuria (sugar in the urine). Here, then, might be a means, thought Banting, whereby an extract of Langerhans cells could be obtained that would not be inactivated by the digestive ferments of the rest of the pancreas. For if the rest of the pancreas had degenerated, following ligation of the duct, the digestive juices would not be present to affect the hormone. This was the idea that now possessed Banting.

"We do not know," he said later, "whence ideas come, but the importance of the idea in medical research cannot be overestimated. From the nature of things ideas do not come from prosperity, affluence and contentment, but rather from the blackness of despair, not in the bright light of day, not the footlights' glare, but rather in the quiet, undisturbed hours of midnight, or early morning, when one can be alone to think. These are the grandest hours of all, when the imagination is allowed to run riot on the problem that blocks the progress of research, when the hewn stones of scientific fact are turned over and over, and fitted in so that the mosaic figure of truth, designed by Mother Nature long ago, be formed from the chaos."

In May 1921 Dr. Banting began to put his idea into concrete terms. Along with his young assistant, Dr. Charles Best, he worked in Professor Macleod's physiology laboratory at the University of Toronto, tying off the pancreatic ducts of dogs. The animal experiments continued and, after several setbacks, proved successful. Less than a year later the two doctors had obtained an extract and were ready to use it on patients at Toronto General Hospital. Soon after, they had in their possession quantities of this extract (insulin) that were sufficiently large and pure to be of indisputable benefit for many diabetic patients. Emaciated men and women began to recover.

Until then doctors had been trying to keep diabetics alive, trying to prolong their lives by restricting their sugar intake, sometimes starving them, in the hope that a new advance against the disease would be discovered in time. Dr. F. John Poynton was but one physician who had under his care diabetic children in a ward of a London hospital. For those youngsters the discovery of insulin came too late. "We had all, according to our lights, worked most diligently at them," wrote Dr. Poynton in *The British Medical Journal* of February 1923, "yet all died. . . . In all the cases of any duration we invariably went through three stages of thought: first the belief that we were succeeding—a belief that was never confident: then the uneasy feeling that we were losing ground: and finally the realization that our efforts were fruitless. We protracted the illness, but nothing more, and this very partial success was so unsatisfactory from the children's point of view that had not there been always a hope that some new advance might appear, or some unexpected improvement arise, it seemed hardly worth while."

Children died and adults died. All over the world, in quiet surgeries, serious doctors had been saying, "I am sorry but your son (your daughter, your husband, your wife) has diabetes." The patient had left the surgery doomed. A death warrant had been pronounced that would, too soon, be executed. Now, insulin had changed the prognosis radically. The dying were beginning to be plucked from the grave.

No wonder Banting and his colleagues rejoiced. They had uncovered one scientific truth that would result in treasure for millions—

the treasure of life itself. H. G. Wells, a diabetic who eventually benefited from insulin injections, wrote: "Scientific truth is the remotest of mistresses; she hides in strange places, she is attained by tortuous and laborious roads, *but she is always there*! Win to her and she will not fail you; she is yours and mankind's forever. . . . You cannot change her by advertisement or clamour, nor stifle her in vulgarities. Things grow under your hands when you serve her, things that are permanent as nothing else is permanent in the whole life of man. That, I think, is the peculiar satisfaction of science and its enduring reward." The Nobel Prize that Banting received in 1923 was a reward paltry in comparison.

Since 1923, purer and longer-acting preparations of insulin have been manufactured, such as Protamine-zinc Insulin developed in 1938 by Scott and Fisher in Toronto. Unfortunately, insulin of whatever kind has to be given by injection, for if taken by mouth it is destroyed by the digestive juices. In recent years, however, hypoglycemic agents other than insulin have been discovered, which can be taken orally. Certain sulfonamide drugs like carbutamide, tolbutamide, chlor-propamide, and one with the formidable name of paraaminobenzol-sulphonamideisopropylthiodiazole, reduce the sugar in the blood by stimulating the islets of Langerhans to secrete more insulin. Such oral insulin stimulators have only limited practical value. During the last few years over a thousand of these sulfonamide derivatives have been developed and other kinds of oral hypoglycemic substances are being evaluated. So in this connection it is probable that, sooner or later, a more effective oral agent will be discovered.

Diabetes, however, is much more complicated than was at first thought. Clinicians became baffled when they observed that insulin requirements in different diabetics varied to a greater extent than they expected. It would appear that diabetes should not be regarded as one disease but rather a syndrome, a consequence not only of a dysfunction of sugar metabolism but of the metabolism as a whole. After all, the pancreas is an endocrine gland and the endocrines can be thought of as an orchestra whose conductor is the pituitary gland. Interference with any one member of the orchestra—the pancreas, the sex glands, the adrenals, the thyroid, or whatever—causes a general disharmony. Moreover, it is now known that hormones are secreted not only by the endocrines, as was formerly taught, but by other cells also. In short, apart from insulin, there are a legion of hormones. Yet Starkey coined the name "hormone" only some 60 years ago, when but two hormones were available to clinicians: adrenalin and thyroid extract.

With such increased knowledge of hormones and the endocrine system, therapeutic advances have been made against diseases other than diabetes. Still, in the public mind, hormones are too often thought to be substances related only to sex. People have read, in large circulation newspapers, stories about men and women who have changed their sex. The Greeks, as usual, had a word for it: hermaphrodite—the name given to the bisexual child whose father was Hermes and whose mother was Aphrodite. Representations of Hermaphrodite can be seen in the Greek sculptures of beautiful youths with marked breasts or of females with male genitalia.

People have read, too, of male and female hormones. These have been used—for the most part without effect—like quacks' nostrums to cure this or that. Thus testicular hormones have been given to arrest the aging process and to promote male sexuality, while the female estrogens have been prescribed to promote Hollywood bosoms for the self-conscious underdeveloped. In any case, it is inaccurate to think that either male or female hormones belong exclusively to one sex. To a degree we are all androgynous, as Freud, in a psychological context, has pointed out. Nor are sex hormones produced only by the gonads, for the adrenal glands also secrete them. Tumors of the adrenal cortex can lead to virilism, where masculine characteristics develop in the female so that pseudo-hermaphroditism results. *True* hermaphroditism is not infrequent in the animal kingdom—goat and pig hermaphrodites abound and hens have had chicks and then subsequently changed their sex to father another brood—but in human beings it is a comparatively rare phenomenon. Only some 40 true cases have been reported in the medical literature.

The female and male hormones do, though, have proper therapeutic uses in medicine. Most recently they have been prescribed to combat certain kinds of malignant growth. Hormones are not, in general, anti-cancer drugs, but the "sex" hormones have a limited value in treating cancers of the breast and of the prostate. Such lines of treatment followed the report of the American surgeon Charles Huggins in 1941 that removal of the testicles had arrested cancer of the prostate. It was this discovery that stimulated a great deal of research into the relationship between hormonal imbalance and cancer. This research continues, but until more is understood about the action of hormones on cells there is very little likelihood of any important progress being made in this particular field.

Recently, also, sex hormonal steroids in pill form have been, and are being, taken by large numbers of women as a contraceptive. In the U.S.A. more than three million women now rely on "the pill," which contains a mixture of these synthetic steroids. The numbers are liable to increase despite the fact that all women using them are really acting as human guinea pigs. No one can be really sure yet what the

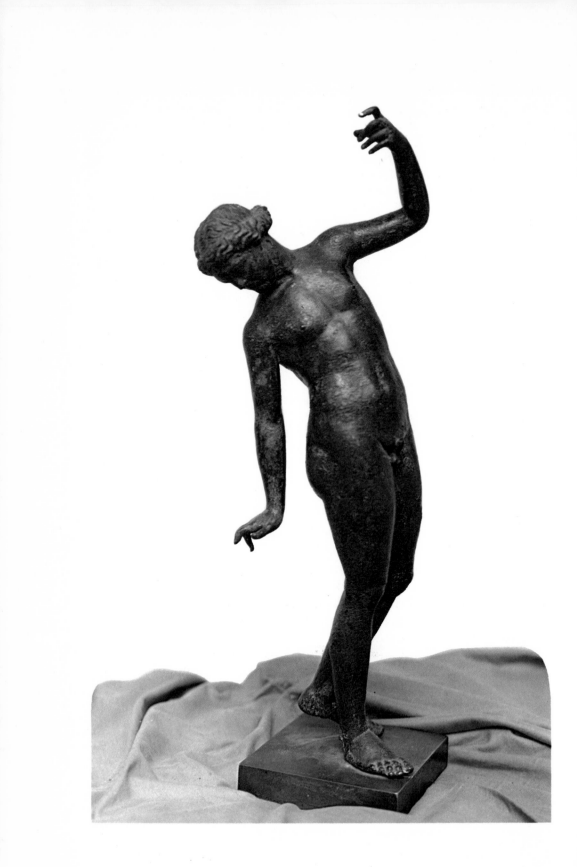

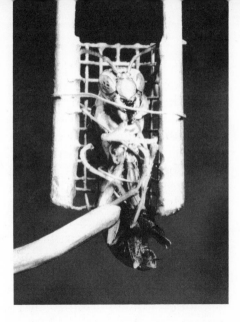

This bronze statuette, the *Hermaphroditus of Mirecourt* (left), shows the extreme of hermaphroditism—a female body with male sex organs. Hermaphroditism is caused by hormonal imbalance. Right, as part of research into hormones at the National Heart Institute in America, wasps are induced to sting by electric shocks so that the hormone in their venom may be extracted for examination.

long-term effects will be and already many complications have been reported—as I shall show in Chapter 4.

Birth control, in the past, has not always been effective or aesthetic. Its history makes strange reading. Devices used have included rags, seaweed, chopped grass, lemon juice, and elephants' dung. Japanese men, before rubber condoms reached the East, used to wear hard sheaths made of tortoiseshell, horn, or leather. If the pill does prove to be safe the discovery of these synthetic steroids will be seen as a most important advance in medical science. Fear of pregnancy leads to all kinds of somatic symptoms, not all of them gynecological. In a world that faces population explosions, where millions face a shortage of food each day, where the same millions each night go to bed with empty stomachs, the value of an easy, cheap, and effective oral contraceptive is inestimable. In India alone 50,000,000 people already exist at a level below the World Health Organization's minimal standards for human subsistence; and without planned populations countless future millions, it would seem, will be doomed to starvation.

Whatever the final verdict on the present mixture of hormonal steroids used in the pill, the research, and the new knowledge that becomes available as a result of it, will surely lead to yet safer contraceptive methods as well as to valuable therapeutic discoveries.

Other powerful hormonal steroids are secreted from the cortex (rind) of the adrenal glands, endocrine organs that lie above each kidney. In the 1940s these adrenal cortex steroids were found to be related chemically not only to the sex hormones but also to Vitamin D, bile acids, and to the active principle in digitalis leaves or strophanthus seeds. One of these steroids was known as cortisone, a drug that doctors were soon (in 1949) to welcome deliriously as a wonder antidote to severe rheumatoid arthritis.

Dr. Philip S. Hench of the Mayo Clinic in Rochester, U.S.A., like many other clinicians interested in rheumatic disorders, had observed how the painful symptoms of rheumatoid arthritis abated when a patient became pregnant, or even when he or she fell ill with jaundice. Moreover, Hench knew that in pregnancy and jaundice the steroids in the body increased considerably. He now logically asked himself whether the symptoms would be alleviated if, by administering cortisone, he increased artificially the amount of steroid in the patient's body. Scientific advances are often made because research workers ask themselves the right questions. It seemed Hench's probings were most pertinent, for when (on September 21, 1948) he gave cortisone to a bedridden woman crippled by rheumatoid arthritis, her recovery was spectacular. Within a week she was happily walking down the main streets of Rochester on a shopping expedition.

The implications of this cure, if truly it was a cure, were enormous. Consider for a moment the painful statistics of rheumatic disease as given in Rudolph Friedrich's book *Medizin von Morgen* (*Frontiers of Medicine*):

"In Europe as well as in the United States of America there are about eight times as many rheumatics as tuberculosis victims. One out of every ten patients suffers from rheumatism. In the United States one hundred million man-days are lost year after year because of rheumatism. (Actually the medical profession in the U.S. has discarded this term as meaningless. It is a 'waste-basket term' including pathological conditions in bones, joints, muscles, and connective tissue.) Two hundred million dollars are spent for treatment and medication. Seven million people are permanently disabled.

"In Germany rheumatism is the main cause of lost time and disability. In Switzerland this disease causes an annual damage of 300 million francs, while the damage caused by tuberculosis is only 60 million francs. England annually loses three million man-weeks and the government pays untold amounts in disability benefits and for treatment and medication. The economic loss caused by rheumatism in the civilized countries is incalculable. The number of rheumatics on earth is estimated at 100 millions, most of them in the cooler regions. Rheumatism rarely turns up as cause of death in statistics, but it kills indirectly through heart disease and other after effects. . . ."

Later, in 1949, when Dr. Hench tried out cortisone on 14 other rheumatoid arthritic cripples at the Mayo Clinic, similar alleviation of symptoms occurred: wheelchairs were discarded, crutches thrown away, sticks waved in the air triumphantly. Cortisone seemed to be the name given to the chemistry of a miracle. When Hench and his colleagues Edward Kendall and Tadeusz Reichstein received the Nobel Award for 1950 President Truman said: "This [cortisone] will be to chemistry what the atom bomb was to physics." Moreover, cortisone and other corticosteroids, along with adrenotrophic pituitary hormones (which stimulated naturally the release of cortisone into the blood stream) benefited patients suffering from diseases other than rheumatoid disorders. All kind of ailments, some of which had hitherto driven doctors to despair and patients to their grave, appeared to respond to the new hormonal drugs. The tapping noise of sticks on the road to Lourdes would perhaps be silenced forever.

As more people received cortisone, however, it was found that the drug did not cure: it merely relieved symptoms. When the drug was discontinued, the crutches had to be taken out again from the attics and the old wheelchairs oiled. Worse, grave and unpredictable side effects appeared with mounting frequency. There were flare-ups of quiescent tuberculosis and of dormant peptic ulcers. Dangerous hormonal imbalances resulted and incipient diabetes became frank. Even mental changes followed the use of the drug. Cortisone was not a "cure-all" but a dangerous drug.

Valuable new corticosteroids were chemically manufactured, such as hydrocortisone and prednisolone, which seemed even more effective in relieving symptoms and were somewhat safer; but the pendulum of medical opinion had swung from a starry-eyed optimism to its opposite extreme. Indeed, the Medical Research Council in Great Britain announced that cortisone was no more effective than aspirin in the treatment of rheumatoid disorders.

Today it is known that the corticosteroids are dangerous drugs. Their employment might prevent an inflammation and pain; it might prevent a permanent deforming disability; but the drugs remain agents that significantly affect biochemically and physiologically *all* the systems of the body. Yet the discovery of cortisone can still be classed as a real advance in medical science providing the drug is used selectively and judiciously. For, despite its side effects, despite the fact that the mode of its action is still not altogether understood, it continues to have valuable widespread uses in dermatology, in ophthalmology, and in a variety of other conditions that include status asthmaticus (a critical form of asthma) and sarcoidosis (a condition of unknown cause previously thought to be due to a benign form of tuberculosis). In selected cases it is still used in certain rheumatoid disorders. Corticosteroids have saved lives, they continue to save lives, and they will save lives in the future. Any drug that can do that, as well

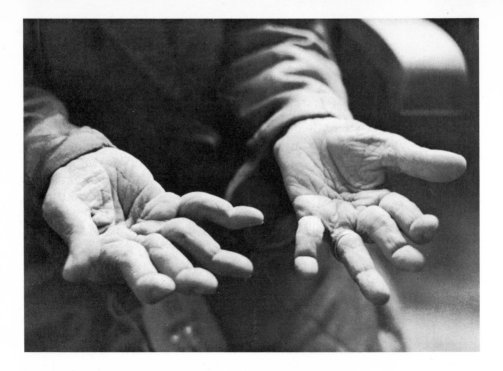

Above, the hands of a woman suffering from rheumatoid arthritis. Right, *Symphony in Red and Blue*, painted by Raoul Dufy in 1952. In 1950, Dufy—whose own hands were crippled by arthritis—went to America for cortisone treatment. It enabled him to complete some 200 pictures in the remaining three years of his life.

as alleviate suffering, cannot be discounted. In any case the story of the corticosteroids, almost certainly, is not yet concluded.

Nor for that matter is the story of other hormones. As recently as January 1966, a British medical journal (*The Lancet*) reported that a new thyroid hormone, thyrocalcitonin, had been discovered. The thyroid gland lies in the neck. It is essentially H shaped, the verticals of the H lying on each side of the windpipe below the Adam's apple. The main function of the thyroid gland is to regulate the body metabolism. Thus if too much of its iodine-containing hormone, thyroxin, is poured out into the bloodstream the heart beats faster, the body fires are stoked up, and a greater amount of energy is used. From time to time one comes across thin, jittery people with protruding, Bette Davis eyes. Unlike Bette Davis, however, these people may be suffering from thyrotoxicosis, a condition in which the thyroid gland is too active. Occasionally this overactivity may be a consequence of an emotional shock.

When I was a medical student I read in one of my textbooks a case history I have never forgotten. A woman was cycling through a dark tunnel at night when suddenly she heard behind her the noise of an automobile, then her moving shadow was thrown onto the walls of the

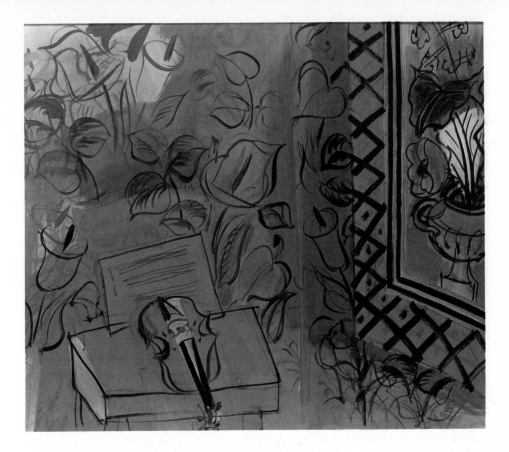

tunnel by the oncoming headlights. In panic she cycled faster and faster and, eyes wide, she glanced backward. The dazzling headlights blinded her. The woman now began to scream with fright as, desperate, she pedaled on even more rapidly. Cyclist and automobile emerged from the tunnel simultaneously. The automobile raced on, its red tail-lights disappearing around the far curved hedge. The woman stood beside her bicycle at the roadside, her heart beating fast and her hands trembling. As time passed her heartbeat did not resume its normal rate. If it went on beating with such rapidity she would die from heart failure. When she visited a doctor he found that her thyroid gland was enlarged. She had cycled into the tunnel essentially healthy: she had come out the other side suffering from thyrotoxicosis.

Such a history is rare; but emotional factors, less dramatic and more insidious, frequently do play a major part in the causation of thyrotoxicosis. Fortunately, today, anti-thyroid drugs are available that often can control the illness. Yet removal by surgery of part of the thyroid may well be called for to reduce its activity. Underactivity of the thyroid also causes illness. Deficiency of thyroxin may be a consequence of a congenital defect or it may be acquired. In the former case, it leads to cretinism; in the latter to myxedema. The famous

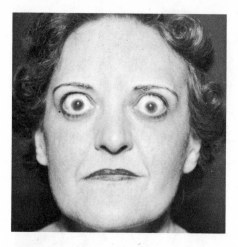

Left, an example of thyrotoxicosis: the wild, protruding eyes are a characteristic feature of this disease of the thyroid glands. Right, a 19th-century etching of a father and son shows two diseases of the thyroid glands—the father is affected by goiter; the son is a cretin.

Canadian pathologist Professor Boyd has described the cretin vividly: "The cretin," he writes, "is a dwarf physically and mentally. The mind, the skeleton, and the sexual organs do not develop. Like Peter Pan, the cretin never grows up, but he has none of Peter's activity for the vitalising influence of the thyroid is lacking. He is a sad, old child. The stature is stunted, the head large, the face broad, the features coarse, the arms short and curved, the sexual organs underdeveloped and the mental powers little better than those of an imbecile. What was intended to be created in the image of God had become what has been called the Pariah of Nature. . . ."

Myxedema occurs in middle life. Deficiency of thyroxin leads to a low body metabolism so that the heart beat becomes slow, the skin dry, the mental powers seemingly sluggish, and the patient probably obese. In fact, in 1874 Sir William Withey Gull described myxedema as, "a cretinoid state supervening in adult life in women." In 1891 the British pathologist Professor George Redmayne Murray treated the condition effectively by injecting a glycerin extract of sheep thyroid beneath the skin, so initiating one of the most important discoveries of endocrinology.

In our time, more and more has been discovered about the hormones of the thyroid gland. Synthetic thyroxin, for example, is now available, as is triiodothyronine (thyroxin in the body cells is changed by enzyme action into triiodothyronine), and diseases like myxedema can be treated as a result. Even infant cretins, if treatment is begun early enough, respond remarkably. Nowadays, too, cancer of the thyroid can be treated with radioactive iodine, taking advantage of the fact that the thyroid gland is remarkably thirsty for iodine and indeed stores that element in its cells: thus the cancerous thyroid cells avidly

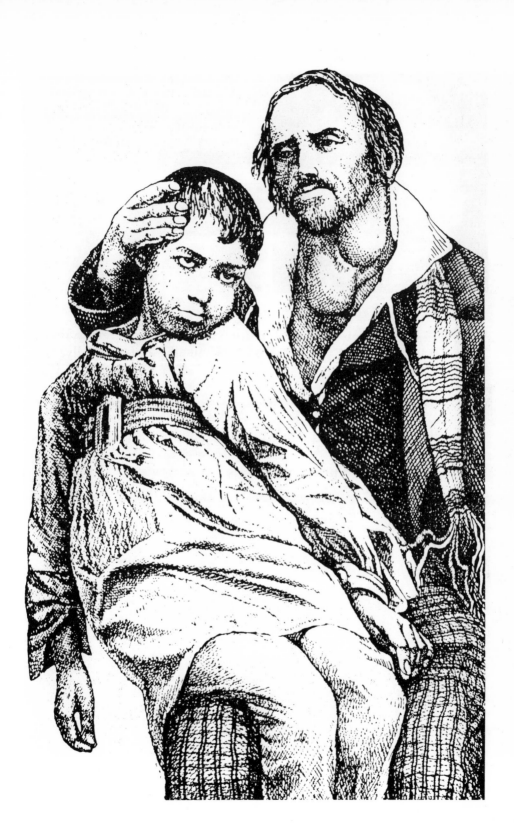

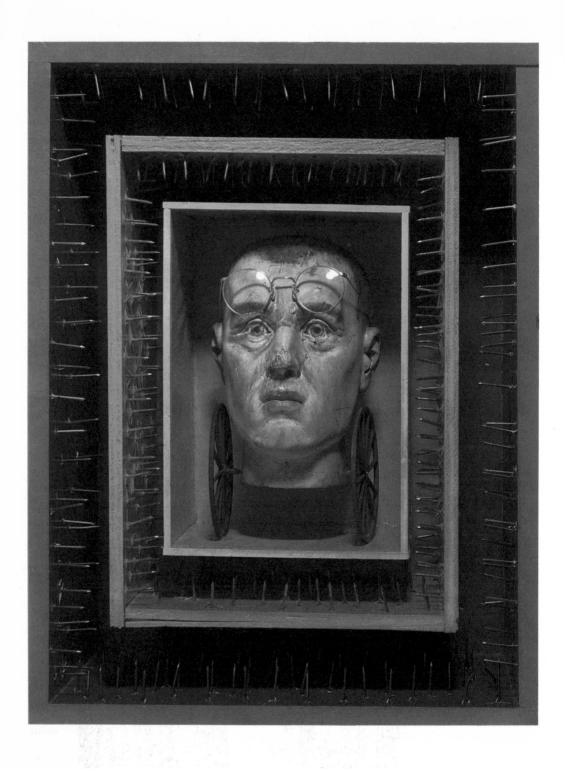

take up the iodine, whereupon the radioactivity kills them. And now comes news of the new hormone called thyrocalcitonin. Let me quote direct from the *Lancet*:

"Thyrocalcitonin is probably involved in clinical bone disease, and there may well be unrecognised syndromes of excess and deficiency. If thyrocalcitonin deficiency is a factor in osteoporosis [rarefaction] the hormone might be useful in treatment. We also want to know whether thryocalcitonin secretion is altered in thyroid or parathyroid disease and, if so, whether this has clinical effects. . . .

"Thyroid physiology, too, needs radical revision. The discovery of thyrocalcitonin means that the thyroid contains not only the familiar iodothyronine-secreting cells but also a separate endocrine system which produces an easily extracted and potent hormone. A new field of research has been opened up, and significant advances in treatment should follow."

Enough has been said to show how, year by year, month by month even, new discoveries about the hormone system are being made that will lead to even more important repercussions in the field of drug therapy. Discussion of hormonal therapy, though, cannot be concluded without some reference to the work of Dr. Hans Selye at the University of Montreal. Dr. Selye, who was encouraged early in his career by no less a person than Frederick Banting, has been working now for many years on the remarkable biochemistry of stress.

That psychological stress factors play a large part in the production of disease is recognized by doctors and laymen alike. Thus the medical profession knows that psychological stress can lead to diverse organic

Left, a "pop art" assemblage entitled *The Ulcer Life,* by American painter Bob Sullivan. The stresses and pressures of 20th-century urban life are strongly suggested by the walls of nails closing in on the subject. Right, an illustration from Hans Selye's *Second Annual Report on Stress* shows "fright thyrotoxicosis" in the wild rabbit. The left-hand rabbit is normal; the right-hand rabbit has been subjected to fright (a barking dog), and the effects can be seen in its eyes. The lower half of the picture shows the respective thyroids of the two rabbits—normal (left) and agitated (right).

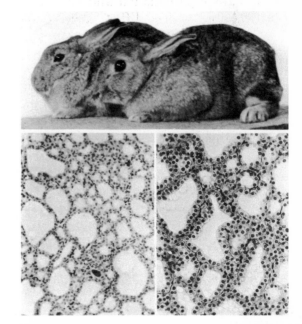

ailments. Not only conditions like thyrotoxicosis, but also duodenal ulcers, certain varieties of hypertension (high blood pressure), and even feverish colds and inflamed tonsils may result from a psychological irritant, as novelist Christopher Isherwood infers in his autobiographical *Lions and Shadows*:

"Something inside me wanted to stand up . . . to astound them all. And because I wouldn't, couldn't, I sat and sulked. . . . I returned to London next day, with the beginnings of a violent attack of influenza. Gargling my swollen throat, I cursed the Oxford climate: but Oxford wasn't to blame—it was Weston himself. Henceforward, I caught a bad cold nearly every time we met: indeed, the mere sight of a postcard announcing his arrival would be sufficient to send up my temperature and inflame my tonsils."

It is easy to say vaguely that stress can produce organic ailments. Doctors in New York remark that, "When stocks on Wall Street go down, sugar in the urine goes up." However, it is difficult to know how, chemically, diseases are produced in the body by psychogenic factors. Hans Selye's rather revolutionary work on complex hormonal imbalances has begun to explain this process. It must be said, though, that the deranged biochemical mechanisms involved are still not completely known so that one can see the answers only "through a glass darkly."

In 1925, while Selye was a medical student, his professor of medicine demonstrated several patients suffering from the earliest effects of various infectious diseases. In his book *Stress of Life*, Hans Selye recalls this demonstration:

"As each patient was brought into the lecture room the professor carefully questioned and examined him. It turned out that each of these patients felt and looked ill, had a coated tongue, complained of more or less diffuse aches and pains in the joints, and of intestinal disturbances with loss of appetite. Most of them also had fever (sometimes with mental confusion), an enlarged spleen or liver, inflamed tonsils, a skin rash, and so forth. All this was quite evident, but the professor attached very little significance to any of it.

"Then, he enumerated a few 'characteristic' signs which might help in the diagnosis of the disease. These I could not see. They were absent or, at least, so inconspicuous that I could not distinguish them; yet these, we were told, were the important changes to which we would have to give all our attention. At present, our teacher said, most of the characteristic signs happened to be absent, but until they appeared not much could be done; without them it was impossible to know precisely what the patient suffered from; and hence it was obviously impossible to recommend an efficient treatment against the disease. It was clear that the many features of disease which were already manifest did not interest our teacher very much because they were 'nonspecific' and hence 'of no use' to the physician.

"Since these were my first patients, I was still capable of looking at them without being biased by current medical thought. Had I known more I would never have asked questions, because everything was handled 'just the way it should be,' that is, 'just the way every good physician does it.' Had I known more, I would certainly have been stopped by the biggest of all blocks to improvement: the certainty of being right. But I did not know what was right.

"I could understand that our professor had to find specific disease manifestations in order to identify the particular cause of disease in each of these patients. This, I clearly realized, was necessary so that suitable drugs might be prescribed, medicines having the specific effect of killing the germs or neutralizing the poisons that made these people sick.

"I could see this all right; but what impressed me, the novice, much more was that apparently only a few signs and symptoms are actually characteristic of any one disease; most of the disturbances are apparently common to many, or perhaps even to all, diseases.

"Why is it, I asked myself, that such widely different disease-producing agents as those which cause measles, scarlet fever, or the 'flu, share with a number of drugs, allergens, etc., the property of evoking the nonspecific manifestations which have just been mentioned? Yet evidently they do share them; indeed, they share them to such an extent that, at an early stage, it might be quite impossible, even for our eminent professor, to distinguish between various diseases because they all look alike."

Ten years later Selye was doing research work in endocrinology. He had qualified as a doctor meantime, gained experience, and now possessed the essential qualifications of a scientific investigator. But he was still interested in curative, nonspecific therapies. Certain measures, like ordering the patient to go to bed, to keep warm, to eat digestible food, were to the point whatever ailment the patient suffered from. And by now he had learned through experiments with rats that the body always reacted physically to stress situations in the same, non-specific way, though the noxious stress irritants themselves were very different: thus poisons, infections, drugs, heat or cold, X-ray radiation, or mental frustration and anxiety always led, at first, to an enlargement of the cortex of the adrenals, shrinkage of the thymus, spleen, and the lymph nodes, changes in the blood count, and gastrointestinal ulcers.

Selye referred to this first nonspecific response to stress-invoking irritants, infections, nervous strain, or whatever, as the "alarm reaction." His subsequent experiments on rats and mice revealed that the alarm reaction was but the first stage of what he described as a much more general *adaptation syndrome*. For the alarm reaction could be a response to a stressor that in itself was hardly harmful: a game of tennis or even a passionate kiss would probably cause the same initial body response. But if the stress-invoking irritant continued unabated further changes in the body became evident, as Selye's rat experiments proved. There was loss of weight, disappearance of the eosinophil cells in the blood, and chemical alterations in the constitution of the body fluids and hormones. This second stage, which followed the alarm reaction, Selye called the "stage of resistance." Eventually, if the irritant stimuli were not removed, the animal fell ill and might even die. This third and final phase was named by Dr. Selye "the stage of exhaustion."

During the latter phase it was found that an imbalance of the hormones of the adrenal-pituitary axis had occurred. Such hormones are soluble chemicals, poured into the bloodstream from the endocrines. These chemicals then travel, as blood-borne messengers, to all parts of the body. "Each hormone," explains Selye, "carries instructions in a code which only certain organs can interpret." But Selye found that several of the hormones of the pituitary-adrenal axis were antagonistic to each other. For example, deoxycortisone acetate (abbreviated to DOCA), an adrenal hormone discovered in 1938, promoted inflammation, whereas cortisone, another adrenal hormone, inhibited that process. Again, one hormone of the pituitary gland (a gland lying in the skull just below the brain) promoted inflammation, while another pituitary hormone had the contrary effect. Normally all the hormones are in an exquisite balance, but as a result of too much stress a derailment of the hormonal complex occurred. The messages they sent to different cells went "mad" and Selye postulated that disease resulted—in some cases nephritis perhaps, in others rheumatic disorders, ulcerative colitis, and so on. Perhaps the hormonal imbalance caused other kinds of disease also: heart disease, hypertension, and many different conditions of unknown etiology? Why one disease should be engendered in one person and a different one in another is a question that remains unanswered.

But Selye's work and theories provide a chemical, hormonal basis to psychosomatic disease, and give new meanings to various dicta in medicine—such as Rudolf Virchow's "disease is life under altered conditions," or the old remark that "health is harmony, disease discord." Whereas Louis Pasteur introduced the idea of specificity into medicine—each clearly defined disease being the sequel of a specific cause (thus rabies results from infection by the rabies virus, tuberculosis

Gigantism, a condition caused by over-production of the growth hormones by the pituitary glands in early life.

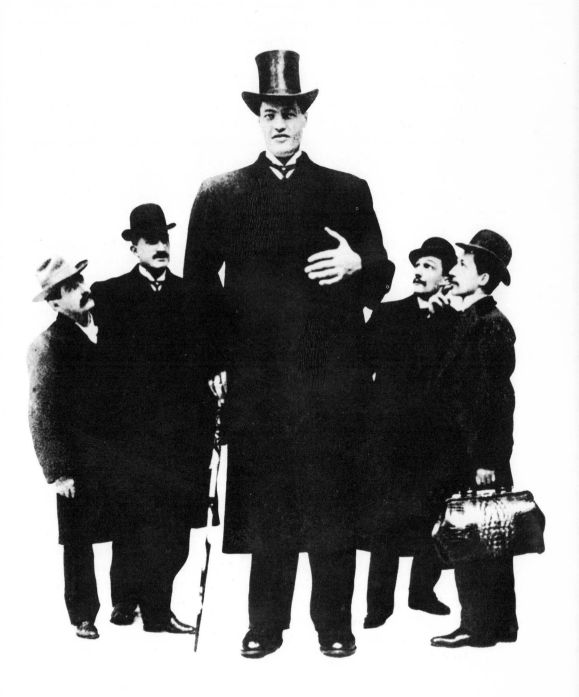

follows the ravaging effect of the tubercle bacillus)—Selye would insist that many diseases have no specific pathogen, but follow on from inappropriate hormonal responses resulting, in turn, from unspecific varieties of stress, emotional or physical.

This revolutionary thinking may be valuable in future research projects. The British surgeon Sir Heneage Ogilvie has said that "Dr. Hans Selye's contribution—perhaps the greatest contribution to scientific medicine in the present century—is that he has taken stress as an entity that enters into the life process of all living creatures, indeed that is inseparable from life itself, and he has studied it objectively by the scientific methods of observation, analysis, and experiment." Other authorities are altogether more cautious and skeptical of Selye's postulates. In his *Textbook of Pathology* Professor Boyd quotes a distinguished colleague, George W. Pickering, as saying: "The history of medicine shows how great is the tendency for the tentative hypothesis to assume the guise of a so-called fundamental principle"; and he reminds us that Selye's experimental work has been performed on rats and not on human beings. Hans Selye himself is very conscious of the opposition he has received from many eminent, orthodox, medical men. Perhaps to support and console himself against such attacks he has written:

"Very few fundamentally new ideas manage to by-pass the heresy stage. Among the really outstanding discoveries, only procedures which have immediate and important practical applications are relatively immune to violent criticisms from the start. This is illustrated by the discovery that penicillin (Fleming, Florey, and Chain), streptomycin (Waksman), and the sulfonamides (Domagk) have marked antibacterial actions, that antihistamines can suppress allergies (Halpern), or that ACTH and cortisone are useful in combating arthritis (Hench and Kendall). Although all these were truly great contributions to knowledge, they have stimulated only minor debates, mostly about limitations of the usefulness and about the damaging side effects of these remedies.

"On the other hand, a new concept in biology, such as Darwin's theory of evolution, is almost certain to provoke what Huxley called a 'public war dance.'

"When Pasteur proclaimed that infectious diseases were due to germs, when Clemen P. Pirquet and Charles R. Richet discovered allergy, the literature was full of biting, hostile remarks, in which those who did not have the originality of creating—or even understanding—new concepts . . . tried to compensate by displaying their wit.

"In his biography of Freud, Ernest Jones points out that the psychiatrist Walther Spielmeyer had, at first, denounced the use of psychoanalysis as 'mental masturbation.' Indeed, by 1910 the mere mention of Freud's theories was enough to start Professor Wilhelm Weygandt—then chairman of a medical congress in Hamburg—to banging his fist and shouting, 'This is not a topic for discussion at a scientific meeting; it is a matter for the police.'"

Much of Hans Selye's work has already led to fruitful speculation; but let us turn back now to an outstanding modern discovery that had and has immediate concrete applications. I refer to the work that in 1948 ended the long search for the anti-pernicious-anemia factor, vitamin $B_{12}$ (cyanocobalamin). Banting, as a man and as a scientist, encouraged Hans Selye; but Banting did more for another scientist, Dr. George R. Minot. For the discovery of insulin allowed Minot, a diabetic, to remain alive, and he in his turn, repaid this debt—if one can call it a debt—by preserving the lives of countless others suffering from pernicious anemia.

The prognosis of pernicious anemia prior to Minot's happy discoveries was as sinister as the name of the condition implies. Then, patients suffering from this form of anemia died within a few years of its onset, despite occasional and temporary remissions. Pernicious anemia, "a most continuate and inexorable malady," was first described in 1849 by Thomas Addison, who pointed out that it affected people mainly between the ages of 40 and 70. People suffering from it exhibited not only the usual features of a *profound* anemia—shortness of breath, headaches, palpitation of the heart, and anginal pain—but also presented more characteristic symptoms. Their skins assumed a lemon-yellow tint, their tongues became smooth, red, and sore, they suffered intermittent fever, and, worst of all, the distressing signs and symptoms of a nervous condition, subacute combined degeneration of the spinal cord, often intervened. In this latter condition the patient complains of subjective feelings of numbness or tingling of the hands and feet, and pain along the nerves; or painful muscular spasms manifest themselves with paralyses that progress until the sufferer, in time, becomes bedridden, and sometimes mentally disordered.

Not surprisingly, pernicious anemia was greatly feared, especially since no effective treatment for it existed. It is instructive to turn the pages of old medical textbooks to see how pernicious anemia was treated in the recent past. Here is a paragraph from a textbook published in 1924: "Pernicious anemia . . . is not very amenable to treatment. A few cases of very bad anemia recover for some years, but as a rule, only temporary improvement can be looked for. It might be supposed that the injection of blood from a healthy person would be a benefit, but this is not the case, since all extraneous blood corpuscles are rapidly broken up. Still, it is worthwhile trying in cases when a thoroughly healthy person can be found to consent to the withdrawal of a few ounces from his body. The remedy which has been most successful is arsenic in large doses; salvarsan has been recommended; whilst bone marrow is sometimes helpful. Attention to the teeth is of the utmost importance."

Injunctions to attend to the teeth or to administer arsenic seem, in retrospect, terribly pathetic. However, even as that medical textbook appeared in the scientific bookshops, events that would lead to a momentous advance in treating this "continuate and inexorable malady" were quietly taking place in Boston, Massachusetts. There, Dr. Minot was advising patients suffering from pernicious anemia to eat a quarter of a pound of liver each day. Such advice hardly sounded scientific. Minot's patients may well have felt they should be given doses of arsenic rather than these liver prescriptions of a food fad. Certainly George Minot was obsessed by diet. As a diabetic he had to be. But why did he choose liver as the special article of diet to be recommended to his pernicious anemia patients?

Kenneth Walker in *The Story of Blood* recounts how once a certain English lady, desperate with her sufferings from pernicious anemia, given up as hopeless by her European doctor, traveled to the East to consult a Chinese healer, who gave her pills that miraculously restored her to health. This Chinese medicaster concocted the pills from the livers of dead birds. But Minot did not know about this fragment of esoteric knowledge. He had read, though, of Dr. George Whipple's work in Rochester, Minnesota. He knew how Whipple had bled dogs until they were profoundly anemic, and then given them different foods. Whipple had found that the dogs recovered most rapidly, that

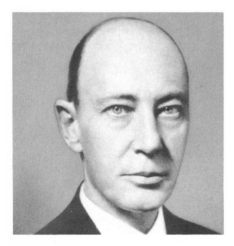

Dr. George Minot, whose experiments with liver therapy completely revolutionized the treatment of pernicious anemia.

the red cells in their blood increased most rapidly, when he fed them with liver. Ordinary anemia, as Minot well knew, was not pernicious anemia. It was hardly scientific, on the basis of Whipple's work, to prescribe liver to patients suffering from pernicious anemia. Yet he gave liver a try. "Eat liver" he had said to his patients, knowing they would die anyway. "Eat grass like Nebuchadnezzar, eat filth, eat dandelions, eat liver." What was the difference when they were all doomed anyway?

Surprisingly, his patients responded to such dietary advice. Minot, without great expectations, recommended his liver therapy to more of his pernicious anemia patients and afterward they returned to his surgery springier in step and happier by far. Dr. Minot examined slides of blood taken from the patients who had been given liver and noted how the red blood cells had increased. All 10 of the patients he was treating with liver were still alive by the end of the year—1925. According to his own experience, according to everybody else's experience, these 10 people should have been dying by then, their blood thin, their skins deep yellow, their tongues red and sore, their spinal cords perhaps affected irrevocably. On the contrary, they seemed remarkably fit. So Minot encouraged them to eat more and more liver, and told a young colleague, William P. Murphy, who worked at Boston's Peter Bent Brigham Hospital, about his discovery.

So, in 1926, Murphy too began feeding pernicious anemia patients half a pound of liver a day. Of course many could not bear eating so much. Fortunately, Murphy found that liver mashed into a fresh pulp and given with orange juice had the same miraculous result. People dying from pernicious anemia, who had been brought to the Peter Bent Brigham Hospital unconscious, now had this pulp poured into them through stomach tubes. In this way they were given liver, more liver, and always liver, until gradually they revived. Like Lazarus they opened their eyes, they moved their heads, they spoke. Within a week they sat up in their beds, recovered.

Gradually, the pages in medical books about the "continuate and inexorable malady" changed their text, for pernicious anemia was no longer pernicious in the old sense. In 1934, Whipple, Minot, and Murphy were awarded the Nobel Prize "for their discoveries concerning liver therapy against anemia." By then, Professor Edwin J. Cohn, at Harvard, had managed to isolate an extract of liver that contained the anti-pernicious-anemia particles. Soon such extracts could be given by injection; and later it was discovered, through the initial work of William B. Castle at Harvard, that gastric tissue in the form of dessicated, defatted hog's stomach contained an agent as powerful as liver to combat pernicious anemia.

Castle observed an absence of hydrochloric acid in the gastric juice of people suffering from pernicious anemia. He put forward the hypothesis that two factors existed to form the active anti-pernicious-anemia principle in the liver. One factor, the extrinsic factor, could be found in certain articles of diet. The other, the intrinsic factor, could be in the gastric juice. To prove his intrinsic factor theory he gave some meat to a normal person and then, before it had become digested, he removed it from that person's stomach. Afterwards, he gave this semi-digested meal to a pernicious anemia sufferer to eat. Repeated ingestions of this half-digested meat improved the clinical condition of the patient as effectively as liver did. His experiments led to the use of dessicated hog's stomach, which contained the intrinsic factor, as an alternative to liver extract.

But in 1948 the red crystals of cyanocobalomin, vitamin $B_{12}$, the active anti-pernicious-anemia principle in the liver, were at last isolated. Nowadays this vitamin, which, unlike other vitamins, contains cobalt, is used to treat pernicious anemia sufferers, and although they have to take it for the rest of their lives, they remain healthy. The dreadful, lemon-tinted skins of patients doctors used to despair of, the smooth, red, sore tongues that used to be seen in hospital out-patients, the secondary spinal cord lesions that were so feared, are now basically things of the past—old doctors' stories in unread pages of old medical textbooks. That such textbooks become out of date so quickly is one index of the advance of medical science.

Vitamin $B_{12}$ is but one vitamin that has practical modern therapeutic uses. For example, vitamin A prevents night blindness; one of the six different substances that make up vitamin B protects man against beriberi; vitamin C wards off scurvy; and vitamin D prevents rickets. The curative value of vitamins can be spectacular. It is nearly 400 years since the explorer Jacques Cartier described how his crew, suffering from scurvy, were treated with vitamin C. Of course, Cartier did not know the disease in question was scurvy nor that the vegetable extract recommended as a cure by a native contained vitamin C. His crew had been prostrate with swollen legs and were too weak to move; their skins were spotted with blood of a purple color, and their mouths "became stinking, their gummes rotten that all the flesh did fall out." After the juice and sap of "a certain tree" were given to the stricken sailors they revived. As Cartier said: "If all the physicians of Montpellier and Louvaine had been there with all the drugs of Alexandria they would not have done so much good in one year as that it did in six days: for it did prevail that as many as used of it, by the grace of God, recovered their health." In affluent societies today, one might assume there would be no need to prescribe vitamin C for scurvy. Alas, there is always a submerged minority, often old people, who cannot afford to buy and eat fresh fruit, and who, as a result, suffer from the disease.

There is still an important place in developed societies for vitamin therapy: babies and pregnant mothers require vitamin supplements; those who have had abdominal surgery, whose digestive systems have been upset as a result, also need to be prescribed vitamins; while those whose blood will not clot efficiently because of a lack of prothrombin require vitamin K to prevent excessive bleeding. In short, modern nutritional knowledge has still an important part to play in the prevention of diseases other than pernicious anemia.

On the whole, though, the real wonder properties of vitamins have little relevance to the *majorities* in affluent countries. Yet, despite the fact that they need no extra vitamins, many still succumb to the blandishments of pharmaceutical vitamin advertisements. An experiment carried out in the U.S.A. in 1944 involved feeding 1242 children and 214 adults a variety of vitamins in addition to their ordinary diets. This vitamin therapy was found to have little or no effect. Such findings were confirmed when a similar extensive experiment was conducted on school children in Britain. The *British Medical Journal* reported: "The vitamins had no statistically significant effect on the rate of growth, nutritional status, muscular strength, condition of the teeth and gums, or absence from school on account of illness."

It seems ironic that overfed nations should take extra vitamins they do not need, while so many who hunger elsewhere must go without, despite international agencies that strive to raise the nutritional status of the less privileged. In an editorial headed "Towards a Starving World?" the British weekly periodical *The New Statesman* commented in January 1966: "The facts are brutally simple. When Africans have no milk to drink, they live solely on maize and quickly contract deficiency diseases. When they have no cattle, they are reduced to penury. When they have no maize they die. . . . A hungry year also faces India. Here as in most of Asia, the intractable factor is the unchecked rise in population. Until 1962, Indian food production generally increased by 2 per cent each year and the population by $1\frac{1}{2}$ per cent. The improvement was thus barely measurable and any projection showed the mass of Indians still undernourished in the year 2100. But, in the race, India was slightly ahead of the grim horseman. Now, after a few poor crop years, she has fallen behind. There is no prospect of a spurt sufficient to make up lost ground. We are in the presence, perhaps, of a turning-point in human affairs so immense that we do not perceive it: 1966 may be the year in which sufficiency in food disappears from the world and famine becomes a recurrent and habitual condition."

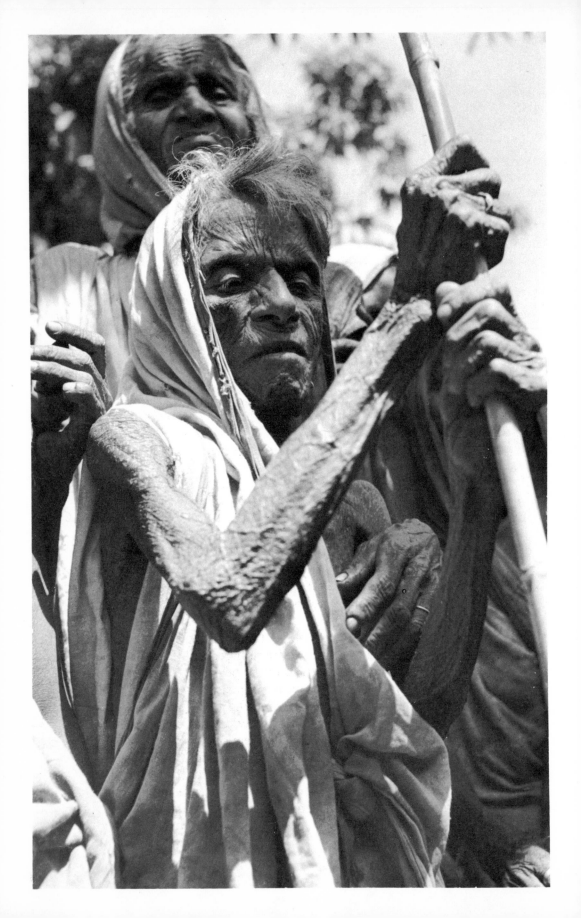

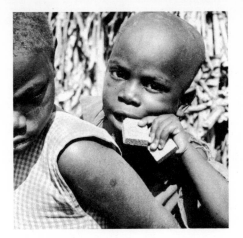

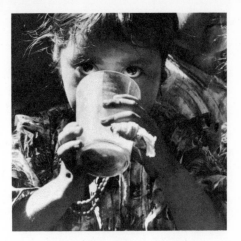

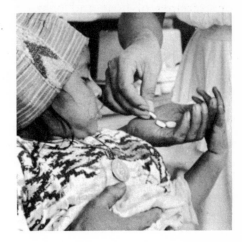

The effects of malnutrition can be seen (left) in this photograph of two Indian women. Despite the new vitamin discoveries, malnutrition remains widespread in many areas of the world. The distribution of high-protein foods is one way in which the WHO is tackling the problem. Above, Congolese child eats his ration of "fishmeal," a concentrated protein product five times richer than fish or meat. In Guatemala (above right), school children are encouraged to drink Incaparina, a high-protein drink developed by the Institute of Nutrition of Central America and Panama (INCAP). Right, at an INCAP clinic in Guatemala, medicine is handed to the mother of a child suffering from an inflamed tongue due to malnutrition.

If there is to be prevention of death and disease from famine it can only come now from the major efforts of the statesmen and politicians of the richer countries. Medical science, which has no nationality, by revealing the secrets of nutritional diseases and by discovering new methods of contraception provides those who have the power and the money (and the agricultural know-how) with means to check "the grim horseman" from riding through less fortunate countries.

The grim horseman is being unseated not only through medical advances, but through the wealth of new surgical techniques also. Operations have become possible that could hardly have been considered a short while ago. Thus, through the invention of the heart-lung machine, open heart operations can take place—the machine taking over the function of the heart while the heart is operated on. Children once doomed by congenitally deformed hearts to lead the lives of invalids and to die early, now as a result of heart surgery may grow up to lead comparatively normal lives. The case of Barry Butler, discussed in the British *Sunday Times* recently, is not a unique instance of a patient who has benefited from the astonishing advances in heart surgery of the past 12 years. Barry Butler suffered from Fallot's tetralogy—a congenital multiplicity of defects in the heart. (Fallot was a French doctor who first described this condition.) As the *Sunday Times* reported: "He was a blue baby. He had a hole in one of the walls of his heart where no hole should have been. Thus deprived of oxygen he was unable, as he grew up, to walk or even stand properly. He spent a great deal of his time squatting on his haunches like a dog. He was unable to dress himself and needed help even to go to the lavatory. He suffered terrible headaches and was easily upset by noise or extremes of heat and cold. At first the doctors said that nothing could be done for him, and it seemed to his parents as though they must look after him as best they could until he died. By the time he was seven, he was deteriorating rapidly; but by then open heart surgery was fast coming into its own. Barry was taken to Hammersmith Hospital where an operation was performed. The operation was successful and after convalescence a remarkable change came over him. His appetite increased, he put on height and weight; his headaches disappeared, he learnt to walk, to ride a bike, to swim." Yet as long ago as 1896 Stephen Paget, the British surgeon, wrote, "Surgery of the heart has probably reached the limits set by Nature to all surgery."

An eminent surgeon of Polish origin once said to me as we stood beside a weak and deaf patient at a London hospital, "This is inoperable. I will operate." The surgeon smiled encouragingly at the patient who faintly smiled back. Then we moved on to the next bed, which was occupied by a diabetic. Once diabetics were at risk when surgical intervention was necessary but thanks to insulin this was no longer the case. Other "inoperable" conditions are rapidly becoming operable. But one of the goals of medicine is to obviate, for the most part, the need for surgery at all. Sometimes, it is true, the surgeon is called in when the physician has failed.

In any event, new drugs to bring down blood pressure, new drugs to aid respiratory cripples, new nonirritant anesthetics and pain killers, have allowed surgeons to operate with greater safety. New intricate methods of diagnosis, new intricate radiological techniques, new intricate biochemical assessments, new intricate electrical tests—all help operations to be performed with greater accuracy. On the other hand the very intricacy of this new knowledge deepens the division between the specialist—the surgeon, the radiologist, the biochemist— and the general physician, as well as widening the gulf between the practitioners of the different specialities themselves. Specialist journals naturally cater for specialists but even the general medical journals consist, for the most part, of highly specialized papers that presuppose a knowledge in their readers that often they do not own. Those doctors who endeavor to read these expositions often find themselves befogged. Many more, lazier, do not even try. I know doctors who freely admit that they carefully read medical articles in the large circulation newspapers rather than those in the professional journals. They plead, "I haven't the time to read anything else," or "I have to read them otherwise I won't know what my patients are talking about."

In an essay, "Unrelated Knowledge," the British author Charles Morgan once wrote: "In a desire to grasp at something, men have specialized more and more. Where great minds, which in the sixteenth century might have aspired to universal knowledge, have specialized, there has been produced in them that humility, that humane, and indeed holy gentleness, which, when we encounter it in men of science, we love as being perhaps the first gleam of the Reenlightenment, the radiance beyond the dark wood. But specialization can be also an ambuscade of charlatans and faithless men, who cling to the wood for the importance that the darkness lends to their little torches. . . ."

Whatever defects are inherent in specialization, with the deepening of knowledge and the seemingly endless proliferation of facts it could not help but be, in medicine, as in other fields, inevitable. It has allowed men to probe deeper into this particular cause and that particular effect. True, the specialist, who does not know the patient, may advise the general practitioner—who does know the patient—to prescribe blindly a drug that he has scarcely used before. The drug may palpably prove to be a failure. Specialists' high expectation of drugs has often proved to be ill-founded. Cortisone is but one spectacular example. One could ascribe blame, too, to doctors—many of them—hopelessly out of touch with indisputable medical advances; but the accent of the previous pages has been on the brighter and more positive aspects of modern medical practice. Other chapters can dwell on the less happy consequences of modern medicine. Meanwhile, I hope the reader who has followed the text so far will agree that demonstrably, in our time, such has been the distinction of medical and surgical progress that much disease has been prevented or overcome, lives have been prolonged, distress and agony relieved.

# 3 Drugs for the Sick Mind

Lately, in popular scientific journals as well as in the orthodox medical press, there has been much discussion about the new drugs now available to treat the sick mind. Many writers speak with unbounded enthusiasm of these drugs, and announce that a revolution is taking place in the treatment of the insane. The implications of such a revolution, if it should turn out to be a successful one, would be far-reaching indeed. Mental illness is, unhappily, widespread. It is not simply that, as T. S. Eliot put it, "The whole earth is our hospital," or that everybody is crazy except you and me, but that, factually, the real wards of the world are filled with the mentally sick. According to the most recently published census of the World Health Organization there are 781,847 beds in mental hospitals in the U.S.A. (about half the total number of beds in all hospitals); in Great Britain 239,998; in Germany 90,541; in France 94,057; in Sweden 33,765; in Holland 26,987; in Japan 106,265. And these figures are on the increase.

New drugs, alas, often turn out to be less valuable than early assessments promised. Pharmacological history teaches us how often a particular drug is thought of as a magical panacea. Then with experience of its practical use the "great" drug becomes "a great drug *but*"; later still it is thought of as a "useful" drug; and finally, as

A mental patient's psyche is projected in her painting of a recurring dream—she is naked, drowning, unable to save herself.

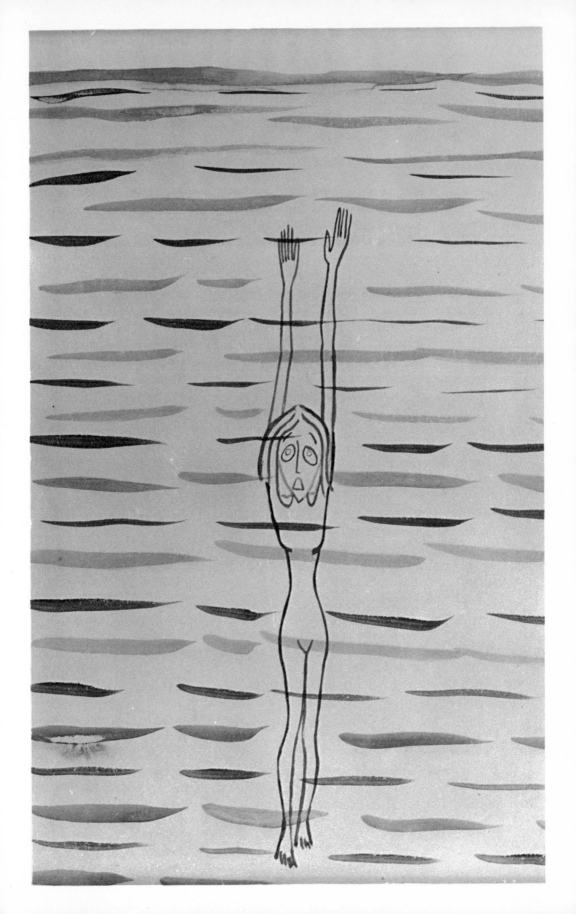

its miracle effects occur with diminishing frequency and the catalog of alarming side effects is compiled, its true value is recognized and the revolution, once heralded with such optimism, becomes aborted.

Will the new revolution in treating the mentally ill conform to this pattern? Will the optimistic dreams of some sanguine psychiatrists prove to be equally illusory? One drug that recently achieved a big commercial success was the tranquilizer meprobamate. A year after its introduction, over a decade ago, Dr. Louis Lasagna of the Johns Hopkins University School of Medicine, Baltimore, carried out a controlled trial of the drug. He wrote in *Medical Letter* that meprobamate was not "qualitatively different in its clinical effect from a number of other hypnotics including barbiturates." Moreover, he pointed out that allergic reactions frequently followed the use of the drug and that some people could even become addicted to it. In 1958 B. Weiss and V. T. Laties, who had used meprobamate in treating anxiety conditions, inferred in *The Journal of Chronic Disease* that the "great drug" was no more efficacious than a placebo. In short, the large claims for this drug (which is infinitely more expensive than the barbiturates) can hardly be supported.

Physical methods of treatment in psychiatry are empirical and seem particularly subject to fashion. Thus, the once popular measure of treating schizophrenics with insulin-coma therapy is now rapidly on the wane, while the operation of prefrontal leucotomy is gradually being relegated to the grim museum of past surgical procedures—such as the Victorian practice of removing the ovaries of women in the treatment of hysteria, and female circumcision as a cure·for other kinds of neurosis in young girls. On the other hand, it would be patently absurd to dismiss all modern physical methods of treatment as having little value. Simply, one should examine with some suspicion the high claims that are made for mind-drugs by certain psychiatric specialists.

There are many psychiatrists who remain deeply committed to drug medication and they would not agree, for example, with Professor Neil Kessel of the University of Manchester, who wrote in *The Practitioner* of May 1965: "It would take a pharmacological zealot to claim that the drugs at present available have done much to reduce or to alleviate neuroses other than depression. Moreover, those milder depressive illnesses which can be classed as neurotic are notoriously unresponsive to psychotropic preparations. One cannot fail to be unimpressed by the results of careful, controlled, clinical trials of drugs for neurotic illness. It is doubtful if, had the millions of pounds worth of pills poured down the throats of neurotics consisted of nothing but starch, they would have been any less efficacious. Certainly they would have been much safer." And in the same paper Dr. Kessel says pithily: "Three important things have happened to neurotics in the past fifteen years. They have been counted; they have been enormously prescribed for; they have had, a miniscule minority, psychotherapy. The first has illuminated the problem they pose; the last may have done some patients some good. The second has been very expensive."

To be just, let me present the opposite view. Dr. William Sargant, physician in charge of psychological medicine at St. Thomas' Hospital, London, and a noted exponent of drug therapy, read a paper at the 1965 British Association meeting at Cambridge, England, and said: "While most of the publicity in psychiatry in recent years has centred around psychoanalysis and the Freudian, Jungian and Adlerian metaphysical theories of the mind's function, and about new environmental and occupational techniques of rehabilitation of the mentally ill, yet going on quietly and almost completely unaided by any government research money, has been a tremendous revolution in the use of physical and drug treatments of the brain in mental illness. This has occurred simply because some psychiatrists decided it was more practical and likely to produce real results if one did treat the brain as the organ of thought and of the mind and soul, and to try to find drugs which can specifically alter recently acquired abnormalities of thought, behaviour and belief so as to make them more normal again. Because of these advances in the drug and physical treatment of the brain of man, nearly everybody of good previous personality who gets mentally or neurotically ill can now be got back to normal again."

As can be seen, then, psychiatrists are divided among themselves about the problem of how to treat the psychologically ill. On one extreme wing, there are those who resort to physical methods; on the other, there are those who believe in psychoanalysis or its derivative methods and delve into the mind in order to cure the mind. The latter often provoke much hostility. It could hardly be otherwise when the theories of Sigmund Freud are, for many, so uncomfortable (as I shall try to show later). However, in attacking Freud's views many, not only psychiatrists, feel obliged to construct their own theories. They cry "balderdash" and then present their own half-baked postulates, which derive from a physical view of mental disease.

A prime example of such thinking is to be found in an essay by Aldous Huxley entitled *The Oddest Science*. He aggressively attacks Freud, Carl Jung, and Otto Rank, and then lamely suggests that psychologists should primarily consider the physical makeup of the patient before treating him. He recommends that doctors should ask: "How much did Mrs. X weigh—ninety pounds or two hundred? Did

Mr. Y have the physique of an ox or a daddylonglegs, of a panther or a jellyfish?" Aldous Huxley complains: "To these questions most psychologists never vouchsafe an answer—presumably because, unlike the rest of mankind, they have never thought of asking them." Huxley's thinking derives partly from Dr. William Sheldon, who related psychic qualities to the constitutional makeup of the body. Now such simplistic views, in Aldous Huxley, are unlikely to be the result of a monumental ignorance, as they appear to be. It seems more likely that, finding dynamic psychiatry unpalatable and perhaps even disturbing, Aldous Huxley, like so many others—artists, priests, *and* psychiatrists—must turn to "physical" considerations for the interpretation of the symptoms of mental disease.

To complicate matters further, even some psychiatrists not physically orientated take exception to the dogmas of psychoanalysis. Thus the late Dr. E. B. Strauss, formerly a consultant in the psychiatric department of St. Bartholomew's Hospital, London, wrote in an introduction to Roland Dalbiez's *Psychoanalytical Method and the Doctrine of Freud*: "The psychoanalytical movement, itself, has developed on extraordinary lines. It has come to resemble a cult more than a scientific discipline. It has its canonical literature, its apocrypha, its orthodoxies and heterodoxies, its inquisitors and its apostolic succession. Orthodox psychoanalysts are compelled to submit their will and reason to as stern a discipline as any members of a Religious Order. Thus it comes about that many psychoanalysts cohabit a little world of their own that is apt to be quite out of touch with systems of thought which are foreign to them."

Whether or not these strictures are justified, the uncommitted reader will note how the language used is emotionally loaded. Dr.

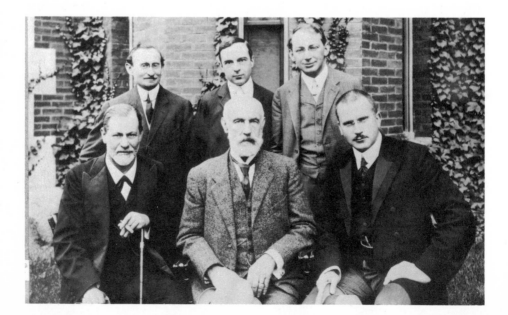

Strauss's feelingly expressed hostility is self-evident, and here I quote him merely to demonstrate at what heat arguments are debated between the various schools of psychiatry—a heat more appropriate to warring politicians or theologians than to scientists of the 20th century.

The two alternative methods of treatment (physical and non-physical) have existed in an embryo form ever since the mentally ill were regarded as sick. Thus it was, primitively, in Greece. An example of one physical form of treatment can be found in the therapeutic armamentarium of Siranus of Ephesus (c. first century A.D.) who, confronted with a "manic" patient, would apply warm poultices of oil to his head. After a few days Siranus would proceed to bleed and cup his patient before scarifying the skin. Nonphysical means of combating disease found expression in those temples of healing that existed in classical Greece. In these early "rest homes" the patient was encouraged to sleep and dream. The dreams that visited the patients were believed to be sent by the gods, and the priests helped to interpret them. Such temple therapy has been compared with modern psychoanalysis. This is a very extravagant analogy since the priest in no way laid bare the patient's delusions or demonstrated their causes.

Modern man is inclined to shrug off these antecedents of scientific medicine as nothing more than superstitious nonsense, but there is no reason to suppose that ancient peoples were any more or any less frightened, or emotionally disturbed, or intelligent than we are. Magic served many purposes, an important one being the means by which man tried to gain control of his environment. The objective of contemporary science is precisely the same. Just as today the prescription of drugs is the province of the doctor, so in former times drugs were dispensed by the man defined by society as being in control of the

Left, a photograph taken in 1909 at Clark University, U.S.A., where Sigmund Freud gave an early account of the subject-matter and development of psychoanalysis. The group includes Freud (seated left), Carl Jung (seated right), and Sandor Ferenczi (standing right).

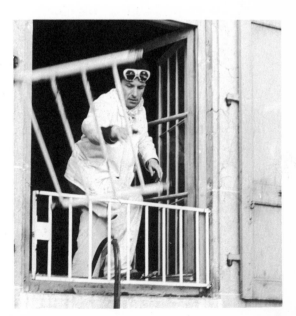

Right, the bars are removed from the windows of a French hospital—symbol of the new attitude to mental illness.

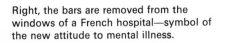

forces of sickness, or for that matter of any undesirable event. North American Indian tribes knew the magician, as is still the case in modern African jungle societies, as the medicine man. Even in our present, sophisticated Western world the links between medicine, drugs, and magic have never entirely disappeared.

In medieval Europe the connection between magic and drugs was a curiously complicated one. There is no doubt that the magicians or witches not only employed drugs, which often consisted of very unpleasant substances, but also consumed them. Perhaps some features of witchcraft can be related to the side effects of drugs. Many witches, for example, genuinely believed they could levitate and could see the devil. At meetings of the coven there would be a cauldron in which sundry substances were cooked and eaten or rubbed into the body. This was followed by ritual dancing. Now, there is a group of substances, of which atropine (still widely used in connection with anesthesia) is the best known, that, when taken in excess, produce a delirious state. Illusions of flying readily occur. Among the symptoms that may be produced are disorientation of time and place, so that anyone consuming the drug in an appropriate mood of expectancy could subsequently believe he had been to a different place. Hallucinations often occur, and convulsive movements, sometimes rhythmical in nature. It seems, therefore, that there may have been a pharmacological contribution to the visions of the devil and to the dancing. Atropine-like drugs can also be absorbed from ointments rubbed into the skin, as was the "witch's unguent." And there would have been no difficulty in procuring the substance: it abounds in numerous wild berries, the deadly nightshade being one of the commonest.

Whether such visions were atropine-induced or not, many witches were mentally unbalanced anyway and would not have needed to resort to drugs to envisage the devil, or to imagine they could fly omnipotently, or to believe they could be changed into animals. Witchcraft, if not always practiced by psychotics, was often the resource of the lonely, the lovelorn, the sexually deviant. Nowadays, doctors would consider that numbers of them needed to consult a psychiatrist, but at that time the Church assumed the authority to diagnose their derangement. "All witchcraft comes from carnal lust which in women is insatiable," averred two Dominican monks, Heinrich Kraemer and Jacob Sprenger, in a notorious and authoritative 16th-century textbook, *Malleus Maleficarum*, designed for magistrates and inquisitors. The treatment was to torture such witches and burn them alive.

It was not until the late 17th century that the mentally sick ceased to be the victims of priests to become, instead, the martyred patients

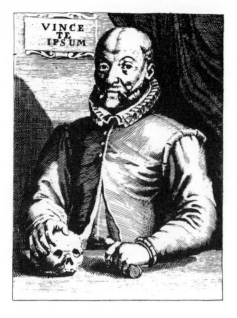

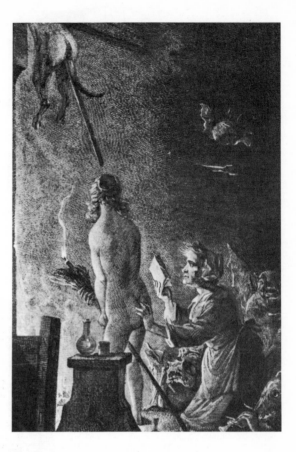

Right, a detail from *The Departure for the Sabbat*, by the 17th-century Flemish painter David Teniers. Above, the enlightened Belgian physician Johann Weyer (1516–88), who held that witches were not evil beings, but mentally disturbed women suffering from hallucinations.

of doctors. For though the insane were no longer burned at the stake they were banished (unless they came from rich families) to Auschwitz-like institutions presided over by brutal wardens, where they were stripped naked before being led to a cell or dungeon. Here they were tied down to a bed for the night, their cell door locked. For almost 200 years the medical treatment of these unfortunates consisted of "Reducing the Patient by Physic." Again I should like to quote Aldous Huxley, this time without quibbling, for he vividly describes this method of treatment:

"Over a period of eight or ten weeks the victim was repeatedly bled, at least one pound of blood being taken on each occasion. Once a week, or if the doctor thought it advisable at shorter intervals, he or she was given an emetic—a 'Brisk Vomit' as our ancestors, with their admirable command of English, liked to call it. The favourite Brisk Vomit was a concoction of the roots of black hellebore. Hellebore had been used in the treatment of the insane since the time of Melampus, a legendary soothsayer, first mentioned by Homer. Taken internally.

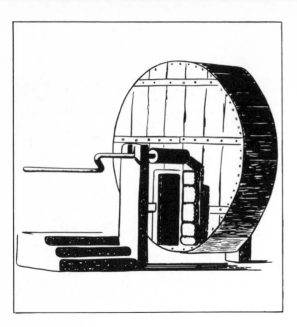

Left, the "wheel," an 18th-century machine used to "calm" mentally disturbed patients. The patients were strapped to a seat inside the drum, which was then rotated. Below, the "douche" (19th century), another method of treating the mentally disturbed.

Right, a 17th-century German cartoon depicts a fictitious Dr. Würmbrandt and his assistant "curing" mental patients. The doctor is thrusting a madman's head into a kiln to drive out demons: his assistant is administering a purge.

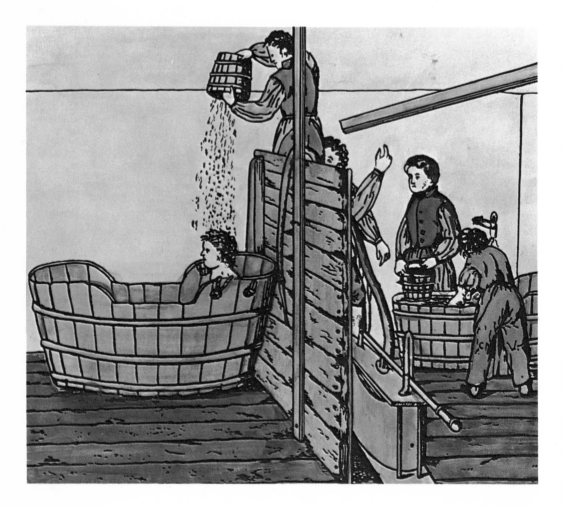

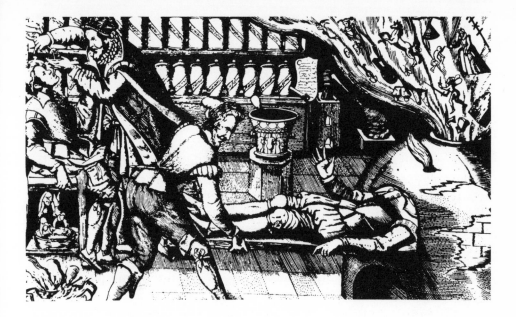

the toxicologists tell us, hellebore 'occasions ringing in the ears, vertigo, stupor, thirst, with a feeling of suffocation, swelling of the tongue and fauces, emesis and catharsis, slowing of the pulse and finally collapse and death from cardiac paralysis. Inspection after death reveals much inflammation of the stomach and intestines, more especially the rectum.' The doses prescribed by the old psychiatrists were too small to be fatal, but quite large enough to produce a dangerous syndrome, known in medical circles as 'Helleborism.' Every administration of the drug resulted in an iatrogenic disease of the most distressing and painful kind. One Brisk Vomit was more than enough: there were no volunteers for a second dose. All the later administrations of hellebore had to be forcible. After five or six bouts of helleborism, the time was ripe for purgatives. Senna, rhubarb, sulphur, colocynth, antimony, aloes—blended into Black Draughts or worked up into enormous boluses, these violent cathartics were forced, day after day, down the patient's throat. At the end of the two-month course of bloodlettings, vomits and purges, most psychotics were 'reduced by physic' to a point where they were in no condition to give trouble. These reductions were repeated every spring during the patient's incarceration and in the meantime he was kept on a low diet, deficient in proteins, vitamins and even calories. It is a testimony to the amazing toughness of the human species that many psychotics survived under this treatment for decades. Indeed, they did more than survive; in spite of chronic undernourishment and periodical reductions by physic, some of them still found the strength to be violent. The answer to violence was mechanical restraint and corporal punishment." Apart from "reducing the patient by physic" more "psychological" principles of treatment governed the behavior of the medical attendants. It was believed that mental disease could sometimes be cured by engendering a keen sense of terror in the patient. Such was the rationale for the snake pit used in 18th-century Germany. The lunatic was tied up with a rope, elevated to a great height before being rapidly plunged down, down, down, into a lightless cellar preferably "stocked with serpents." More common and universal were less technical mechanisms for inducing terror such as the whip. The "certifiably sane" therapists could beat their crazed victims or threaten them with more exotic forms of torture. Whatever refinement was used—ducking the patient under water for hours on end, or producing vertigo by means of a ceaselessly circulating swing—could be justified as part of the therapy necessary to bring the patient back to normal health.

Such hospitals or prisons were not secret places on the map, hidden behind barbed wire. Unlike the concentration camps of our own time many were open or partly open to the public who, for entertainment, would flock to, say, Bedlam (Bethlem)—the name given to one of these "hospitals" in London. Here they could watch the chained inmates who were naked or smeared with their own feces or covered with rags. They enjoyed observing the pale, haggard faces of the lunatics, their grimaces, and their strange antics. It was a good laugh, a good belly laugh.

Not all people, however, acted so insensitively to the plight of the mentally sick. In France, in England, in America, and elsewhere, eventually reforms were instigated that led to a much more humane treatment of "the prisoners." In 1793 Philippe Pinel, who was the medical superintendent of the Bicêtre hospital in Paris (and later consulting physician to Napoleon) unchained his patients, not because of any theories about insanity but because of the compassion he felt for their miserable condition. An account of the first unchaining in that Paris hospital makes heartening reading:

"The first man on whom the experiment was tried was an English captain, whose history no one knew, as he had been in chains for forty years. He was thought to be one of the most furious among them. His keepers approached him with caution, as he had in a fit of fury killed one of them on the spot with a blow from his manacles. He was chained more rigorously than any of the others. Pinel entered his cell unattended and calmly said to him. 'Captain, I will order your chains to be taken off and give you liberty to walk in the court, if you will promise me to behave well and injure no one.' 'Yes, I promise,' said the maniac. 'But you are laughing at me. . . .' His chains were removed and the keepers retired, leaving the door of his cell open. He raised himself many times from the seat, but fell again on it; for he had been in a sitting posture so long that he had lost the use of his legs. In a quarter of an hour he succeeded in maintaining his balance and with tottering steps came to the door of his dark cell. His first look was at the sky, and he exclaimed, 'How beautiful, how beautiful!' During the rest of the day he was constantly in motion uttering exclamations of delight. In the evening he returned of his own accord to his cell and slept tranquilly."

Pinel's action to free the insane from oppression was born of the spirit of Liberté, Egalité, Fraternité, and it found an echo in the minds of those concerned with humanitarian reforms in Britain. Thus in 1796 William Tuke, the Quaker, founded the York Retreat, the first humane asylum in Britain. Seventeen years later his grandson, Samuel Tuke, published a detailed account of how the patients at the York Retreat responded favorably to a "mild system of treatment." Tuke's treatise, in turn, influenced others to abandon their old terrific methods of management. About this time, George Rose, a member of parliament, took up the cause of the neglected insane, though he failed repeatedly to persuade parliament to pass his bills. It was not until 1815 that a Select Parliamentary Committee was appointed to inquire into the lamentable conditions still dominant in the vast majority of public and private asylums. Its important report uncovered so many appalling injustices that it touched the conscience of a larger body of progressive public opinion. Even so, 13 more years had to pass before (in 1828) some of the reform measures recommended by the Parliamentary Committee became part of British legislation.

In America, Dorothea Lynde Dix (1802–1887), a Sunday-school teacher, devoted herself to the cause of the mentally afflicted and prepared a memorial to be presented to the state legislature. This was voiced by her friend Dr. Samuel Howe in 1843:

"I come to present the strong claims of suffering humanity. I come to place before the legislature of Massachusetts the condition of the miserable, the desolate, the outcast. I come as the advocate of helpless, forgotten, insane and idiotic men and women.... I proceed, Gentlemen, briefly to call your attention to the *present* state of Insane Persons confined within this Commonwealth, in *cages, closets, cellars, stalls, pens! Chained, naked, beaten with rods*, and lashed into obedience...."

Dorothea Dix referred to the condition of one young woman who "stood clinging to, or beating upon, the bars of her caged apartment, the contracted size of which afforded space only for increasing accumulations of filth, a *foul* spectacle; there she stood with naked arms and dishevelled hair; the unwashed frame invested with fragments of unclean garments, the air so extremely offensive.... Irritation of

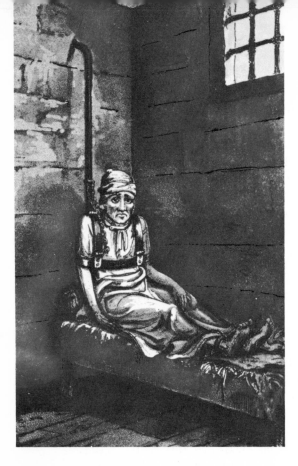

Left, a drawing from life of William Morris, a 55-year-old mental patient discovered in one of the "cells" of Bethlem (Bedlam) Hospital, London, in May 1814 by reformer Edward Wakefield. Morris had remained riveted in irons and strapped to the wall by 12-inch chains for 10 years. He was released within weeks of his discovery, but died in 1815 "from a very considerable disease of the lungs."

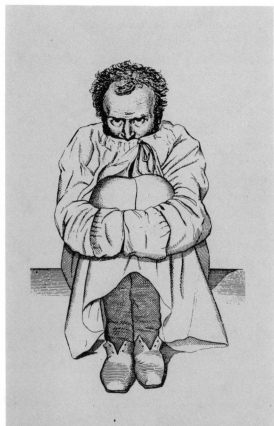

Left, a straitjacketed patient, shown in a French engraving of 1838—one of a series illustrating the main types of insanity known in French asylums at the time.

Right, Philippe Pinel supervises the unshackling of mental patients at the Salpêtrière hospital, Paris, in 1796— a contemporary painting.

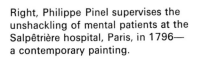

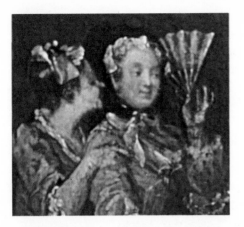

Left, a detail from a painting in the *Rake's Progress* series by the 18th-century British artist William Hogarth. Hogarth has his rake committed to Bedlam to illustrate the final degeneration after a life of sin. The contemporary association of lunacy with possession by evil spirits, and hence sin, goes some way toward explaining the appalling treatment suffered by the insane—and the attitude of a public that would go to be entertained by the amusing "antics" of the inmates of an asylum.

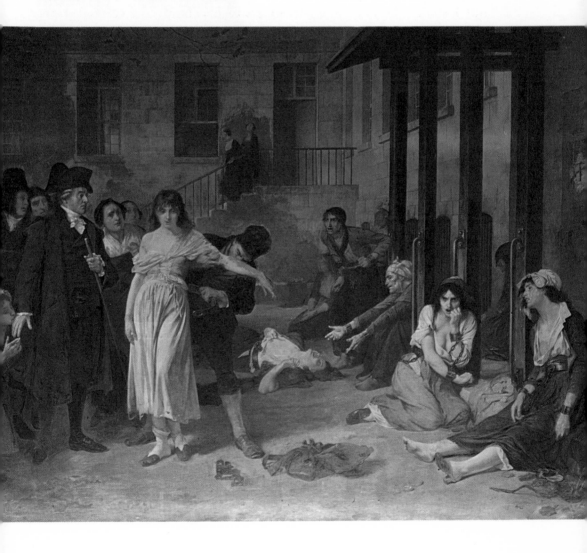

body, produced by utter filth and exposure, incited her to the horrid process of tearing off her skin by inches. . . ."

Knowing that most medical men believed little could be done for such maniacal outcasts and that they felt there was no point in bettering their conditions, Dorothea Dix cited how one raging maniac had benefited simply by kindness. "A young woman," she continued, "a pauper, in a distant town, Sandisfield, was for years a raging maniac. A cage, chains, and *the whip*, were the agents for controlling her, united with harsh tones and profane language. Annually, with others (the town's poor) she was put up at auction. . . . One year, not long past, an old man came forward in the number of applicants for the poor wretch; he was taunted and ridiculed: 'what would he and his old wife do with such a mere beast?' 'My wife says yes,' replied he, 'and I shall take her.' She was given to his charge; he conveyed her home; she was washed, neatly dressed, and placed in a decent bedroom, furnished for comfort and opening into the kitchen. How altered her condition! As yet *the chains* were not off. The first week she was somewhat restless, at times violent, but the quiet, kind ways of the old people wrought a change; she received her food decently; forsook acts of violence, and no longer uttered blasphemous or indecent language; after a week, the chain was lengthened, and she was received as a companion into the kitchen. Soon she engaged in trivial employments. 'After a fortnight,' said the old man, 'I knocked off the chains and made her a free woman.' She is at times excited, but not violently; they are careful of her diet; they keep her very clean; she calls them 'father' and 'mother.' Go there now and you will find her 'clothed,' and though not perfectly in her 'right mind,' so far restored as to be a safe and comfortable inmate."

The reforms initiated by Pinel in France, by the Tuke family in England, by Dorothea Dix in America, can be accounted as real clinical advances, for in mental disease the chances of recovery are, in part, dependent on the conditions in which the patient is kept. But no further progress in treatment was evident until psychiatrists began to discover the cause of mental disorder.

In Germany the so-called psychicists considered mental disease to be a disease of the disembodied soul in sin. Of course there were many other fanciful theories. One of these, popular in France about 100 years ago, was called the "theory of degeneration." It was held that mental affliction was congenital and would in succeeding generations become worse and worse. Thus a degenerate family would be saddled with a nervous disposition; their children would be frankly neurotic, and the children's children psychotic. The final progeny would be idiots. This pessimistic doctrine of congenital degeneration was believed in by many psychiatrists until the end of the century. Nor was it confined to 19th-century France. It held sway among many prominent mental specialists in Germany too, one of whom was R. von Krafft-Ebing, remembered today for his studies of sexual perversion.

It was Sigmund Freud, the founder of psychoanalysis, who liberated psychiatry from its state of pessimistic helplessness. Already in 1885, when only 30 years of age, he had traveled to Paris to study under the great neurologist and head of the Salpêtrière clinic, Jean Martin Charcot (1825–1893). Charcot was experimenting with hypnosis in treating patients suffering from hysteria, and on his return to Vienna the young Freud himself tried out this technique on his neurotic patients. He found he could not hypnotize all of them and in any case those who could be hypnotized often did not benefit as a result. So Freud evolved the technique of free association, which was later to become a basic maneuver in the psychoanalytic approach. He invited his patients to relax on a couch. They were then encouraged to say spontaneously whatever came into their heads. Many painful and hitherto forgotten memories surfaced, which Freud noted owned a sexual connotation. At first he collaborated with Dr. Joseph Breuer, a Viennese colleague who had also been using hypnosis, but when Freud resolutely emphasized the significance of sexuality in the etiology of neurosis their collaboration collapsed. The antagonism toward Freud's theory of sexuality displayed by Breuer was a precursor of what was to come.

Freud's habit of seeking for a cause to account for an effect—his basic training after all was as a neurologist—led him to evolve over many years a complicated doctrine of psychological determinism. This doctrine revolutionized for all time the whole approach to normal and abnormal psychology. But, after his break with Breuer in 1894, Freud stood alone for 12 years and had to endure much hostility from medical colleagues. They did not find comfortable Freud's theories of unconscious motivation, repression, resistance, and transference. They mocked his view that dreams and even slips of the tongue were unconsciously motivated. They were utterly shocked by his conception of dynamic infantile sexuality and rejected with horse laughs the idea that the latter could deeply influence mental development.

Until then it was believed that our sexual instincts originate at puberty. Freud noted how several sexual components—the cutaneous, the muscular, the oral, the anal—revealed themselves before passing under the primacy of genital impulses. Moreover, these components became confluent with aggressive and destructive tendencies and this led to various forms of sadism—for example, oral and anal sadism. Once these primitive components come under the primacy of the

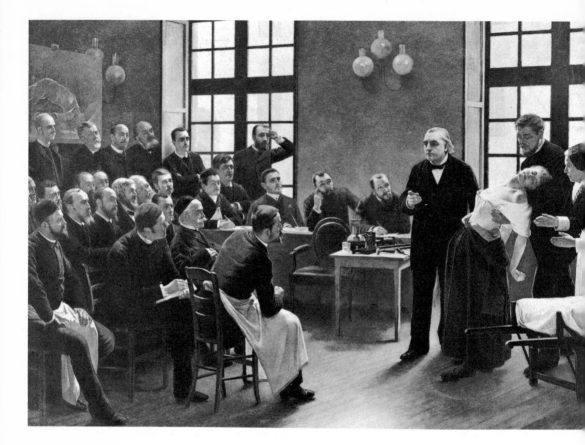

genital zones the infant's sexuality is directed toward obtaining gratification through his or her parents (or their most important surrogates). This represents the Oedipal phase of emotional development, which reaches its height between the third and fifth year of life. The Oedipus complex is named after the king of Thebes in Sophocles' trilogy. Oedipus killed his father and married his mother, not knowing their identity. Later a terrible plague ravaged Thebes and the oracle declared that only the banishment of Oedipus would bring it to an end. When the truth of his "sin" became evident his mother took her own life and he put out his eyes and roamed about the earth in misery. The punishment meted out to Oedipus—the putting out of his eyes—was in Freudian terms symbolically one of castration. In reality, too, the young four- or five-year-old boy, because of unconscious desires for his mother, fears that he will be punished by his castrating father.

As the boy's sexual interest becomes focused on his penis, so the phallic orientation in a girl is toward her clitoris. According to Freud the Oedipal strivings are given up because of castration anxiety. The

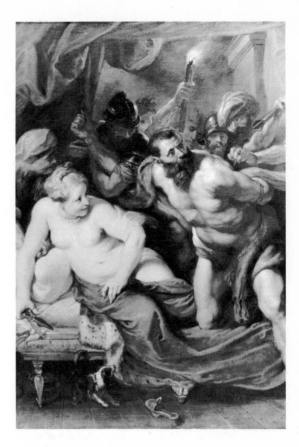

Right, Rubens' *Samson and Delilah.* In the biblical story, Delilah deprives Samson of his strength by cutting his hair. Unconscious representations of the castration theme occur frequently in both art and literature.

boy fears that he *may* be punished in this way. The girl, who directs her desire towards her father, cloudily comes to believe, because of her "anatomical deficiency," that she has already been castrated. The resolution of Oedipal strivings is necessary to attain normal adult sexuality. In the neurotic, Oedipal tendencies unconsciously remain.

By postulating that infants are not "innocent," as was formerly supposed, but own strange sexual strivings and suffer from an unconscious anxiety of being sexually mutilated, Freud, as has been said already, shocked many people. It was one thing for dramatists, poets, novelists, to bear witness to the truth of incestuous longings, as Stendhal, for example, confessed in his autobiography: "I was in love with my mother. I must swiftly add that I lost her at the age of seven. . . . I always wanted to kiss my mother and wished that there were no such things as clothes. She loved me passionately and often took me in her arms; I kissed her with so much ardour that I was sometimes forced to turn away. I detested my father when he came and interrupted our kisses. I wanted to lie for ever on her breast." But it was another thing for a doctor, a scientist, to make a law of such matters and elevate them into universal truths.

Indeed, Freud's views disturbed many inside, as well as outside, the psychoanalytical movement. Some of his own disciples found his views intolerable and attempted to discover other dominant drives—other, that is, than sexual ones—to account for nervous breakdown. Alfred Adler believed that individuals thirsted for power. Otto Rank recanted his earlier Freudian beliefs to propose that normal and abnormal development was related to "birth trauma." Carl Jung, another ex-pupil of Freud, delved into medieval alchemy after postulating mystically that there existed a collective unconscious that had at its command psychic experience perhaps a million years old, which had been passed down from generation to generation. Its unguarded emergence, Jung believed, could lead to severe, aberrant, psychotic symptoms.

Views of men like Adler and Jung are much less disturbing than those of Freud, not only medically but also in their wider, sociocultural and religious implications. Thus the American magazine *Pulpit Digest* could comment: "Dr. Jung presents a sane and practical psychology, and is fair and sympathetic in his attitude towards religion. There is probably no modern psychologist whose writings are of more significance and value to the minister than the writings of Carl Jung." It is evident that all Freudian schismatics, Jung or whoever, labored ceaselessly to produce a theory of the mind's workings that was contradictory to the Freudian system, though they all used his terminology in a manner that divested it of its original meaning. There are those, too, who have taken what they imagine to be most valuable from the teachings of Freud, Adler, Jung, Rank, etc. They call themselves "eclectic analysts"; but how they arrive at their individual jigsaw theoretical constructs is an enigma, since the views of Freud and his wayward disciples are ultimately contradictory.

So much for analytical theory, which here, I am afraid, is necessarily incomplete and oversimplified. How though, in practice, can modern psychoanalysts apply Freud's theories and cure mentally ill patients? In the course of analysis a dynamic relationship ensues between the analyst and the "analysand," the person being analysed. The patient, lying on the couch, relaxed, gives vent to his feelings and thoughts without evident selection, while the psychiatrist records and studies the material uttered, keeping in mind its possible symbolic significance. Soon, ambivalent emotions—love and hate, dependence and revolt—become released and are "transferred" onto the analyst, who has become identified with one or other of the important figures of the patient's childhood. Hence the term "transference." Since the analyst represents one or other of the patient's parents or surrogates, the patient's attitudes become neurotically and sexually overdetermined. The presenting neurosis becomes converted into a "transference" neurosis. It is the existence of this transference that permits the analysand to reveal to himself the real nature of his underlying feelings and to resolve them.

A full analysis may last as long as four years and the patient is required to visit the analyst some four times a week. It is, then, a time-consuming treatment and, necessarily, an expensive one. Moreover, in order to benefit, the patient must be intelligent and determined to go through with his analysis—for it is often a painful experience. As many hitherto mentally unbalanced people can testify, a full analysis is worth every penny spent and the years involved in its application. All the same, it is not surprising that numerous people opt for shorter forms of analytical psychotherapy where the psychiatrist directs the patient more actively and forces the pace of the analysis.

Obviously any analysis will depend in part on the character and ability and the emotional maturity of the analyst. Psychoanalysts are rigorously selected and have to undergo full analysis themselves before they are recognized by the official institutes of psychoanalysis. After all, the doctor-patient relationship is loaded even in other spheres of medicine. One hears, often enough, of the eccentricities of psychiatrists. Like other people they are fallible. A novelist friend of mine sent his wife who had been displaying neurotic symptoms to see a psychiatrist (not an analyst). The "transference" in this case occurred in more senses than one, for my friend's wife ran off with the man she had consulted. No doubt such instances are rare, but one is reminded of how even Freud's most brilliant pupil, Sandor Ferenczi, introduced into his psychoanalytical technique an addition best left to a loving mother. Freud rebuked Ferenczi for this in a letter he sent to him on December 13, 1931:

"I see that the differences between us come to a head in a technical detail which is well worth discussing. You have not made a secret of the fact that you kiss your patients and let them kiss you; I had also heard that from a patient of my own. Now when you decide to give a full account of your technique and its results you will have to choose between two ways: either you relate this or you conceal it. The latter, as you may well think, is dishonourable. What one does in one's technique one has to defend openly. Besides, both ways soon come together. Even if you don't say so yourself it will soon get known just as I knew it before you told me.

"Now I am assuredly not one of those who from prudishness or from consideration of bourgeois convention would condemn little erotic gratifications of this kind. And I am also aware that in the time of the Nibelungs a kiss was a harmless greeting granted to every guest. I am further of the opinion that analysis is possible even in Soviet Russia where so far as the State is concerned there is full sexual freedom. But that does not alter the facts that we are not living in Russia and that with us a kiss signifies a certain erotic intimacy. We have hitherto in our technique held to the conclusion that patients are to be refused erotic gratifications. You know too that where more extensive gratifications are not to be had milder caresses very easily take over their role, in love affairs, on the stage, etc.

"Now picture what will be the result of publishing your technique. There is no revolutionary who is not driven out of the field by a still more radical one. A number of independent thinkers in matters of technique will say to themselves: why stop at a kiss? Certainly one gets further when one adopts 'pawing' as well, which after all doesn't make a baby. And then bolder ones will come along who will go further to peeping and showing—and soon we shall have accepted in the technique of analysis the whole repertoire of demiviergerie and petting-parties, resulting in an enormous increase of interest in psycho-analysis among both analysts and patients. The new adherent, however, will easily claim too much of this interest for himself, the younger of our colleagues will find it hard to stop at the point they originally intended, and God the Father Ferenczi gazing at the lively scene he has created will perhaps say to himself: maybe after all I should have halted in my technique of motherly affection *before* the kiss. . . ."

As has been indicated, one of the drawbacks of analysis is the long period of time necessary for the patient to uncover his unconscious conflicts and resolve them. Lately, drugs have been discovered, notably lysergic acid diethylamide (LSD 25) that, when taken by human beings, stimulate the midbrain in such a way that the forgotten experiences of infancy and childhood can be recalled. When LSD is used as an adjunct to psychotherapy, some authorities maintain, the patient can be cured in a much shorter period than was hitherto thought possible. Dr. R. A. Sandison, a noted psychiatrist who works in Worcester, England, asserts that with successful LSD psychotherapy there is "a broadening of the personality, greater resistance to stress and therefore less likelihood of a return of symptoms."

LSD is one of the hallucinogenic or psychotomimetic drugs—so called because the drug stimulates hallucinatory, or rather pseudo-hallucinatory, visions and the mental state produced is akin to that met in a psychosis such as schizophrenia. Apart from releasing repressed memories, LSD, like mescaline and marihuana (hashish), can strangely interfere with sense perception. In fact, this group of drugs is wrongly named because the mental state induced does not truly mimic schizophrenia; nor are the "hallucinations," when experienced, true ones. A truly hallucinated person believes that what he perceives exists in reality and not merely in his imagination, whereas under LSD the critical ability of the patient usually remains sufficiently unimpaired for him to evaluate the hallucination for what it is—an imaginary or memory artefact. Perhaps, in some ways, then, though I know of no authority who has put this forward, the patient perceives something comparable to an eidetic image (ghost image).

Many normal people, not under drugs, are capable of experiencing such eidetic visions, particularly children and those adults who are endowed with an artistic temperament. Some artists, indeed, appear to have had eidetic personalities, among them Sibelius and William Blake. It is said that when Blake wished to draw portraits of historical characters, he could conjure up at will, in absolute detail, an eidetic

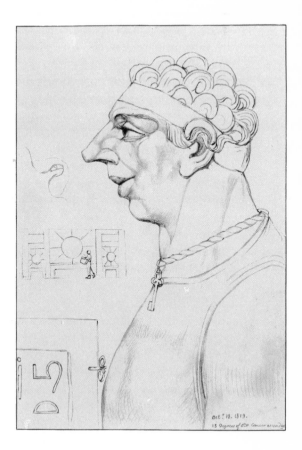

*The Man Who Built the Pyramids* by William Blake—a portrait done from an eidetic image conjured up in the artist's mind.

projection of one of them before his eyes and then use his ghostly image as a "living" model.

Again, other experiential states that sometimes follow the taking of LSD, such as the oceanic feeling of being transcendentally identified and at one with the universe, can also be experienced by people who are not drugged—as it was, for example, by the great mystics.

The mind-transforming properties of LSD were discovered in 1943 at Basel, Switzerland, by Dr. Albert Hofmann, an analytical chemist, when he accidentally inhaled a small amount of the drug and, as a result, sank "into a not unpleasant delirium which was masked by an extreme degree of fantasy." Dr. Hofmann, remembering his intensely colored, fantastic visions, then deliberately took what proved to be rather a large amount of the potent LSD and, within an hour, experienced mild dizziness, restlessness, inability to concentrate, visual disturbances, and uncontrollable laughter. Hofmann observed how the faces of the people about him were transformed into grotesquely-colored masks. His description of the way everything seemed to undulate with brightly changing colors has been corroborated by many others who subsequently took the drug. But LSD has not a uniform effect: some experience pleasurable sensations, others feel great anxiety and terror, as, for example, when they lose their sense of time and imagine they will never return to a normal perception of it, or when they feel they are being born or actually dying.

Subsequent to the discovery of LSD, experiments on animals were carried out. Thus spiders built more perfect webs under LSD—under mescaline, by the way, the spiders' webs were much more disarranged. Carp, which normally hug the bottom of their watery ambience, became surface swimmers when influenced by LSD. In man, apart from the mental changes already related, dilation of the pupil occurs, stronger knee-jerk reflexes are noted, and so on; but, most important, no grave physical side effects have been observed, though the major mental dangers in the therapeutic use of the drug are considerable, for it can induce psychosis or a depression that may lead to suicide.

A decade passed before LSD psychotherapy was tried out in the U.S.A., Germany, and Britain. Early reports confirmed that patients under the influence of the drug regressed to childhood and revealed more quickly their repressed infantile memories. In reverting to infantile ways of thinking patients would often feel themselves to be once again babies at the breast. They would be subject to impulses that, for instance, drove them to suck at the doctor's or nurse's fingers. Dr. H. Leuner, who works at Göttingen University, Germany, believes, along with other workers, that therapy can be considerably aided by allowing the drugged patients to satisfy such infantile cravings. Thus, during the reliving of the oral phase, Dr. Leuner gives his patients an apple, "as the mother's breast itself and not just as a symbol of it," and also feeds his patients liquids at these times. During the anal phase of regression the patients were permitted to smear with paste and paint the walls of an adjoining room. When aggressive impulses emerged the patients were encouraged to tear large quantities of newspapers and to throw "cardboard boxes, tins, and bottles at hallucinatory figures which they had painted on the walls of a room specially adapted for acting-out." By 1959 the possibility that LSD, sometimes augmented by other drugs such as Ritalin and Methedrine, could help to cure intractable neuroses and also shorten the period of psychotherapy necessary, had alerted psychiatrists the world over.

Patients, themselves, often testify to the value of the drug as can be learned from listening to tape recordings made of conversations between them and their therapists. Let me give but one example of a 32-year-old man, a "case of anxiety" who had been attending the Marlborough Day Hospital in London and who, before treatment with LSD, had had about 200 hours of psychotherapy spread over the preceeding six years. "Psychotherapy kept my head above water and helped me to cope with my anxiety. However, the anxiety neurosis remained and I did not know what happiness meant," stated the patient. After 65 sessions under LSD and continuing with interpretative psychotherapy the patient maintained that he had matured since he started on LSD. "I think it's a wonderful drug," he said. "It has completely made my life worth living which it certainly wasn't before."

However many people praise the marvels of LSD it should be noted that the testimonials of patients can be notoriously misleading, and hardly prove anything. Every faith healer, every acupuncturist, will pull out of his briefcase letters, sincere letters, from his patients, that testify to cures and which display gratitude for the method of therapy adopted. While LSD may have a limited value when used by skilled therapists it should be noted also that many doctors using the drug are not in fact so skilled. Indeed, sometimes "fringe" therapists are attracted to using LSD because of its dramatic effects and possibly also because it gives the dispensing therapists an enormous sense of power over their patients.

Dr. Sidney Cohen of Los Angeles reports in his book *Drugs of Hallucination* on the curious condition of "therapist breakdown": "A strange malady which has not yet been described elsewhere is an affliction, not of the receiver, but of the giver of the hallucinogens. This peculiar disorder might be called therapist breakdown. An unusual number of those dispensing these drugs have themselves come down with psychiatric disturbances. Research personnel seem immune

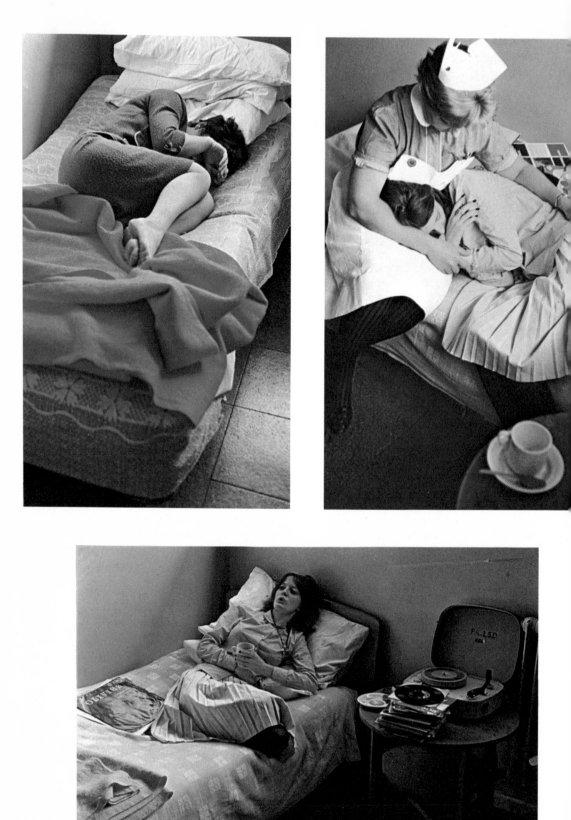

to the disease: it is the therapist or quasitherapist who suffers the affliction. The manifestations are variable. After intensive, though sometimes only after brief, contact with the drugs, a few have gone on to a psychotic breakdown or to megalomaniacal ideas of grandeur. Marked depressions and even a suicide in which these agents played a role are known. A couple of practitioners have found themselves in legal difficulties because of antisocial practices. This is an impressive morbidity, in view of the relatively small number of American practitioners using the hallucinogens. It constitutes a substantial minority of those dispensing the drugs. Of course, not all are stricken. The majority of therapists using LSD remain intact and in good health. How can it be that so many have fallen prey to these mental ailments? True, doctors also become patients, and psychiatrists and psychologists are not exempt from the very ills that they treat, but hardly in the numbers seen in those involved with the hallucinogenic drugs."

During the last 14 years psychochemicals, other than the hallucinogenic agents, have been introduced into psychiatric practice. These include the neuroleptics, which in small doses act as tranquilizers, the tranquilizers themselves, and the antidepressants. Their introduction has led to therapeutic gains that some authorities label as modest while others, agreeing with the pharmaceutical companies, make much greater claims for them.

Just as the LSD group of psychochemicals induce psychotic-like states, the neuroleptics, in large enough doses, act to some extent as "antipsychotics." One of these neuroleptics named chlorpromazine, a phenothiazine derivative, heralded the commencement of the new psychochemical therapy when it was introduced in 1952. Chlorpro-

At some hospitals the drug LSD is given in carefully selected cases to facilitate the release into consciousness of repressed memories and relationships from early childhood. These photos of patients at Powick Mental Hospital, England, were taken at various stages of LSD treatment. Above left, a patient adopts the fetal position while reliving the actual birth experience. In regression to childhood (above right), a patient substitutes a nurse for her mother: she has painted her nails black in her anxiety to conceal unacceptable feelings—symbolized for her by the fingers. Left, a patient's attention is totally engaged by the sound of a record turntable revolving: under LSD auditory acuity is heightened considerably. The fear and guilt associated with many repressed traumatic experiences can make their release extremely frightening (right). For this reason, nurse therapists remain with the patient throughout the period of treatment.

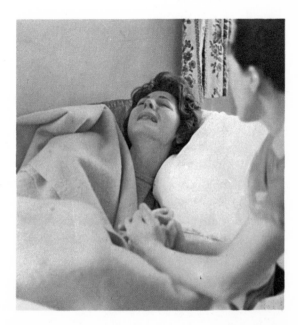

mazine was discovered in France by Delay and Deniker. They knew how patients under this drug became indifferent toward surgical procedures while remaining aware of what was happening all around them. Accordingly, they tried out chlorpromazine on patients suffering from acute episodes of schizophrenia, and such was its antipsychotic, dampening effect that it allowed a number of such patients to lead a relatively normal life.

Indeed, nowadays, many psychotic patients can be treated in general hospitals and then allowed, sometimes, to go home rather than be committed to a mental institution. Most of these patients need to take chlorpromazine for the rest of their lives. Unfortunately the drug can, on occasions, lead to unhappy side effects and when chlorpromazine is stopped by the general practitioner, for these or other reasons, disaster can fall upon the patient and his family.

Chlorpromazine, then, does not cure the patient. In or outside hospitals it can, in some cases, reduce excitement and other disturbing symptoms to make the illness more bearable. Even in normal subjects chlorpromazine, and the many other neuroleptic drugs introduced during the last 10 years, blunt the imaginative process. They also inhibit psychomotor activity so that it becomes a conscious effort, for example, for a patient to move his limbs. This neuroleptic inhibition of psychomotor activity is often remarked on by patients treated with such drugs. They say: "My arms feel as if they don't belong to me though I'm not nervous any more," or "I've slowed up so that when I'm dressing and undressing everything is a bit heavier. I'm not so tired and sleepy as I was."

Such complaints become more pronounced with high doses and sometimes, too, the patients incorporate this action of the drug into their delusory system of thinking. Here are some actual quotations from patients of H.-J. Haase, professor of psychiatry at Düsseldorf:

"Do you think this crippling will get better? I notice that eating and walking are so very slow."

"Doctor, please help me! I can't sit down. I can't lie down. I can't walk. I don't know what to do. Please help me!"

"My entire nervous system is being held up. My eardrum has gone slack and it sends out sounds of its own accord. It still vibrates, and that's how the radio signals get in, and then they can stop my whole nervous system."

"As you know, I'm the victim of a tragedy that they want to cover up. Now that everything's alright again, they shouldn't go and block my whole nervous system, so that I'm completely helpless. I'm held back in walking and eating. In the morning I have to let myself be washed, like a little child."

114

Other patients welcome the neuroleptic action of such drugs and bear witness to its beneficiary effects. Two further quotations from patients of Professor Haase will have to suffice here:

"The tablets calm me down so that my nature doesn't come out. Everything is so unimportant to me. I couldn't care less where I am, whether I'm here or somewhere else. I used to say I was a 'Royal Charlady,' but that was all madness. I only imagined it."

"I feel lighter and freer, the tablets have loosened the inner tension and that has got my thoughts in order again.

"Do you know what else the tablets have done—at least I think so—they have made me less sensitive when anybody says anything to me. I used to be so sensitive before."

Though it is in the treatment of schizophrenia that the neuroleptic drugs have had their widest application, they have been administered in maniac syndromes, in alcoholism, and in the psychoneuroses. Doctors who, by using a neuroleptic drug, rapidly end a period of psychotic disturbance naturally experience deep satisfaction. They have the gratitude of the patient and his relatives; but frequently those psychiatrists committed to physical methods of treatment and basically ignorant of psychodynamics, imagine they have brought about a cure when, in fact, they have only masked symptoms. After all, the causes that triggered off the mental disturbance generally persist. The discharge rate from mental hospitals today may be unprecedentedly high but so, also, is the readmission rate. Treatment based on giving neuroleptics may, for patient and doctor, be a godsend, but it is not the miracle answer.

The same is true for the new tranquilizers—that is, the mild, nonbarbiturate sedatives such as meprobamate and chlordiozepoxide, which have been prescribed for patients displaying neurotic symptoms. Meprobamate may allay anxiety but the causes of the anxiety remain. Nor do patients always welcome the removal of their anxiety symptoms. One New York analyst, Dr. Louis Linn, cites the case of a woman who had fantasies that she might be compelled to indulge in exhibitionistic sexual behavior in public. Given meprobamate to reduce her anxiety she compared the effect of the drug with the cutting of the wires of a fire alarm. "The clamor of the fire alarm is silenced but the fire goes on unabated, and nobody is warning me to fight it." Her anxiety, in short, had been replaced by worse feelings of dread.

Patients are too often given tranquilizers mistakenly; they present symptoms of agitation or anxiety when, in fact, inwardly they are depressed. True, tranquilization whether by these new, nonbarbiturate sedatives or by neuroleptics in small doses, can open the door to psychotherapy. But many psychoanalysts maintain that the use of the

Three paintings by mental patients. Left, the disordered image of faces within a face reflects a patient's own disordered reality: the concept of a disordered body is common to many psychiatric patients. Below, a room as seen and "felt" by a victim of psychosis. The actual world of solid objects has been transmuted into a swirling, impermanent miasma. Describing his experiences, the patient exclaimed, "The walls are moving and I am unable to control them." Right, a characteristic eye motif drawn by a schizophrenic represents the cold, calculating look of an all-knowing accuser. In this case, the effect is emphasized by the face reflected in the eyeball.

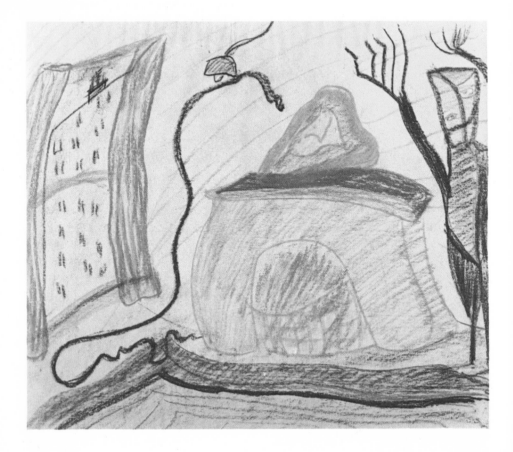

tranquilizers militates against a successful analysis. Given on their own, tranquilizers such as meprobamate may to some extent relieve anxiety, tension, and phobic ideas, but whether they are superior to the cheaper barbiturates is doubtful.

Finally, there is the group of antidepressant drugs that includes imipramine and phenelzine. The treatment of depressive illnesses by physical methods has sometimes been most helpful. As long ago as 1935, Ladislos Jos Meduna of Budapest introduced convulsive therapy into psychiatry. In those days convulsions were induced by injecting into the veins cardiazol, a camphor derivative, and this rather crude and frightening treatment helped many patients who displayed a depressive mood that exceeded customary sadness and was accompanied by deep feelings of guilt. It may be that unconscious masochistic strivings were satisfied by such convulsive therapy. That some quick method to combat morbid depression had become available was important, for almost all depressive illnesses are dangerous in that most suicides are associated with them.

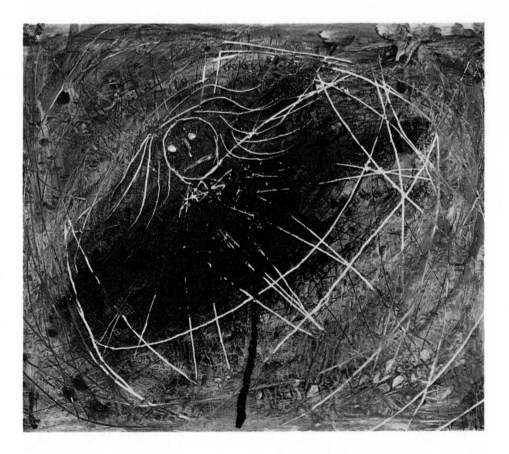

After 1938 electro-shock replaced cardiazol as a means of producing convulsions. At present, modified electric convulsion therapy (ECT) is widely given to depressive patients. (Patients are anesthetized before being given the electric shocks.) Though ECT is a relatively safe form of therapy it does not always work and sometimes can affect the brain cells and cause memory defects. The new antidepressant drugs therefore, if efficacious, must be recognized as a great step forward in physical therapy. Certainly there are psychiatrists who have implicit faith in these new drugs. For example, Dr. John Pollitt of St. Thomas' Hospital, London, maintains that they are effective in two thirds of depressive cases of all types. He believes, in addition, that such drugs do not merely alleviate the depressive syndrome but actually cure it. There are many psychiatrists on both sides of the Atlantic who would not quarrel with Dr. Pollitt's statistical assessments and who would believe that, by restoring sleep patterns in patients and by promoting their appetite etc., they allow the previously depressed patient to relate to other people normally and that this very adaptation begins to reverse the complicated depressive process.

Other psychiatrists are not so sanguine, disagreeing with such statistics and pouring scorn on such superficial interpretations of psychodynamics. Recently a clinical trial tested the merits of imipramine, phenelzine, ECT, and a placebo in the treatment of depressive illness. The subsequent report to the Medical Research Council of Great Britain by its clinical psychiatry committee was published in the *British Medical Journal* of April 3, 1965. Its conclusions were that both on a short term basis (after one month's treatment in hospital) and on a long term basis (up to six months) ECT and imipramine increased the frequency of recovery over and above the spontaneous rate shown

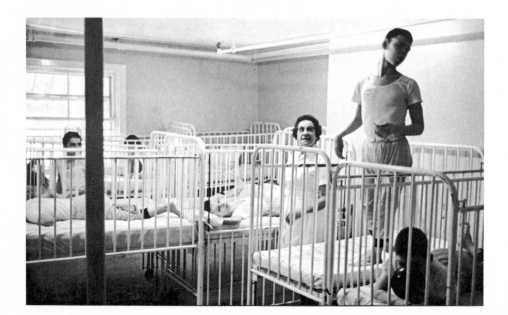

by those patients taking an inert substance—that is, a placebo. Phenelzine, on the other hand, had no advantage over the placebo. True, the number treated—some 250 patients—was not statistically large, but the results were nevertheless melancholy as regards the much used antidepressant, phenelzine. These and other drug trials tend to undermine statements like those of Dr. William Sargant who has said that within the next 25 years most mental illnesses will be as easily treated with drugs as are physical illnesses at present. Such optimism seems unwarranted; but the value of drugs, and of other physical methods of treatment, should not be underrated—when they are used propitiously and with a keen appreciation of their very definite limitations.

That mechanistic psychiatrists tend to exaggerate the potentialities of the psychochemicals is understandable. The wish is there. All of us, perhaps, as children, imagined that a magic elixir might exist to transform the raving, ugly beast into a rational, handsome prince. The shadows of adults can still be seen on the road to fairyland. In our century, too, it has been demonstrated that some psychoses have an organic genesis. General paralysis of the insane, for instance, results from syphilis contracted years before, and now can be dealt with by penicillin. Certain psychotic symptoms may follow on decades of alcoholism. Mental disturbances or deterioration may be a sequel to arteriosclerosis. Some psychiatrists reason that since certain forms of "insanity" result from organic pathogens others might too. They argue that, as the years pass, other as yet unknown organic causes of mental disease may be uncovered. Even before the introduction of the tranquilizers the value of certain chemical restraints such as the barbiturates had been verified. To think in these terms, moreover,

Left, mentally retarded children at the Butler's Memorial Home near Montreal, Canada. As yet, drugs and physical treatment can do little to improve the mental condition of the retarded. Right, measuring a patient's IQ at St. George's Hospital, London.

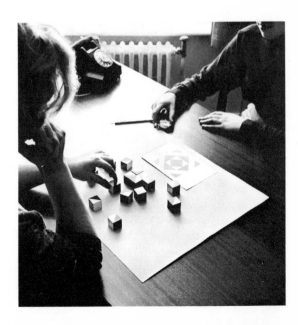

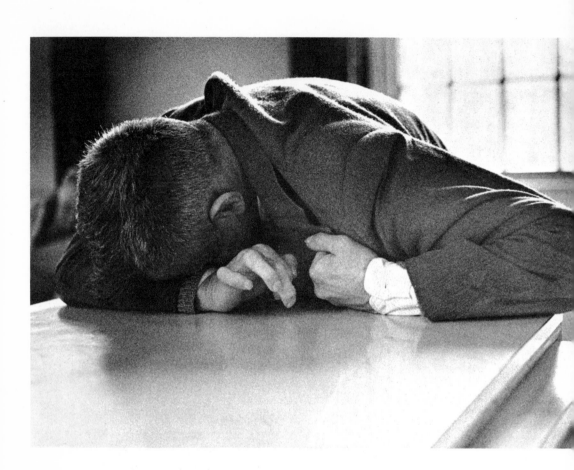

allows a psychiatrist to retreat from Freudian sexual psychodynamics.

Conversely, there is no virtue in the fact that many Freudian therapists profess with pride that they are ignorant of the action of the new drugs—though there are analysts, a minority, who do not eschew the new psychochemicals and who believe that these drugs, far from interfering with analysis, allow many more people to become analyzable. They argue that if the administration of drugs to a patient under analysis has unconscious significance for that patient, then perhaps these implications themselves can be analyzed.

The debate continues, sometimes with great heat, between the psychiatrists of the many different schools. To give drugs or not to give drugs is but one dispute. Perhaps where so many medical authorities differ as to the effect and value of drugs for the sick mind it might be appropriate to conclude this chapter with a testimony of a patient (an engineering draftsman) who suffered a nervous breakdown and subsequently spent several weeks in hospital, where he was given electric shock treatment and drugs. The patient claimed to recall

Left, the isolation and despair of the mentally depressed patient. Right, electric convulsion therapy (ECT), still commonly used in cases of severe depression. The protective gag placed in the patient's mouth is to prevent him damaging his teeth or biting his tongue.

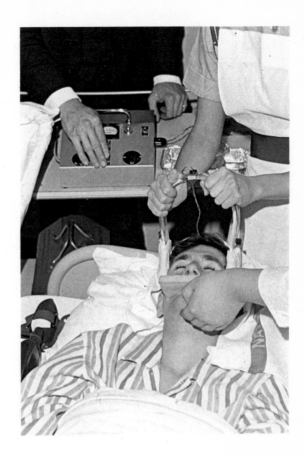

almost every detail of his experience, and described it vividly in *The Lancet* of February 12, 1966:

"I was chiefly struck by the godlike detachment of the hospital psychiatrist. To be fair, this varied from man to man, but I got the impression that, by and large, they thought they could cure anything with drugs and shock, in much the same way that a mechanic tackles engine repairs. The atmosphere of the place was such that once I began to recover, I tried to get out as quickly as possible, even though I was conscious of not being myself. I did sign myself out for a few days, but I was persuaded to go back. Perhaps this attitude to the medical staff was a symptom of my illness.

"On the effect of the drugs I was given, I am more sure of my ground. The worst part of the experience was when I began to recover. I could not concentrate for two minutes together. I could neither read nor follow the television. Occupational therapy needed a tremendous effort—not the actual work, but to take an interest in it. On the other hand, just sitting doing nothing brought no relief. The days dragged terribly. Normally I am quite happy just dabbling about doing nothing in particular. I have been in hospital on my back with a slipped disc and remained cheerful. It is very hard to describe the feeling. It is not depression, it is not pain. The drugs were apparently tranquillizers, but I certainly did not feel tranquil. . . .

"Eventually I found that the best thing was to be doing something which needed absolutely no mental effort. I got into a ritual which seemed to help. I voluntarily mopped out the w.cs and washrooms every morning, polishing the taps, and so forth. I made a point of washing and drying the cutlery. I went for frequent walks. We were supposed to stay in the grounds, but I got several miles away at times. I became quite fond of certain walks on the moors. Looking out for certain objects seemed to engage my attention. . . .

"When I was discharged I still had this terrible feeling. Quite how the doctors decide you are 'cured' is a mystery to me. It seems to depend on how many electric shocks you have had. How they decide the particular number of shocks is also a mystery. It seems an arbitrary, ritualistic system to me. Once a week the head doctor came round, an occasion of some importance in the hospital life. Since I wanted to get out quickly I never answered anything but 'fine' when asked how I felt. This was my only direct contact with the medical staff. I knew fairly well one patient who had had the maximum number of shocks. He was worried that he still did not feel right, and he said so during the doctor's round one week. The doctor just shrugged, saying they had done their best, which was no great help to the man.

"When I got home I occupied myself cleaning up our cellar workshop and tidying out cupboards. . . .

"I was eager to start work because I thought it would help. My firm was very good and allowed me to start on short time for a fortnight, and then I worked full-time. I was much better by then, but I still had this terrible feeling, this lack of concentration. I was not very effective at work, I could not read a book nor follow even the simplest of the orchestral music in my collection. Everyday life required a tremendous effort. . . .

"From the time I went into hospital I had been taking some 16 pills a day. After 6 weeks at home I suddenly decided that I would stop taking pills and see what happened. I had a few rough nights, but there was an immediate improvement. I felt more like my old self. Within a week I could read for pleasure. I could just jog along as of old without having to force myself into taking an interest in life. Perhaps this would have happened anyway. Perhaps I did a dangerous thing and got away with it. Perhaps this feeling was some peculiar reaction to the drug not experienced by others, but I don't think so.

"Relatives and friends all remarked on the sudden improvement in my manner—some without knowing the reason. Although I felt so much better, I could not understand why it was so noticeable to others until I met other patients at the clinic who had been in hospital with me. They had a bloated look about the face and a vacancy of the eyes which I had not noticed when we were all together. Their manner was faraway; it obviously was an effort for them to answer simple questions. When I got home I discussed this with my parents. They said that I had been exactly the same till I stopped taking the pills. . . .

"I hope you don't feel I am making a specific complaint against the hospital. I was in a very bad way and I am grateful to the people who looked after me. It cannot be an easy job. But I feel that I have had to drag myself back into normal life in a way that would not have been necessary if there had been more sympathetic contact with the doctors and less blind faith in drugs and shock. . . .

"All in all, I am doubtful whether these drugs are really understood. Certainly a drugged patient behaves very quietly and appears very calm, but in my experience the mental torment is worse than at the height of the delirium. Then your thoughts race, but you are only half aware that you are ill. Later, you are fully conscious of your illness but can do nothing about it. You have no thoughts; you lead a sort of suspended, frustrating existence. The only reason you are quiet is because you don't know what the devil to do with yourself. Some sign from the doctors that they understand how you feel would be a great help. As it is, it seems that they have no idea—and if so how can they really know what they are treating? No doubt many of these impressions were affected by my illness and were illogical. None the less it is how I felt which matters."

# 4 The Human Guinea Pig

The responsibility of the doctor is primarily to the patient under his care, but from time to time what is best for the patient conflicts with the interests, and occasionally with the health, of the patient's immediate family. The moral dilemma for the doctor becomes even more complex when the interests of the patient conflict with the needs of society at large. Thus a patient may be a diabetic or an epileptic who drives an automobile, having concealed his disability from the licensing authorities. The doctor, then, may feel that the legal claims of society should take precedence over the individual's right to privacy.

When society allows its representatives to pervert humanistic conceptions of justice so that its laws grow unarguably evil, as in Nazi Germany, the crisis of conscience for the doctor becomes even more imperative and marked. The possibility that, in the future, outrageous conduct by perverted powers and acquiescent doctors may occur cannot, alas, be discounted; and the recent advances in pharmacology—the development of the mind drugs in particular—as well as the future discoveries that are bound to take place, allow us to envisage the existence of a situation whose nightmare aspects could make the world of 1984, as depicted by George Orwell, pale into timid insignificance.

The medical block at Auschwitz; many of the Nazis' experiments were carried out—by doctors—behind this door.

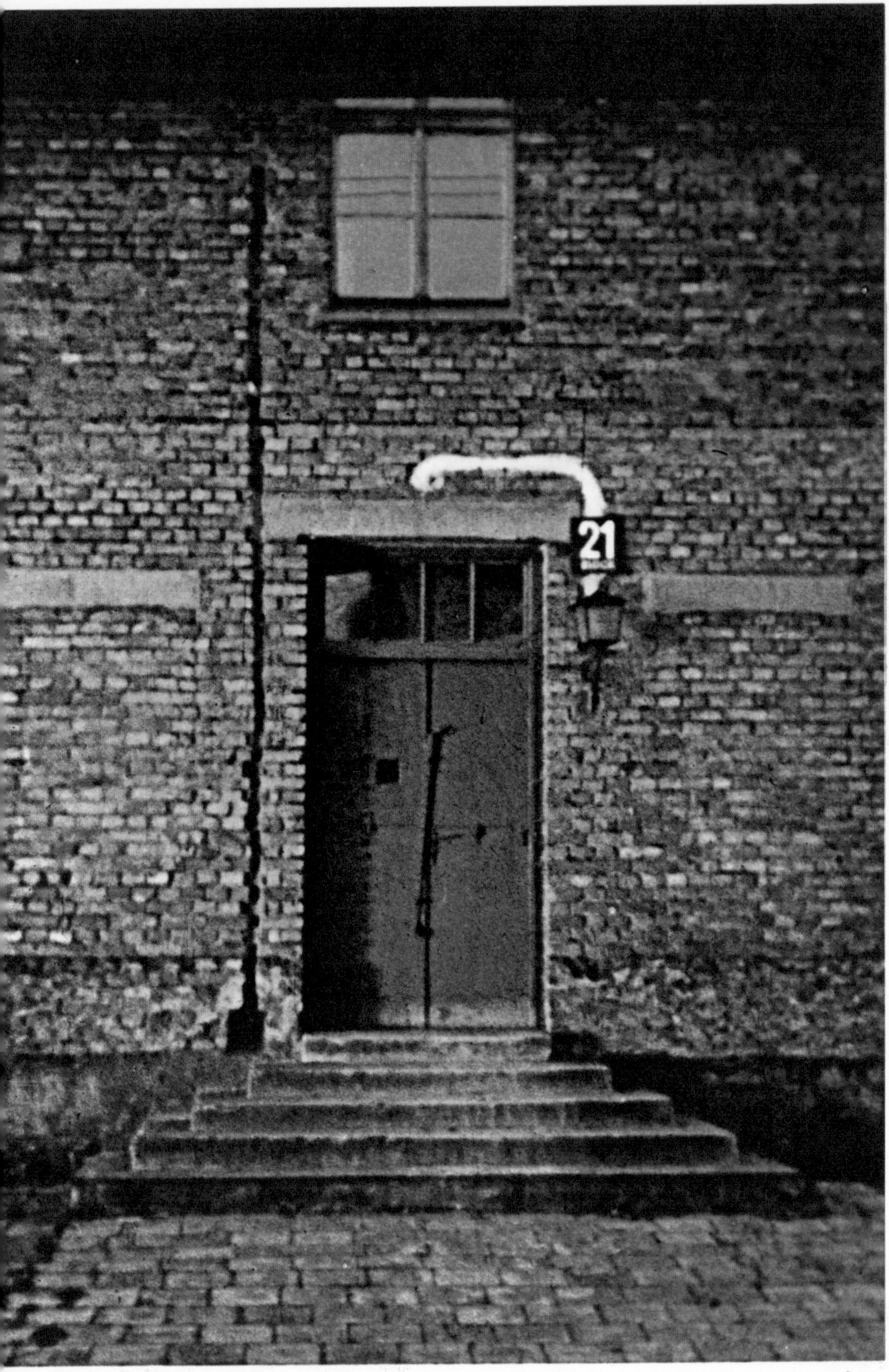
21

When the state cultivates, or a majority group attitude permits, the paranoid notion that certain members of the community are dangerous, degraded, and subhuman—be they Jews, the insane, or criminals—then the likelihood that doctors will be pressed into the service of demoniacal agents becomes a real possibility. We have seen, in an earlier chapter, how the mentally sick were wretchedly treated in past centuries; the predicament of the Jew in Nazi Germany is still fresh in many minds; and from time to time profoundly shocking statements are made by "responsible" representatives of different nations on how criminals should be dealt with. As recently as August 1965, the Chief Justice of the Supreme Court of Pakistan said at a Commonwealth and Empire Law Conference in Australia: "Medical science having advanced so greatly, it should be possible now to deprive a criminal of the use of a hand or whole limb by a small piece of surgery."

The hanging, drawing, and quartering advocates abound in the most sophisticated societies, and the definition of what is criminal, and therefore of who is criminal, is not an irrevocable, absolute one: it alters in time and with the nature of the societies, themselves always dynamically changing. In a nation diseased—and no nation, whatever its record, is necessarily immune—doctors are made to obey the dictates of the state even though the commands issued are, by humanistic medical standards, criminal and quite opposed to the Hippocratic spirit. Even the most eminent and internationally respected of doctors find themselves, in such circumstances, obliged to obey or to risk their livelihood, if not their lives.

Consider the quandary of the German professor Gerhard Domagk on October 26, 1939, when he received a long-distance call from Sweden announcing that he had been awarded a Nobel Prize for his discovery of prontosil—perhaps one of the greatest advances ever made in medical science. Written confirmation of this high honor soon followed, and on November 3 Professor Domagk replied to the rector of the Caroline Institute in Stockholm. He indicated in his letter that he hoped he would soon have the opportunity to address scientists in Stockholm and to express his gratitude for the recognition his work had received; but first he had to make sure that Germans were permitted by the government to receive such prizes.

Domagk received congratulations on his award from the United States, where one of President Roosevelt's sons had been successfully treated with prontosil, and from Sweden, Denmark, Norway, the Netherlands, Belgium, and Switzerland. In Germany, however, news of the award was suppressed, and only those who had listened to foreign radio stations were able to congratulate Domagk personally.

"Conform or die." Berlin crowds give a mass salute to their Führer (October 1938).

On November 17 he was arrested at his home by the German secret police. Outside in the street, Gestapo men waited with drawn revolvers. At police headquarters Domagk, whose work had benefited people of all races, religions, and creeds, was relieved of his watch, penknife, pocketbook, collar, and necktie, and locked up in Cell No. 10. Later that month the Caroline Institute in Stockholm received a second letter from the professor. They had no idea that he had been arrested. With consternation they read that since the Führer and Reich-Chancellor had forbidden German nationals to accept Nobel awards and since those in Stockholm knew of the Nazi decree, they could hardly expect him to engage in an act of disloyalty. In short, Gerhard Domagk, under impossible pressures, had to decline the prize.

Later, Domagk was allowed to go home, but he was watched incessantly. "Any new suspicion aroused against me," he said afterward, "might be fatal to myself and family." Conform or die was the dictate of the Nazi regime, an alternative that obtained then for doctors eminent or otherwise, and that can become operative in any

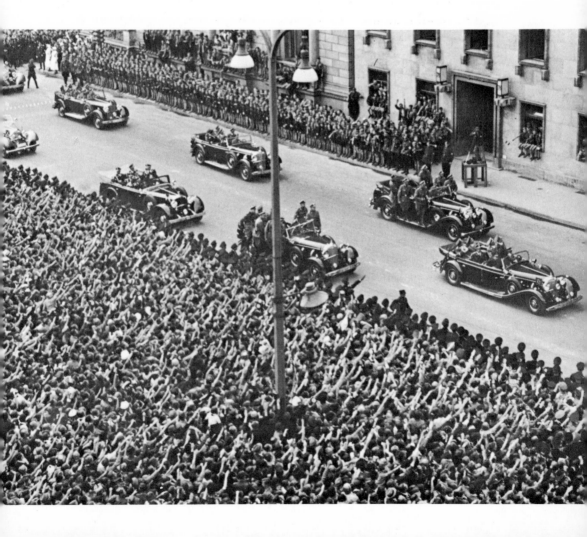

totalitarian country. The majority of doctors in Nazi Germany, in fact, could adapt themselves to the regime without contravening their Hippocratic oath. Most of the 90,000 doctors in Hitler's Germany felt that to protest was useless, and closed their eyes to flagrant medico-ethical abuses; but only some 350 committed medical crimes. The extent of their criminal activities, however, is out of all proportion to their numbers. The amount of suffering they caused was fantastic and horrifying. They engaged in experimental work with drugs and in surgery. They did low-pressure and cooling experiments, frequently killing their human guinea pigs without a qualm. They carried out fearful tests on the possibility of drinking seawater. They experimented with viruses such as those that cause hepatitis (inflammation of the liver), and also with typhus vaccines. They perpetrated unspeakable experiments on Jewish twins. They worked as death doctors with mustard gas. They tried out methods of sterilizing human beings and eliminating human beings. Their blood lust and their capacity for cruelty seems, in retrospect, limitless.

For 2400 years doctors have followed the ethical code of Hippocrates. In all languages they have sworn: "I will use treatment to help my patient according to my ability and judgement, but never with a view to injury or a wrongdoing." They have been committed to the oath: "I will abstain from abusing the bodies of men and women, either free or slave. . . ."

The slaves in Nazi Germany were incarcerated in concentration camps, and the S.S. doctors in charge abused barbarously the bodies and minds of men, women, and children. There were doctors who perpetrated these medical crimes with delight and enthusiasm; there were some who assented to such acts under the excuse of a higher duty to the state; there were others who conformed timidly, fearful that if they disobeyed they themselves would be punished.

It should be remembered that the majority of the "experiments" were performed during the war years, when many German doctors felt themselves to be on a similar footing to soldiers. During the war the idea of command and of obedience to orders became imperative in democratic countries as well. Even in peacetime, army medical officers are exhorted during their initial military training to behave as officers first and doctors second. But the fact that a nation is at war does not release a doctor, even in the armed forces, from his moral obligation to the Hippocratic oath, however many combatant soldiers no longer feel obliged to observe the Sixth Commandment.

Unpleasant though it may be, it is necessary here to particularize and to allow the reader to perceive the quality, if not the quantity, of the crimes committed by the minority of doctors in Nazi Germany.

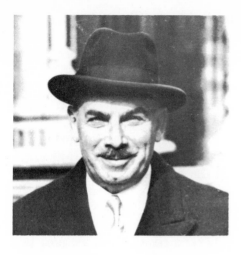

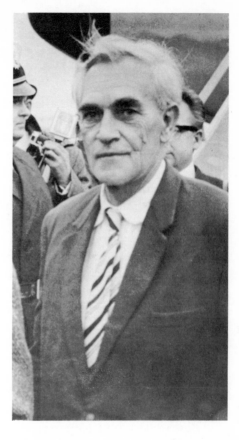

Above, Dr. Wladislaw Alexander Dering, photographed in London in May 1964. Right, Dr. Horst Schumann, deported from Ghana to Germany in November 1966 to stand trial for alleged war crimes.

For to cite, in abstraction, the savagery unleashed on countless human beings by doctors in the Dante's inferno of concentration camps is to defeat any person's imaginative capacity to grasp what the nature of these crimes really was. Perhaps only by feeling the truth of what happened in our own time can we hope to prevent similar bestial acts occurring again in the future.

In 1964, in a libel trial in London, the plight of some of those experimented on in Auschwitz was again revealed. The libel action was brought by a Polish doctor practicing in London, a Dr. Dering, who worked at one time as a "prisoner doctor" at Auschwitz. Prisoner doctors were pressed into service at the camps so that German doctors could be free to serve at the Eastern Front where they were desperately needed. By helping some of the camp inmates to regain a semblance of health the prison doctors allowed such people to be used again as slave labor for the German war effort. Some of these prisoner doctors also engaged in the human experiments required by those in ultimate authority. A record of the libel action brought by Dr. Dering was given in *Auschwitz in England* by Mavis M. Hill and L. Norman Williams. Here is a passage from this abominable record; the witness who speaks (called "the first man") is but one voice that here must speak for innumerable others:

The first man was called. He was now thirty-eight and lived in Israel. He was born in Salonika, and was at High School when the Germans came. They took him to Poland about the beginning of April 1943. He was with his parents in the same wagon until they got to Poland where they separated the men and the women. His mother did not want to be separated from him. He was taken to Birkenau and the next morning they 'made a number in his forearm.'

Undoing his cufflinks—his fingers seemed all thumbs, and he took some time about this—he exposed a tattooed number, which the interpreter read to the court as '114302.'

*Mr. Hirst* [for the defense]: Within a very few days after your arrival at Birkenau did a German officer visit your Block?

*The first man*: Yes. A German officer came. He asked for two men of each age group between sixteen and thirty.

He was chosen as one of two eighteen-year-olds, but had no idea then why he was being selected.

*Mr. Hirst*: Who did the selection?

*The first man*: The German officer gave the orders, and the Block elder had to perform the order—the choice.

That happened after he had been at Birkenau for two days. He did no work there. The next morning he was taken with a group of others to Block 12 at Birkenau. There they were given special clothes, and every morning a doctor took their temperature and pulse. 'They took us to the camp of the women and did irradiations.' The room into which they were taken, one by one, had a table; it was not very dark. An officer of the *Luftwaffe* was in charge and later the first man learned that the officer's name was Dr. Schumann; he was tall and there was a sign—a scar—on his cheek.

When his turn came, he was told to take off his clothes and was naked. 'They told me that I should put my genital organ, together with the scrotum, on a machine.' The machine was over his genital organs. There was the noise of a motor. He stood there, with the motor running, for from five to eight minutes. The machine was directed, so far as he could judge, to the centre. Afterwards he was told to leave the room. All the others stood in front of the machine. When it was over they were taken to

Block 12. He was examined every day afterwards to see if there were any signs on his organs.

His organs were not stained. 'I saw that on the organs of my comrades were dark stains. Generally, after the irradiation, I had not pains specially, but I had a general ill feeling.'

One morning he was taken away with five others by ambulance to a place which, he later learned, was Block 28, Auschwitz. He was taken with another of the men to the first room on the left, a doctor's room.

*Mr. Hirst*: Who was present?

*The first man*: Dr. Dering. *This* Dr. Dering. (The man pointed to the plaintiff.) At that time I did not know his name, but I now recognise him. Dr. Schumann was also there. Dr. Dering had on a white gown.

*Mr. Hirst*: Was anything done?

*The first man*: Yes.

*Mr. Hirst*: Describe what was done.

*The first man*: They told both of us to take off all our clothes. Afterwards they gave us a piece of glass. Dr. Dering came with a sort of club and put it into my rectum.

*Mr. Hirst*: What happened after you were given the glass?

*The first man*: When he introduced the stick into my rectum, some drops came out of my member.

*Mr. Hirst*: Who is 'he'?

*The first man*: Dr. Dering.

He, and the five others were taken to Block 21, to a room with beds. Nobody came to see them that day. He saw Dr. Dering the following morning, and they spoke in French, which the first man then spoke fluently. He had begun the conversation.

*Mr. Hirst*: What did you say?

*The first man*: I did not know what they would do to me. When I came to know that I was to be operated on then I said, 'Why are you operating on me? I am fit, not sick.' He answered me in French, 'If I take not the testicle off you they will take it off me.'

After that conversation they put him on a stretcher and took him to the operating theatre. He was able to walk, and did not want to go on the stretcher because he was afraid; he resisted. Men 'took' him. They were wearing white gowns. He did not remember whether there was one room or two rooms, but there were two tables for operating. He was sitting on the stretcher, and male nurses held him and wanted to give a spinal injection. He resisted; and the needle broke. The first time, when the needle broke, they started to curse in Polish.

*Mr. Hirst*: Who were 'they'?

*The first man*: I could not see who, but I only heard words in Polish. I was bent over.

A further, successful attempt was made to give him a spinal injection. He had 'terrible pains,' which continued until the lower half of his body was paralysed. He had no other injection of any kind in Block 21 on that day. After the lower half of his body went dead they put him on the operating table. He was fully conscious.

*Mr. Hirst*: What happened?

*The first man*: They took off the shirt I had, and put iodine on the skin, the left side of the lower abdomen. I was lying back. I saw the doctor putting the iodine on with a swab. After some minutes I saw Dr. Dering when he had my testicle in his hand and showed it to Dr. Schumann, who was present. I felt no pains during the operation.

*Mr. Hirst*: How, if at all, did you react to the pain at the time of the injection?

*The first man*: What could I do? I felt pains. I continued to speak in French, saying 'Don't do this.'

Since that trial Dr. Dering has died. The other doctor mentioned, the Luftwaffe medical officer, Dr. Horst Schumann, who was in charge of the male castration and female sterilization "experiments" at Auschwitz, lived in the German Federal Republic until after 1950 without any criminal proceedings being taken against him. Since then he has practiced in Ghana and other African states, and the West German government succeeded only recently in extraditing him.

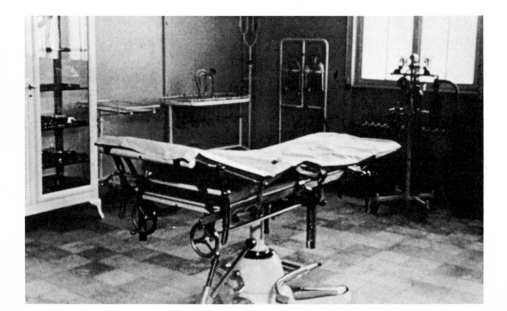

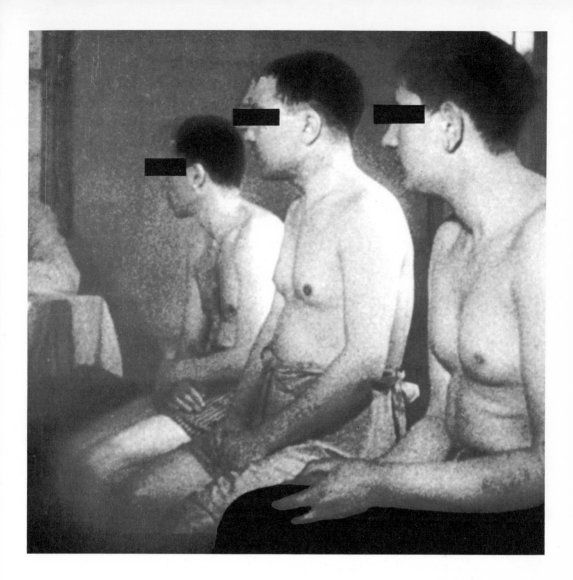

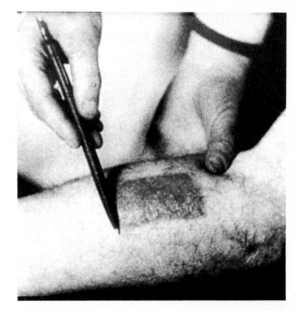

Left, the operating theatre of the medical block at Auschwitz. Above, three of the men selected for experiments in sterilization. Right, a phosphorus burn inflicted by doctors for experimental purposes. (Stills from *Night and Fog,* Alain Resnais' documentary on Nazi atrocities, made in 1958.)

It is difficult, no doubt, for many to understand the mentality of those doctors engaged in such medical atrocities. Yet those superior to them in the medical hierarchy, those nearer to Himmler and Hitler, not only ordered such experiments to be carried out but sometimes urged the doctors engaged in the work to be even more ruthless. Thus Karl Gebhardt, head physician of the Hohenlychen Orthopedic Sanatorium and President of the German Red Cross, began a series of experiments at Ravensbrück concentration camp for women on July 20, 1942, in which he tested the efficacy of the new sulfa drugs on gas gangrene infections. Dr. Gebhardt and his assistant, Dr. Fritz Fischer, inflicted deep surgical wounds on healthy young women and introduced into the wounds a mixed infection containing septic gas gangrene material and earth. The S.S. Professor Dr. Grawitz, who came to the camp to see how their work was progressing, suggested they had been too lenient. Wounded German soldiers on the Eastern Front had developed gas gangrene and he wanted to know whether the sulfa drugs were effective in combating this infection. He told Gebhardt that the wounds they were inflicting did not compare with the extent of the wounds the soldiers had suffered, and urged them to inflict actual bullet wounds on the women being experimented on. Hitler had, after all, decided that when the well-being of the nation was at stake, experiments on human subjects were permissible—and that the persons detained in concentration camps or prisons ought not to remain completely unaffected by the war while German soldiers were subjected to almost unbearable strain, and while women and children too were engulfed under a rain of incendiary bombs. Such was the grim, ironic justification for the sulfa drug experiments. As if, even without the medical experiments, the concentration camp victims were living in some mythical Elysium.

Despite the conditions that prevailed at such camps there were a few doctors who refused to revoke the Hippocratic oath they had taken years earlier. There was, for example, Dr. Adelaide Hautval, daughter of a French Protestant pastor, who was sent to a camp for arguing with the Gestapo about the way Jews were being treated in France. As a prisoner she was made to wear a yellow star and a band with the words "amie des juifs " written on it. Eventually she was transferred to Auschwitz, where she refused to participate in the sterilization experiments. Brought before Eduard Wirths, the garrison doctor, Adelaide Hautval said that what she had been asked to do was contrary to a doctor's ethical code. Wirths tried to persuade her to comply. He argued that the Jewish subjects used for the experiments were people "different from you." Hautval replied that there were several other people different from her, beginning with Wirths himself.

Fortunately Dr. Hautval was not sent to the gas chambers and survived the war. To protest, as she did, was not ridiculous; it was an act of humanity, nobility, and courage.

If the action of individuals such as Dr. Hautval makes heartening reading, so, too, does the behavior of the Dutch medical profession as a whole during this period of its history. The Reich Commissar for the Occupied Dutch Territories, Seiss-Inquart, ordered the Dutch physicians on December 19, 1941, to concentrate their medical efforts on the rehabilitation of the sick, so that the latter could be made to do "useful work." This command may have sounded mild enough on the surface, but from such small beginnings German doctors had progressed to killing the infirm and sterilizing those "racially unfit." When the Dutch doctors resisted Seiss-Inquart's order, he threatened to take away their licenses. The Dutch physicians promptly returned their licenses, saw their patients secretly, and abstained from writing birth or death certificates. A hundred Dutch doctors were then sent to concentration camps. The rest of the medical profession quietly took care of the widows and children of their unfortunate colleagues and still refused to act against the spirit of their Hippocratic oath. As a result no Dutch medical man participated at any time in the amoral experiments of their German counterparts.

Many of the Germans who participated in the criminal experiments maintained that their activities might, in the long run, help alleviate the suffering of soldiers at the front. Today, in many countries, including the U.S.A., Soviet Russia, and Britain, doctors who cooperate in experiments on the efficiency of chemical, bacteriological, and radiological war weapons no doubt also rationalize in similar ways. The U.S. Defense Department may advocate that "many forms of chemical weapons are more humane than many others that exist," but with their training, doctors should be able to question the accuracy of such statements and to recognize that no medical practitioner, in any case bound by his Hippocratic oath, can possibly defend the "bad against the worse."

By "humane" chemical weapons the U.S. Defense Department means those incapacitating psychochemicals that could temporarily paralyze entire populations. Such psychochemicals include LSD, Methedrine, psilocybine, and mescaline. It is known that every month pharmaceutical companies supply the U.S. Army Chemicals Center with 400 different drugs of this kind. According to Dr. M. van Sim, research on these drugs for such purposes has been undertaken ever since 1957. The House Committee on Science and Astronautics reported to Congress on August 9, 1959, that the U.S. was spending between 35

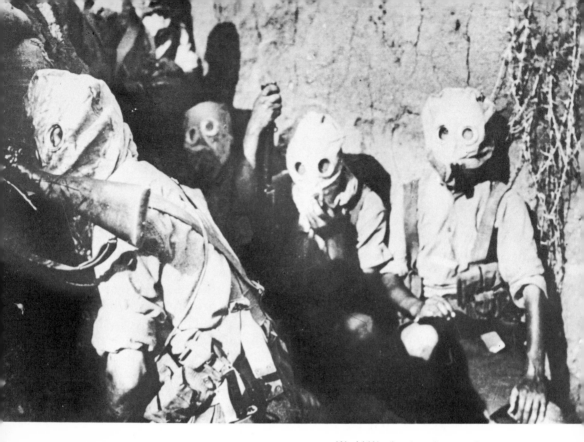

World War I saw various crude attempts at chemical warfare. Above, British troops entrenched on the Salonika front prepare for an expected gas attack.

and 40 million dollars each year on chemical-biological-radiological warfare research, and the committee recommended that, by 1962, 125 million dollars should be spent per year "to put this country on a par with the Communists."

The disabling drugs would not necessarily lead to *temporary* mental confusion, narcosis, blindness, or paralysis, as has been suggested. The psychochemicals notoriously do not have a standard effect on all people. The reader will recall how, in an earlier chapter, I discussed the dangers of LSD, a drug that has caused some people to commit suicide and induced a *permanent* psychosis in others. Moreover, from the point of view of military effectiveness, optimum doses would have to be given through dispersed gas or by pollution of the water supplies. (LSD in solution is tasteless, odorless, and colorless, and therefore particularly difficult to detect.) However, the optimum dose for a grown, healthy adult would be particularly damaging for the infirm, for the pregnant, for children, and for babies. Individual dosage, in short, could not be controlled; so the conception that harmless psychochemicals could render a whole city defenseless and temporarily crazy while the army took over humanely is but a military fantasy—which does not mean, alas, that psychochemicals will never be used in this way as weapons of war. (William Burroughs, the American novelist, declared in the *New Statesman* of March 11, 1966, that U.S. forces are using LSD in gas form in Vietnam.)

In any event, by whatever means LSD were to be disseminated—through the air, through water, or through food—it would not be possible to drug the whole population. As Dr. Sidney Cohen has rightly pointed out in his book *Drugs of Hallucination*, large numbers, safely indoors, would be entirely unaffected; and these, seeing others hallucinated and apparently mad for no evident reason, could easily stampede to cause a general panic, the results of which could be devastating. It is in this critical light that doctors should examine statements made by military authorities like America's General Stubbs, who has said: "We are attempting to completely separate these agents from the lethal agents so that any castigation normally given to toxic agents will not be associated with these agents since these do not maim or kill. As a result we hope to have a weapon which will give the commander much freer rein in its use as compared to toxic agents."

A film has been made recently that shows American troops being used for experiments with one of the hallucinogenic drugs. According to Dr. Sidney Cohen, army personnel were given small doses of the drug in their coffee without their knowledge. One sergeant who by chance did not take coffee shouted orders with increasing perplexity at his men, who began falling about, giggling helplessly. Such an experiment could hardly have taken place without the participation of some doctors, who doubtless felt that the drug dose, being infinitely small and controlled, would cause no permanent damage. Even on this level, in an experiment that some observers might consider no more sinister than a practical joke, it seems to me that the doctors involved acted against their basic medical ethical code. It is useless for such doctors to protest that they hold no authority in policy-making decisions. The death doctors of the concentration camps made that plea during the Nuremberg trials.

Some doctors, particularly those who have specialized in bacteriology, are also involved in biological weapon research. Germ warfare has occupied the minds of military strategists ever since the First World War, when German agents were purported to have inoculated horses and cattle with pathogenic bacteria and to have endeavored to spread cholera in Italy. During the Second World War several nations,

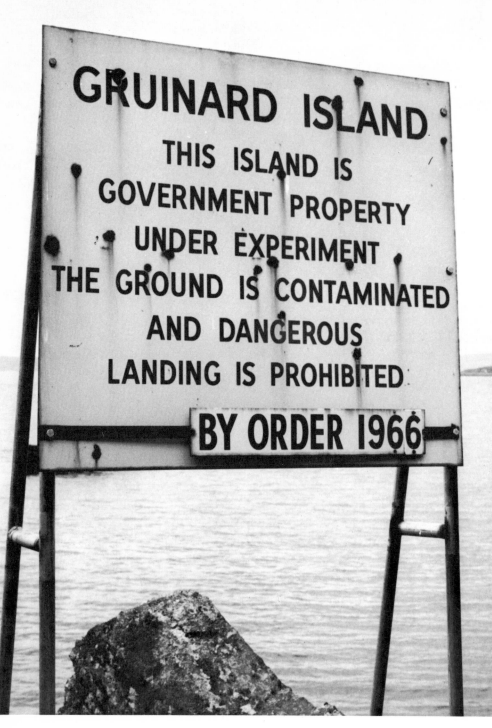

Left, Gruinard Island, used by the British for germ warfare experiments during World War II. The island, situated off Scotland's northwest coast, was sprayed with the germ anthrax, which kills most kinds of livestock and vegetation, and can cause severe fever or death in human beings.

Right, in Vietnam, U.S. military planes spray defoliant chemicals over an area of dense vegetation (September 1966). The chemicals, said to be harmless to human beings and animal life, destroy foliage that may be shielding enemy troops.

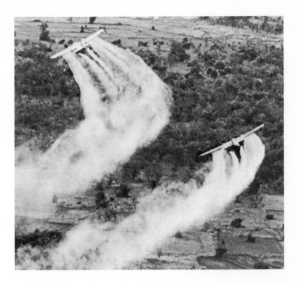

including America, Great Britain, and Canada, carried out experiments in biological warfare without having recourse to such weapons in practice. There have been persistent allegations, however, that the Japanese not only experimented on their own nationals but also actually employed bacteriological weapons. Twelve Japanese, among them the commander in chief of the Kwantung Army, were charged in 1949 at Khabarovsk in Soviet Russia with disseminating plague in China and with using Chinese and Russian prisoners for their preliminary experiments. Japanese pilots are also said to have sprayed cholera, typhoid, and paratyphoid organisms prepared in their biological warfare factory near Harbin, Manchuria. According to the *New York Times* of July 16, 1955, a Japanese writer, Horisha Akiyama, was an eyewitness to Japanese germ warfare experiments that resulted in roughly 2000 human guinea pig casualties.

Documented charges of using germ warfare in the Korean war have also been directed against the Americans by an international scientific commission. These allegations have been denied by the American authorities. The report of the commission, which followed on investigations and epidemiological studies in North Korea and China between June 23 and August 31, 1952, was signed by scientists from Brazil, Britain, France, Italy, Soviet Russia, and Sweden. The commission reported large numbers of plague-infected rodents previously unknown in that area, contaminated clams found close to reservoirs in rural parts of the country, and so on—as well as actual outbreaks of plague, anthrax, and cholera, said to have resulted from the dropping of different containers from American aircraft.

What of the doctors who engage in the experimental work necessary to produce biological weapons? How can they reconcile the principles of medical ethics with such research? It would appear that some have no conflict of conscience, but others have had second thoughts on their moral responsibility. Dr. Theodor Rosebury, for example, who now has a post in the Department of Bacteriology at the Washington University in St. Louis, Missouri, writes admonitory and well-argued articles on medical ethics and biological warfare. At one time Dr. Rosebury worked at the notorious Camp Detrick in Maryland, where "secret work" proceeded during the Second World War. (Camp Detrick is now called Fort Detrick, and similar installations exist in Canada and Britain.) Dr. Rosebury writes:

"Twenty years ago I was in full agreement with a group of physicians and others on the need for BW [bacteriological warfare] research and development in the United States. I reported for work at Camp Detrick in December, 1943, a few months after the installation had been started and just as medical personnel there were beginning to number more than a handful. There was much quiet but searching discussion among us regarding the place of doctors in such work. Most of us were civilians who chose freely to go and work there. Detrick at that time was the kind of technical post in which civilians, in or out of uniform, made all the important decisions; the professional military kept respectfully out of our way. We resolved the ethical question just as other equally good men resolved the same question at Oak Ridge and Hanford and Chicago and Los Alamos. We were in a crisis that was expected to pass in a limited time, with a return to normal values. At Detrick a certain delicacy concentrated most of the physicians into principally or primarily defensive operations—*principally* or *primarily*: the modifiers are needed because military operations can never be exclusively defensive. The point is not extenuating. If extenuation is possible, and I think it is, it depends on the factor of time. We were fighting a fire, and it seemed necessary to risk getting dirty as well as burnt."

In fact I do not think extenuation is possible under any circumstances. The oath of Hippocrates becomes meaningless if medical ethics, with regard to chemical-biological-radiological weapons, becomes diluted with "ifs" and "buts." Unequivocally the doctor must take an absolute, purist attitude on this issue. The issues may be complex but the spirit of medical ethics is simple.

Another grave ethical problem involves the right of police or military personnel, with or without the aid of doctors, to interrogate prisoners under the influence of psychochemicals, which remove inhibitions and promote verbal release. Those who are "drunk" with such drugs, it is commonly thought, sometimes reveal more than they intend. Sobriety disguises the man. It was this kind of thinking that prompted Dr. Robert House in 1922 to question two suspected criminals at Dallas County Jail, Texas, after they had been drugged with scopolamine. His investigations led him to declare that those under the power of scopolamine could not "create a lie." From that time the idea of a truth drug became part of the dark side of 20th-century materia medica. Soon, though, scopolamine was discredited as a truth drug. It failed to produce the desired result and also, on occasions, led to alarming toxic effects. Since 1922 newer drugs have been administered for the same shabby purpose; but psychiatrists know that sedated patients sometimes confess (because of unconscious guilt) to crimes they have never committed in reality. Moreover, experiments conducted at Yale University on volunteers who had lied about certain embarrassing episodes in their past, proved the unreliability of interrogation under truth drugs. Cross-examined stringently, after being given sodium amytal, the majority adhered to their earlier fabrications; others merely substituted one lie for another. Even assuming that some subjects confessed the truth, the investigator would be hard pressed to assess the validity of that confession. Efficacious or not, there is no question that truth drugs have been used for criminal, political, and military investigations in different parts of the world.

Clearly the ethical problems of doctors today extend far beyond the old physician-patient relationship. Provided doctors remind themselves that medicine is an international, not a national, discipline, and that humanity does not mean American humanity or Russian humanity, white humanity or black humanity, healthy humanity or infirm humanity, their guiding lines are clear. More difficult is the problem of ethical experimentation in man, where a new drug is given with the patient's consent during its early clinical trials.

Sooner or later a new drug discovered in the laboratories has to be tried out on a human being. Such drugs are first administered to laboratory animals, but animal tests are not always relevant: an animal cannot explain that drug X has made his ears ring, that drug Y gave him a headache, that drug Z induced sensations of nausea and acute doom. Again, drugs may cause no side effects in an animal but may be toxic for man. It has also been argued that a number of valuable drugs discovered in the past, because they are highly toxic for animals, would not have even reached clinical trials. For example, quinine might well have been dismissed as a drug too dangerous to administer to man, because dogs are inordinately sensitive to it. A number of pharmaceutical research workers suggest that miracle drugs

141

may have been discarded simply because they were never given to human beings. Such a hypothesis cannot be argued against or validated, but one knows that a drug that shows activity in a laboratory animal will also, almost certainly, have some activity on a human being. Animal testing remains a valuable, though unreliable, safeguard.

I have little sympathy with antivivisectionists, but no doubt *unnecessary* experiments are performed on animals. This is lamentable; even more so is the fact that unnecessary experiments are also being carried out on human beings—not by doctors coerced by perverted powers, but by those who are simply obsessed by the spirit of abstract, scientific inquiry. The late Pope Pius XII, who read a report of an experiment in which artificial delirium was produced in 30 healthy subjects and 24 mental patients, was stirred to ask: "Did these 54 give their consent to the experiment, and did they do so in a manner sufficient and valid for natural law? It is the observance of the moral order which gives a value and dignity to human action and which preserves a person's rectitude and keeps him in the place due to him in the whole of creation, that is, with regard to material beings, other people, and God." One does not have to be religious to go along with such sentiments.

Following a human guinea pig experiment in 1965 at Brooklyn, New York, angry exchanges occurred between doctors. Highly qualified medical specialists had injected live cancer cells into debilitated patients without their consent or knowledge. When live cancer cells are injected into a healthy human being the body will expel them as it would any foreign transplant. The researchers wished to know whether a human body, debilitated by chronic disease (other than cancer), would also reject foreign cancer cells. Laudably, the research doctors, one of whom is an expert on cancer and virology and a consultant to the United States Public Health Service, were interested in discovering a means to immunize patients against cancer. The patients injected with the live cancer cells, who naturally would not have agreed to such a maneuver, assumed the injections to be part of the treatment they needed. On hearing of this experiment, three doctors in the same hospital resigned from the staff in protest and an investigation followed. The research doctors were found guilty of unethical conduct and the investigatory committee recommended that their medical licenses be suspended.

The Harvard doctor Henry Beecher, writing in *The New England Journal of Medicine* (June 16, 1966), revealed further abuses of clinical medical experimentation. He told how 11 children had their thymus glands removed while undergoing surgery for congenital heart disease. The thymectomies were proposed as part of a long-range study of "the

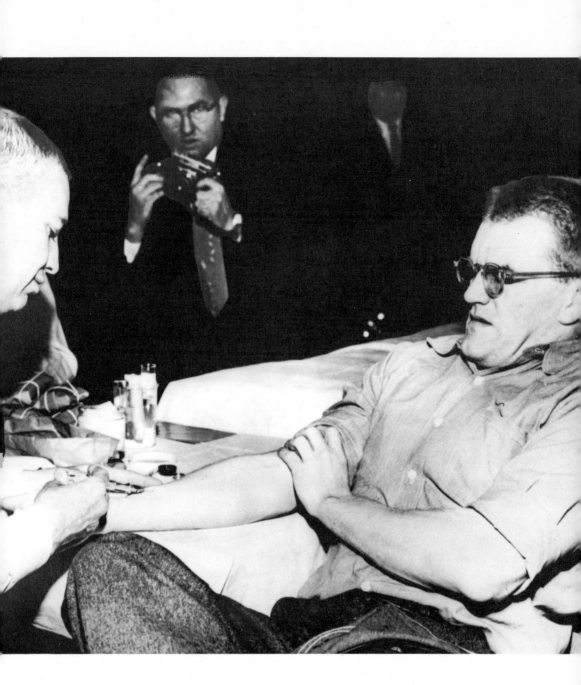

At Ohio State Penitentiary, a prisoner-volunteer is given a cancer cell injection by a doctor. Various aspects of medical research have been undertaken by teams of doctors working with volunteers in American prisons. For the prisoners, the incentive is the hope of either a pardon or a reduced sentence.

growth and development of these children over the years." Dr. Beecher also gave many other documented examples of dubious experimental procedures. Thus in one study, 157 charity patients suffering from typhoid fever were denied chloramphenicol, which can be a lifesaving drug for this disease. Of these 157, as many as 36 died. It is probable that 23 of the 36 unfortunates would have lived if the drug had not been withheld.

Not all such "pure" experiments come to light. In the great teaching hospitals some avant-garde doctors allow their scientific enthusiasm to outrun ethical considerations. A prominent physician of St. Bartholomew's Hospital, London, has pronounced: "The sticking of needles and catheters in patients in guise of treatment when what was done was really in search of knowledge, seems to me to be very near common assault;" and Sir Heneage Ogilvie, consultant at another London teaching hospital (Guy's), writes: "What is new in medicine is research by fraud. The performance on patients who have come to us in good faith for the cure of their ailments of any number of tests and investigations, many of them unpleasant, some of them dangerous, all of them unnecessary for the diagnosis or treatment of their ailment. . . ."

A great deal of disquiet exists, then, and some physicians, like the Harley Street doctor M. H. Pappworth, have made a point of airing publicly human guinea pig experiments in London teaching hospitals. In the British periodical *The Twentieth Century* he pointed out that insulin had been deliberately withheld from diabetics so that they lapsed into coma. He also records several other examples of human experiments that he has discovered through his reading of the medical journals of the last 20 years. Here I shall quote just one of the experiments he cites:

"A professor of a London teaching hospital has described how 66 patients with liver disease, who had previously experienced many unpleasant investigations including liver punctures, were submitted to the following procedures simultaneously:

"(1) A large catheter was passed into the main arm vein and so into the main chest vein and thus into the heart. This procedure is known as cardiac catheterization. But in this experiment the catheter was passed right through the heart and so into the principal vein draining the liver, thus enabling blood samples to be taken directly from the liver.

"(2) With the first catheter still *in situ* another was passed through the main vein of the thigh, and so into the chief abdominal vein, then into the kidney vein, so that blood samples could be obtained directly from the kidney.

"(3) The patients were then given large doses of ammonium chloride. The professor quoted papers previously published pointing out that the administration of this substance to patients with liver disease almost invariably produces profound neurological and psychological disturbances varying from a mild delirium to acute mania with frightening hallucinations, and the likely consequences were therefore known by the doctors responsible. . . .

"Did all the patients really give full consent, after honest and detailed explanation of what was to be meted out to them? Were the complications and dangers even mentioned? How many sane patients would agree to such experiments on themselves if they knew the likelihood of the development of extremely unpleasant happenings, however transient they might be? But it is recorded that half the patients had mental disturbances even prior to the experiment, due to their severe liver disease. How would these be deemed legally to have given consent? And what of one patient who was 16 and another only 8? Did their parents give full consent after full explanation?

"In addition to the 66 patients with liver disease, 33 other patients were used as controls and were submitted to the same unpleasant procedures. Did they also give full consent after full explanation, including the fact that the experiment was neither treatment nor necessary investigation?"

On British television lately, other experiments of a similar nature have been discussed on the program *Man Alive*. It seems that patients suffering from cardiac conditions were artificially put into heart failure, while others with liver ailments were fed with substances that would induce liver failure. Many doctors feel that allegations against the researchers have been exaggerated. Few will deny, however, that such unnecessary human guinea pig experiments have taken place and are taking place. Sometimes such experiments are not done primarily to gain new knowledge but rather to advance the career of the researcher. For by publishing the results, he or she becomes known as an expert in this or that sphere of medicine. The pressures to publish in medical periodicals have got quite out of hand. Candidates for particular jobs are ever more frequently invited to list their publications, so the need to experiment for publication purposes becomes increasingly imperative.

Many readers will be appalled by the clinical experiments related above. Yet some of them may already have taken part unwittingly in a drug experiment. Many adults, at one time or another, have been prescribed a new drug. They have assumed it to be safe. They know that it has first been tried out on laboratory animals, and that no untoward effects have been reported following the usual clinical trials. Although exhaustive precautions have been taken, confidence cannot always be justified, however. From time to time national medical catastrophes occur. The Salk polio vaccine, when first introduced in the U.S.A., was a case in point. The thalidomide disaster was another.

By 1960 thalidomide, under the trade name of Contergan, had become the favorite sleeping tablet of West Germany. It could even be bought over the counter without a prescription. It had been combined with aspirin and other well-known remedies so that it could be taken for nervousness, headaches, coughs, and colds. It was given by doctors to many patients, including pregnant women who were not sleeping well. Why not? The animal tests had been performed on mice, rats, guinea pigs, rabbits, etc., and the clinical trials had been most reassuring. The experimental stage of thalidomide was then for practical purposes over, since the pharmaceutical company responsible for manufacturing the sedative was sure of its safety.

For four years the company marketed thalidomide in West Germany and the results confirmed their confidence in the drug. Indeed, a number of adults and children, either purposely or inadvertently, had taken overdoses of the drug, sometimes large overdoses. The suicide attempts were unsuccessful: the accidental overdoses led to some children sleeping for 16 hours, but they recovered uneventfully. Thalidomide appeared to have a very low toxicity.

Then in 1960 a new clinical syndrome appeared, the outstanding feature of which was phocomelia (seal extremities): in other words, newborn children exhibited arms so short that their hands began almost directly from their shoulders. To a lesser degree, their legs showed defects of growth. There were other congenital malformations also. Phocomelia is rare, so rare that the majority of doctors never see a case during a lifetime of practice; but by the end of 1961 an epidemic of phocomelia had occurred in West Germany.

Soon it was realized that the infants with seal limbs had been born to mothers who in early pregnancy had taken thalidomide under the trade name of Contergan. In West Germany alone 5900 luckless thalidomide babies were born. In Japan also, where thalidomide had been freely dispensed, some 700 cases were reported by May 1962; in Britain 430. Throughout the world, in fact, wherever thalidomide had been marketed under different trade names by different pharmaceutical companies, limbless and deformed children were born to be sorrowed over.

The question arises whether the thalidomide disaster would have been averted if the drug had first been tested on *pregnant* laboratory

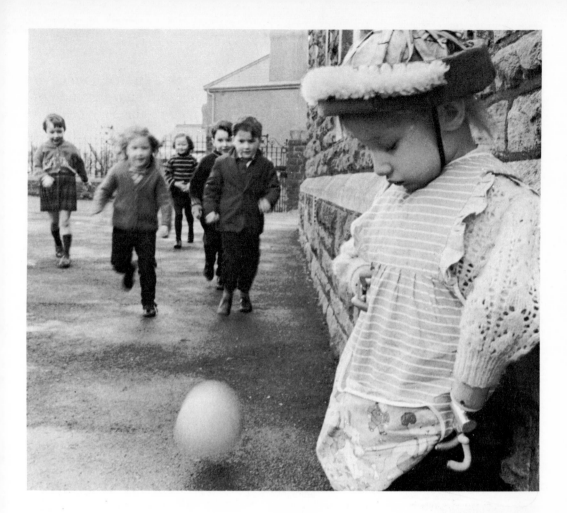

The thalidomide children will always be handicapped, though intensive efforts are made to help them lead as normal lives as possible. Highly complex artificial limbs are produced by skilled craftsmen working in what is virtually a new industry (right). These limbs, made individually to measure, have to be adjusted and re-fitted as the child grows.

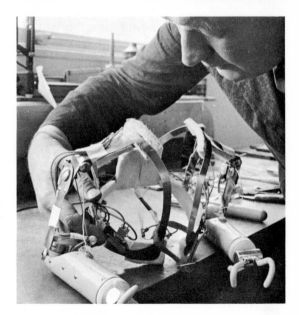

animals. Various scientists have made post hoc tests on thalidomide in this way. Investigations on such animals as mice and hamsters did not yield convincing results. With other species, though—the New Zealand white rabbit, for example—specific doses of thalidomide, administered during a definite period in pregnancy, led to limb deformities in the newborn offspring similar to those seen in human babies. Clearly, a broader scope of drug testing in animals is necessary. No thought had been given, until the thalidomide tragedy, to testing new drugs on pregnant animals for their possible effect on the human embryo. That it had not would seem to most people startling and alarming.

The fact remains that, despite animal tests and human clinical trials, no new drug released for general consumption is absolutely safe. Representatives of the pharmaceutical companies know that the experimental stage of a new drug is by no means always concluded with animal tests and clinical trials. They are aware that general use will often reveal new information about a drug. It is essential that the public be aware of this. It is all very well to administer new drugs that seem to be efficacious, and for which there is no real alternative, to those who suffer from a serious illness. Often, however, drugs are marketed when very reasonable alternatives already exist, and which, in any case, are intended to alleviate only minor ailments. The introduction of such drugs may bring large profits to a pharmaceutical company before a drug becomes discredited. The glossy propaganda the manufacturer directs toward the general physician may lull his critical sense—but the process may yet lead to another thalidomide-type disaster.

It seems to me that one of the biggest experimental surveys now taking place involves the new oral progestin-estrogin contraceptives. Despite reassurances regarding its safety, the final word on "the pill" has yet to be said. Meanwhile millions of women of different nationalities are acting as human guinea pigs in a very real sense. There are, after all, alternative methods of contraception, although it must be admitted that none seems quite as effective and certainly none as aesthetically advantageous as the pill; also, in some countries—including Latin America, Puerto Rico, Ceylon, and Pakistan—relatively few people seem willing to depend on more traditional methods of contraception. The choice in these and other countries, then, cannot be considered a real one. In Western societies, however, there are definite alternatives for most people and a cautious physician would not yet advocate the oral pill.

Many doctors of high integrity may well disagree with this contention, though they are aware that the oral contraceptives produce side effects in many women—among them nausea, breast tenderness (which may interfere with precoital sexual play), increased appetite, weight changes, abdominal cramps, and depression. These side effects, they would justly point out, are usually temporary, and if the subject persists with the pill such symptoms tend to vanish. More alarming are other complications such as liver damage and jaundice, and thrombotic episodes. Even here, it would be argued, there is no hard evidence that such serious complications are directly the result of the contraceptive steroids. Doctors who recommend the pill know there has been widespread concern as to whether the oral contraceptives predisposed some women to thrombophlebitis and pulmonary embolism; but they have been reassured by the conclusion of a committee of nine experts, appointed by the Food and Drug Administration in the U.S.A. to investigate thrombosis, that there is no evidence of any significant increase in this condition among women taking the pill.

This committee worked on retrospective evidence rather than projective studies, which are much more valuable. Indeed the committee itself recommended that critical projective trials should be undertaken. In Britain too, a survey is at present being undertaken by a committee under Sir Derrick Dunlop, which will report eventually on any association between thrombosis and oral contraceptives. It would seem to me that, until this study is concluded, the oral steroids, from this point of view alone, cannot be fully vindicated. As Dr. Alfred Byrne has written in the *Sunday Times*: "Though it may sound harsh to say so, the eleven tablets now on sale will remain on the market during the two or three years taken by the study, for the only satisfactory way to reach valid conclusions is by experience." If Dr. Byrne had wished to be harsher he would have written, "by the experience of human guinea pig experiments."

In any case the question whether or not the oral contraceptives are also carcinogenic is still open, for a carcinogenic effect may not be revealed for as long as 20 years. True, the results so far are highly reassuring: in San Juan, Puerto Rico, none of the 913 women who have been taking the contraceptive steroids for up to 10 years has developed a cancer of any organ of the reproductive tract or of the breasts. Again, massive doses of estrogens given to rhesus monkeys continuously for seven years did not provoke any cancerous change in any organ. Indeed, some authorities would suggest that estrogen and progestogen *prevent* breast and genital cancer to some degree. The fact remains that if estrogen is administered to particular strains of mice continuously for longer than one year, 50 per cent develop cervical cancers.

Let us hope that the oral contraceptives will be proved harmless. Their advantages are particularly pertinent to a world faced with a

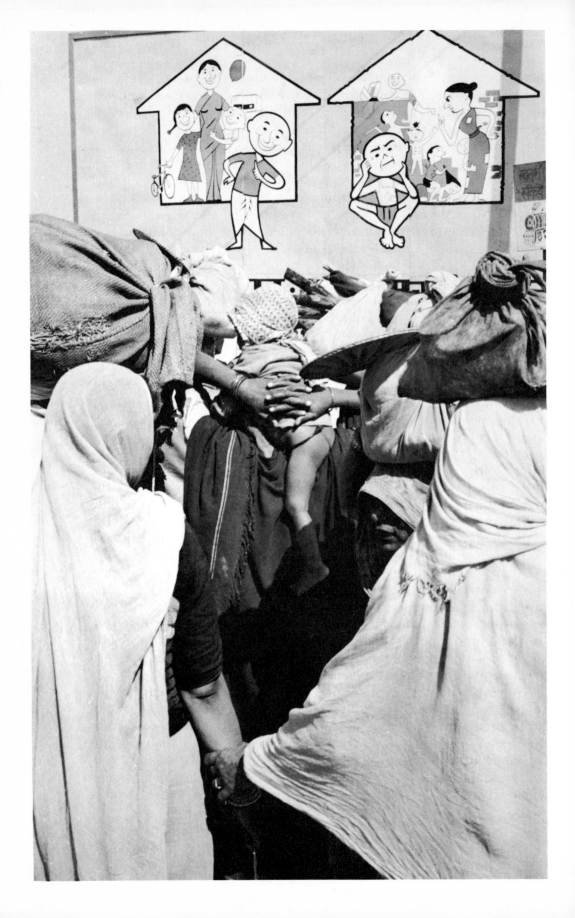

population explosion. In Mexico and Brazil alone, the total population at the present rate of growth will be doubled within 23 years. As Dr. A. C. Crooke, the well-known British endocrinologist, has written in *The Practitioner*: "The advent of a satisfactory method of birth control for the community at large may prove to be one of the greatest discoveries of the century. The accelerating growth of the population, due largely to advances in hygiene and medical science, can only lead to disaster unless some kind of control is accepted by mankind."

The family doctor cannot, however, consider the problem of population explosion when advising his individual patients. Ethically he is responsible for the safety and well-being of the individual under his care, and his guiding light must be: "Do unto others as you would have done unto yourself." Consent to partaking in a human guinea pig experiment is meaningless if the patient is not totally aware of all the dangers involved; nor can consent exist if the patient is unaware that an experiment is taking place. However encouraging the results of the experiment so far, final conclusions cannot be given for another decade yet.

That patients and doctors alike need to be fully aware of the dangers, as well as the advantages, of so many postwar drugs becomes increasingly apparent. Since a "safe" antibiotic like penicillin can cause some 300 fatalities in the U.S.A. alone each year, perhaps it will not surprise some that (according to Dr. Alfred Byrne) as many as "ten per cent to fifteen per cent of illnesses treated in hospitals" are a consequence of doctors and the drugs they have prescribed. But this figure astonishes me. It is recognized that all kinds of miracle drugs, with the passing of years, are found to produce side effects that earlier experiments had not revealed. Chloramphenicol (Parke, Davis called

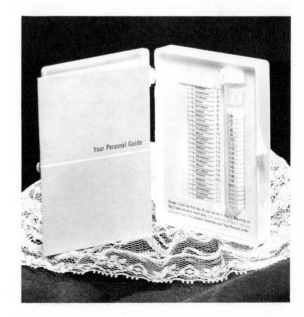

Poster cartoons are used in India (left) to emphasize the need for family planning. In November 1966, the Indian government, faced by severe famine, finally sanctioned the general prescription of contraceptive pills. In the West, attractive, clearly-marked plastic cases (right) help to create public confidence and promote sales.

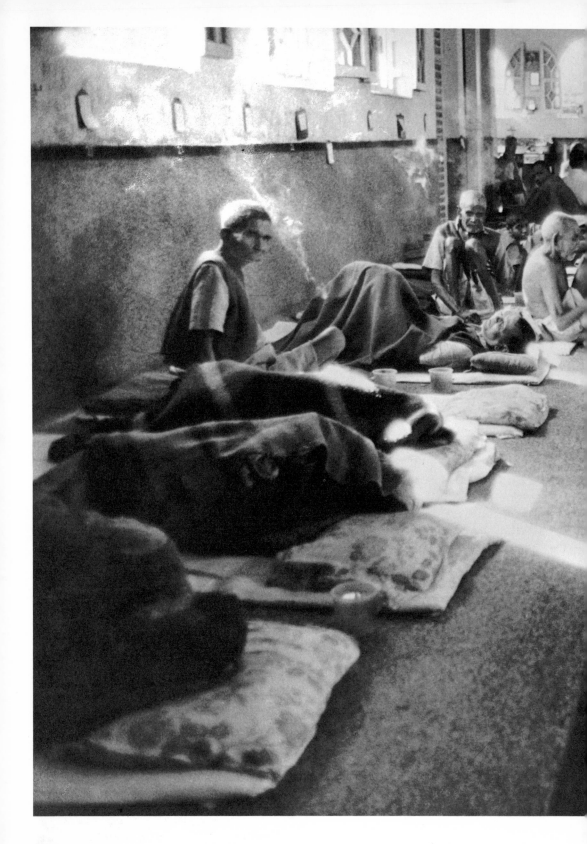

The Death House in Calcutta, where the starving homeless are brought to die. When overpopulation makes such tragedy commonplace, the medical risks associated with the contraceptive pill may well be considered justifiable.

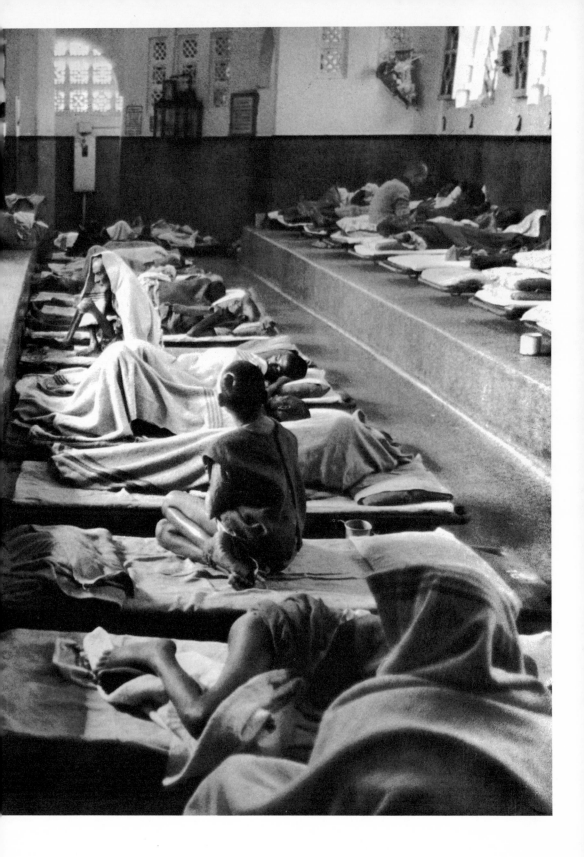

the drug Chloromycetin) is a good example. All over the world it was welcomed as a most valuable broad-spectrum antibiotic. The Kefauver Committee reported that in the U.S.A. "it enjoys a greater sales volume than any other single trade-name ethical drug." It was used for serious and minor respiratory infections, serious and minor gastro-intestinal infections, serious and minor urinary infections, eye and ear infections, and so on. No wonder Parke, Davis sold some $86 million worth of Chloromycetin in 1960. Yet by then the dangers of the drug were known. As far back as 1952 it had been reported in the U.S.A. that grave blood disorders had been associated with Chloromycetin. In that year too the *British Medical Journal* reported that patients had died of aplastic anemia as a result of the drug and warned doctors against its indiscriminate use. They pointed out that "the only absolute and imperative indication for its use is typhoid fever."

The public may well ask whether tests on drugs by the pharmaceutical companies extend over a long enough period to establish the range of their usefulness and their toxicity. If the answer is in the negative then all of us taking such drugs are inadvertently participating in a human guinea pig experiment. Dr. William Bean of the Iowa State University has said: "The richest earnings occur when a new variety or variation of a drug is marketed before competing drugs can be discovered, improvised, named, and released. This bonanza time may last only a few months. Unless there are large earnings, the quick kill with the quick pill, the investment does not pay off. Commercial secrets must be kept dark, lest a competitor gets the jump. Under this system it is impracticable to do tests extending over a long period of months or years to establish the range of usefulness and potential dangers from toxicity. Such tests usually have to be done in hospitals and often in medical schools, where secrecy in science cannot be tolerated. Thus, after extensive laboratory tests on toxicity and pharmacological properties, but sometimes with a minimum of clinical trial, a drug may be marketed."

It seems that the ethical position not only of the doctor but also of the pharmaceutical companies needs redefining. The relationship between the profit motive of such firms and the dispensation of drugs to all and sundry needs closer examination; but this I must leave to another chapter.

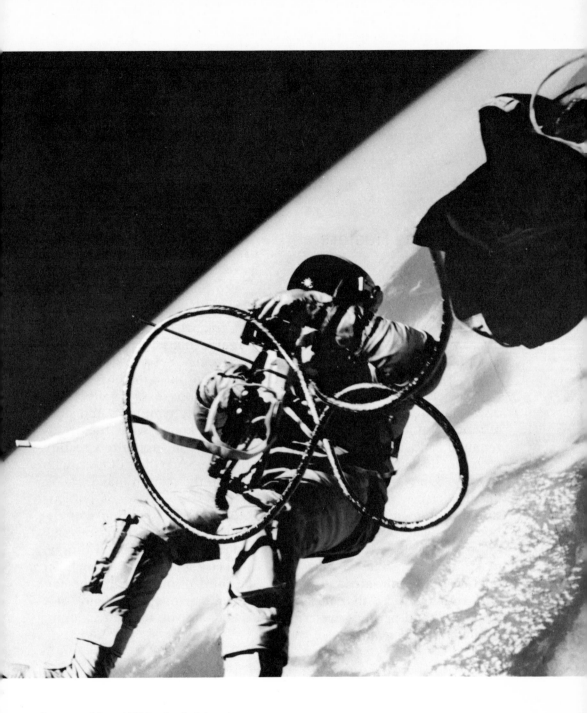

Astronaut Edward White, the first American
to maneuver outside his capsule in space—
a "guinea pig" in both the purely medical
and the wider scientific senses. (White
was killed during a launching-pad test
at Cape Kennedy in January 1967.)

# 5 The Fringe Healers

About one patient in every three seeking advice and treatment from a doctor in an urban practice suffers from a functional or stress disorder. That is to say, he has no organic illness. His symptoms, though, may be distressing and even alarming. Yet the doctor consulted is generally not trained to deal with them. As a medical student the physician will have learned about the diagnosis of, say, gallbladder disease or tuberculosis of the lung. He knows the symptoms and signs of innumerable concrete, clinical entities. He knows what therapy is required, and he knows the prognosis. He would agree too readily with the distinguished British surgeon the late Sir William Osler, who taught: "One finger in the throat and one in the rectum make a good diagnostician." But when it comes to this large group of patients suffering from nonorganic symptoms, the ancient Egyptian conception of a healer may be more to the point: "He who treats the sick must be expert, learned in the proper incantations, and know how to make amulets." The average modern doctor may scoff at such an opinion but, confronted by at least one third of his patients, he can only reassure them that nothing is basically wrong, tell them "not to worry," and perhaps prescribe a placebo, an iron tonic, a vitamin, or some kind of sedative.

A 12th-century miniature shows the Calaarius, the prophetic white bird that (according to medieval legend) visited the sick. It was believed that if the bird looked at the patient, he would recover; and that if it looked away, the patient would die. The sick have always been susceptible to primitive concepts of healing—and still are.

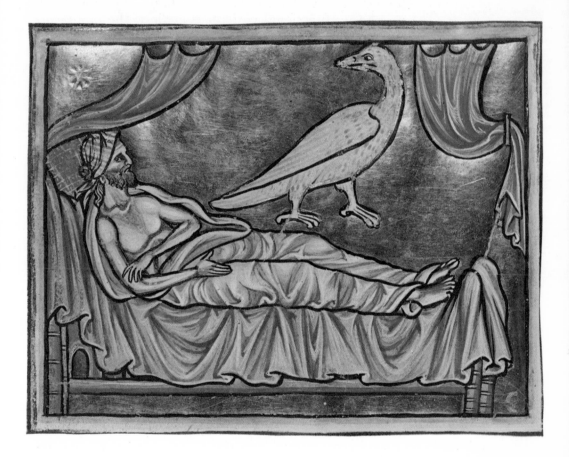

The nature of the symptoms expressed in stress disorders was recently cataloged in *The Practitioner* by a group of British doctors in general practice. One of them, Dr. David Hart, outlined the following main stress symptoms for which his patients sought advice: lassitude, blinking, nausea, headache, heartburn and lump in the throat, palpitation, precordial pain, bad heads and hot flushes, abdominal discomfort, indigestion, dysmenorrhea, sense of suffocation, amenorrhea, anorexia, inability to draw a deep breath.

Other doctors would add to this catalog indefinitely: backache, biliousness, blotches on the skin, fibrositis, insomnia, etc. The list is endless. The number of functional patients is endless; the number of good, honest doctors confounded by such symptoms endless.

It is not always practical or possible for the doctor to refer such patients to psychiatrists—because of the worldwide shortage of psychiatrists, and because the cost of psychiatric treatment can be prohibitive. Besides, the average doctor everywhere, like the average patient, is prejudiced against psychological methods of treatment for apparent somatic symptoms. Plato's remark that "the great error of our day is that physicians separate the soul from the body" still holds.

So, inevitably, more and more people, failed as they are by the medical profession, still suffering despite the iron tonic, the vitamin, and the sedative, grasp at any straw, take cognizance of advertisements for this or that brand of proprietary pill and hopefully engage in self-diagnosis and self-medication. Certainly the vendors of proprietary medicines flourish; and even old wives' tales still work, on occasions, their potent magic. It has been said that "doctors drop drugs of which they know little into stomachs of which they know less." In which case, why shouldn't the owner of the stomach follow his own hunch?

True, from time to time orthodox bodies publish and broadcast their admonitory advice. In 1909 for instance, the British Medical Association published an exposé of the innumerable, secret proprietary remedies, revealing what they cost to manufacture, and analyzing their content. The B.M.A. report, *Secret Remedies*, concluded wistfully: "It is not, however, only the poorer classes of the community who have a weakness for secret remedies and the ministration of quacks; the well-to-do and the highly placed will often, when not very ill, take a curious pleasure in experimenting with mysterious compounds."

Among the proprietary medicines then analyzed by the B.M.A. were the famous Beecham's Pills, which used to be advertised as "worth a guinea a box" though a box sold for only one shilling and three-halfpence (about 14 cents). The B.M.A. pointed out that the prime cost of the pills in this box was only half a farthing (the equivalent of about a tenth of a cent).

Many will remember the circular wrapper around the Beecham's box, which stated that "these renowned . . . pills cure Constipation, Headache, Dizziness, or Swimming in the Head, Wind, Pain, and Spasms of the Stomach, Pains in the Back, Restlessness, Insomnia, Indigestion, Want of Appetite, Fullness after Meals, Vomitings, Sickness of the Stomach, Bilious or Liver Complaints, Sick Headaches, Cold Chills, Flushing of Heat, Lowness of Spirits and all Nervous Affections, Scurvy and Scorbutic Affections, Pimples and Blotches on the Skin, Bad Legs, Ulcers, Wounds, Maladies of Indiscretion, Kidney and Urinary Disorders and Menstrual Derangements." The B.M.A. analysts showed that each pill consisted only of aloes (0·5 grains), powdered ginger (0·55 grains), and powdered soap (0·18 grains).

At least such a formula was simpler than the medicines of bygone centuries—simpler, for example, than the universal elixir prescribed by the London physician Dr. William Salmon in the 17th century, which comprised: "Rex Metallorum [gold], Powder of a Lion's heart, Filings of a Unicorn's Horn [the sea unicorn or narwhal of arctic seas], Ashes of the whole Chameleon, Bark of the Witch Hazel, Lumbrici [earthworms], Dried Man's brain, Bruise wort, and Egyptian Onions." Salmon's mixture was advertised to be taken at certain phases of the moon to open obstructions and to work as a "hypnotick" or "cardiack." Beecham's pills could be taken any time.

The phenomenon of proprietary medicines of course is not one that belongs merely to the past. This morning I counted no fewer than 13 major advertisements for proprietary medicines in one newspaper that lay on my desk. My eyes roved from ARE YOU WORN OUT WITH CATARRH—*don't delay get Mentholatum Balsam today* to JUNO JUNIPAH TABLETS! *You can't even taste them but in no time their gently corrective action means you CAN taste the joy of feeling and looking your old self again.* Wondering what Juno Junipah tablets were really for, I went on to read CONSTIPATION *worrying You?—take Brooklax chocolate laxatives*: and then my eyes escaped, only to read DOAN'S NEW BACKACHE PILLS. *At last something to soothe away the pain.* And so on to syrup, which promised to soothe irritating coughs, to get rid of the phlegm, to promote healthy sleep, and speed recovery.

The advertisements for this or that product are often accompanied by a testimonial. Thus the advertisement for *Phyllosan,* said to "fortify the over-forties," has a statement from an elderly Kent gentleman. He writes happily: "Phyllosan has kept me fit and well." *Why did [he] benefit from Phyllosan?* asks the copywriter. And he thunders the answer himself—certain, dogmatic, oozing with bright confidence: *Because [he] needed what Phyllosan could give him, essential nutrients, iron and B vitamins. These can help the body, form more red blood corpuscles, revitalise the circulation and benefit the nerve tissues. So, if you too have the same need as [he] had, start your health bringing course of Phyllosan today.*

The copywriters' technique seems similar in most of the advertisements, whatever the proprietary product—be it Vitamized Iron Jelloids or Bemax, recommended for those who are nervy, tired, and generally below par. Proprietary drugs are all *potentially* dangerous, if only because they are aimed blindly at an ignorant public. They are at best a palliative not a cure—a palliative moreover for which the public pays too high a price. As for the copywriters of proprietary advertisements, one may recall the words of the poet George Santayana who wrote: "Advertising is the modern substitute for argument: its function is to make the worse appear the better." If doctors labor to destroy the reason for their own existence, then medical copywriters, it seems, labor to destroy the reason!

There is today, both in America and in Europe, a huge proprietary drug industry. It would be even more massive in the U.S.A. without the restraints imposed on the industry by such regulating bodies as the Post Office Department, the Food and Drug Administration, and the Federal Trade Commission. Former postmaster general Arthur Summerfield pronounced that more money is being made today in this kind of fringe-medicine activity than "in any other criminal activity." According to the Arthritis and Rheumatism Foundation practically 50 per cent of the (11,000,000) American arthritic patients spend money on misrepresented drugs, and in a report of the Federal Council on Aging to President Eisenhower in 1954 it was stated that 4000 quack cancer practitioners were cashing in on this particular tragic condition.

In his book *The Toadstool Millionaires* the American author James Harvey Young discusses the economics of medical quackery in the U.S.A. He maintains that the "take" each year to promoters of specious medication exceeds a billion dollars. Of this, half a billion goes into the nutrition racket, wasted on foods and food supplements with therapeutic overtones. "Another quarter billion," James Harvey Young states, "is spent for medicines and gadgets falsely purporting to promote recovery from arthritis and rheumatism. A hundred million goes for ineffective reducing remedies, fifty million for fake cancer cures, and millions more for other panaceas that hold out the vain promise of curing ailments ranging from the common cold to heart disease."

Hippocrates warned: "Wherever a doctor cannot do good, he must be kept from doing harm." What should be true for a doctor should be true also for those commercial firms who make fortunes out of man's maladies and hypochondria. Quite obviously there should be

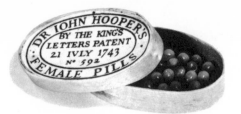

Above, Dr. John Hooper's "Female Pills,"
which (in the words of their patent)
contained "the best purging stomatick
and antihysterical ingredients." Right, a
19th-century advertisement for a popular
patent stomach medicine.

Below, the showmanship associated with
the selling of quack cures is illustrated in
an 18th-century cartoon. A mountebank
and a "minister," working in partnership at
a fair, claim between them a remedy for
all ills—of both body and soul.

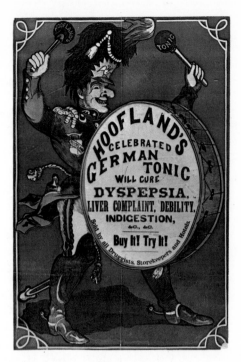

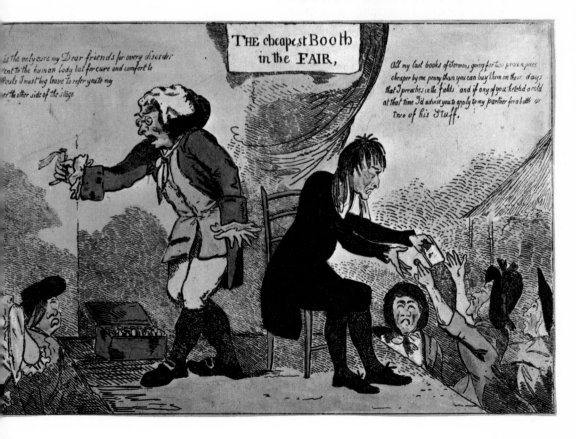

controls to check the exploitation of people who, when unwell, lose their sense of independence and tend to regress into childhood, to the time when they heard and absorbed old wives' tales such as "an apple a day keeps the doctor away," or "eat fish to make your brains grow," or "don't eat the pith of oranges for it destroys the blood."

Doctors may believe that medical science has moved away from the era of magic and of healing by incantation, by astrology, and by touch. The sicker a patient is, however, the more primitive he tends to become: hence the massive sale of patent medicines and the persistence of old wives' tales and health superstitions. Even in recent times the following charm against toothache—written on paper, then rolled up into a ball—was worn around the necks of many in the county of Ross and Cromarty in North Scotland:

> Peter and Paul sat on a marble stone
> Jesus came to them alone.
> "Peter," says he, "What makes you so quake?"
> "Why Lord and Master, it is the toothache."
> Whoever shall carry these words for my sake
> Shall never be troubled with toothache.

Apart from the economic success of the patent-medicine manufacturers and the survival of folk medicine, another concrete sign of the failure of contemporary medicine—not to mention the primitive gullibility of the public at large—is the continued existence and influence of fringe "healers." For hypnotherapy, radiesthesia, acupuncture, faith healing, osteopathy, and homeopathy still thrive.

An anecdote (first recorded in 1787 in the memoirs of Major James George Semple) concerning the 18th-century London quack, Rock, has its sad, modern relevance. "He was standing one day at his door on Ludgate Hill, when a real doctor of Physic passed, who had learning and abilities, but whose modesty was the true cause of his poverty. 'How comes it,' says he to the Quack, 'that you without education, without skill, without the least knowledge of science, are enabled to live in the style you do?—You keep your town house, your carriage and your country house: whilst I, allowed to possess some knowledge, have neither, and can hardly pick up a subsistence!' 'Why, look ye,' said Rock smiling, 'how many people do you think have passed since you asked me the question?' 'Why?' answered the Doctor, 'Perhaps a hundred.' 'And how many out of those hundred, think you, possess commonsense?' 'Possibly one,' answered the Doctor. 'Then,' said Rock, 'That one comes to you; and I take care of the other ninety-nine.' "

That the quacks of past centuries were sometimes more successful than the licensed doctor is understandable. After all, bleeding, dosing, and enemas were once, not so long ago, the main armory of orthodox practitioners. Furthermore the quacks of yesteryear advertised and exhibited a public showmanship (they still do) that most licensed practitioners eschewed. Today, the manufacturers of proprietary medicines sell their products with the help of advertising agencies. The old quacks wrote their own copy—and with much greater verve. Compare, for example, an advertisement for a modern proprietary product with the text of a leaflet by Cornelius of Tilbourne, one of the master quacks of 17th-century Britain. At the head of his handbill was a royal recommendation: SWORN CHYRUGEON TO KING CHARLES II FROM WHOSE HANDS I RECEIVED A GOLD MEDAL AND CHAIN. The text continued: *I recover and give sight to the blind. I restore sight in a moment, I cure deafness (if curable), I cure vomiting, rising of vapour, pain in the milt, stitches in the side, and all scorbutick distempers. . . .* Cornelius then went on to list his other curative powers together with the names of the nobles he had cured and the diseases they had suffered from.

As for showmanship, the 18th century—in Europe the heyday of fringe practitioners—affords many colorful examples: men like James Graham, who was among the first to exploit medico-electrical apparatus, and Anton Mesmer, father of modern hypnotherapy. It would have been instructive to visit James Graham's "Temple of Health" in Pall Mall, or Mesmer's clinic in Paris.

Graham's "Medical Institute" (the Temple of Health) was opened in 1780. It contained various electrical appliances, but the greatest attraction was his magnetico-electric bed—the so-called Celestial Bed. This was a bed, apparently, where those suffering from infertility could "infallibly produce a genial and happy issue." Graham not only maintained that his bed could cure the barren, but that it would also allow them "superior ecstasy." For those procreating on it, he averred, would enjoy prolonged orgasms that could be measured "not in moments but in hours." Here is the contemporary account of a French visitor to Graham's Temple, as quoted in Eric Jameson's *The Natural History of Quacks*:

"Scarcely has one set foot on the first step on the staircase than one hears harmonious strains of wind instruments which reach the ear through hidden openings in the staircase, while the sweetest perfumes flatter the sense of smell till the entrance of a magnificent apartment is reached. This is used for the delivery of lectures, in which the Doctor professes to abolish barrenness. Music precedes each lecture from five o'clock till seven when Dr. Graham presents himself vested in doctor's robes. On the instant there follows a silence which is

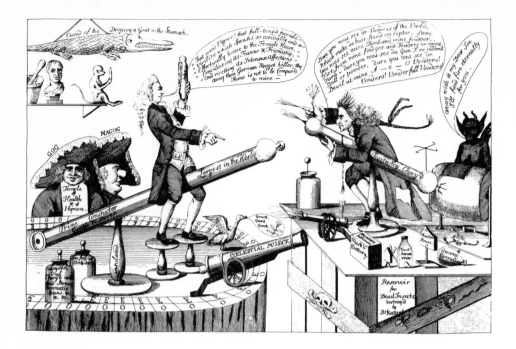

interrupted only at the end of the lecture by an electric shock, given to the whole audience by means of conductors hidden under the cushions with which all the seats are covered. . . . All these details, however, are only accessories of his establishment. The sumptuous bed in brocaded damasks is supported by four crystal pillars of spiral shape. On whatever side one gets into this bed, which is called Celestial, one hears an organ played in unison with three others which make agreeable music consisting of varied airs which carry the happy couples into the arms of Morpheus. For nearly an hour that the concert lasts one sees in the bed streams of light which play especially over the pillars. When the time for getting up has come, the magician comes to feel the pulse of the faithful, gives them breakfast, and sends them away full of hope, not forgetting to recommend them to send him other clients."

It is uncertain whether Dr. Graham ever qualified in medicine. But by all accounts he was an extraordinarily handsome man with a magnetic personality—perhaps the only qualifications he needed. At the height of his career he was charging (on his own claims) £50 ($140) for a night on the bed, though a contemporary recorded that "many a nobleman paid Graham £500 to draw the curtains."

Equally fantastic scenes were enacted in Mesmer's lavish Paris clinic in the 1780s. Here, at the Hotel Bullion in the Rue Montmartre, scores of people could be seen sitting with their feet immersed in a large wooden tub, applying magnetized iron rods and filings to themselves, many moaning piteously or breathing with a sound resembling a death rattle. In the center of this mass of people stood the Viennese

Left, two notorious 18th-century quacks (parodied in an engraving of 1783). Dr. James Graham, celebrated inventor of the "Celestial Bed" is on the left; on the right is his German rival, Katerfelto, who arrived in London in 1782.

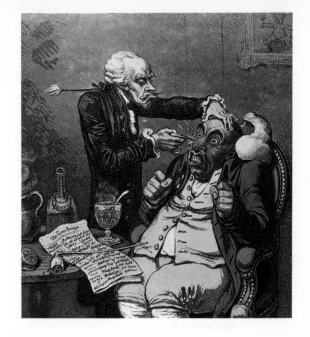

Right, James Gillray's conception of "Perkinsism," a popular form of therapy involving the use of Elisha Perkins's "metallic tractors" (patented in America in 1798). These allegedly "magical" electromagnetic rods were supposed to draw out disease at its source.

physician and showman Franz Anton Mesmer, carrying a wand, and wearing his famous purple cloak. As he darted this way and that, some beat their heads against a wall, others lay writhing on the ground. Occasionally Mesmer would stop, catch hold of a patient's hands, hold them in his while he gazed deeply into wild eyes. Then the purple-cloaked figure would touch the sick person with his wand, and a "cure" sometimes resulted.

Those panting, quivering people were not mad. They were simply in a trance. They had been "mesmerized" by Mesmer's magnetized rods—or so Mesmer claimed, for he ascribed his healing force to "animal magnetism," emanating from the stars, which he believed he had the gift to transmit. Mesmer was a trained doctor and sincere in his beliefs. But he had the fringe healer's intuitive understanding that showmanship and the awe inspired by a reputation could heighten suggestibility and aid the healing process.

Mesmer's activities aroused the anger of orthodox medical practitioners, first in his native Vienna and then in Paris. In 1778, despite some apparently striking successes with hysterics, he was hounded out of Austria. In Paris, where he then settled, he encountered the same unpopularity. He was branded an imposter and charlatan. In 1784 the Académie des Sciences appointed a distinguished commission of physicians and scientists to investigate his activities. Although the commission acknowledged many of Mesmer's cures, it ascribed the phenomenon of mesmerism to "some as yet unknown physiological causes"—not to animal magnetism. Mesmer was discredited. His popularity waned, and it was to be quite some time before any serious medical interest in the therapeutic possibilities of mesmerism or "hypnosis" was revived.

Mesmer is dead these many years and his purple cloak in rags. But he has his modern counterparts—hypnotherapists or hypnotists. These hypnotherapists know that Mesmer's theory of animal magnetism is nonsense. They do not use wands or iron rods or indulge in overt theatricality. The trance that such modern healers induce is altogether a more peaceful one. But some hypnotherapists recognize that the aura of glamor and mystery associated with hypnotism can still aid them. To obtain therapeutic successes they, like Mesmer, need to have their patients in affectionate awe of them. Many medically qualified hypnotherapists, though (and the distinction between lay and medical hypnotherapist is important), find their occupational aura of mystery and glamor irksome. Those of them who own a scientific seriousness naturally wish to dissociate themselves from a tradition of theatricality—from the old abracadabra "turn" on the music halls; from the "mystery item" that used to appear on television variety programs. Such hypnotherapists would agree with Dr. Richard Asher, who, during a lecture demonstration at a London hospital, said: "The less ritual and the more straightforward the procedure the better. The patient should not be made to feel that there is elaborate ceremony or mystery or be given the idea that the hypnotherapist has any special power over him. . . ." Dr. Asher recommended a commonplace atmosphere. The patient, he felt, should regard the procedure as no more impressive than a visit to the dentist.

In 1952 it was made illegal to practice hypnotism on the stage in Britain for entertainment purposes. In the same year the British

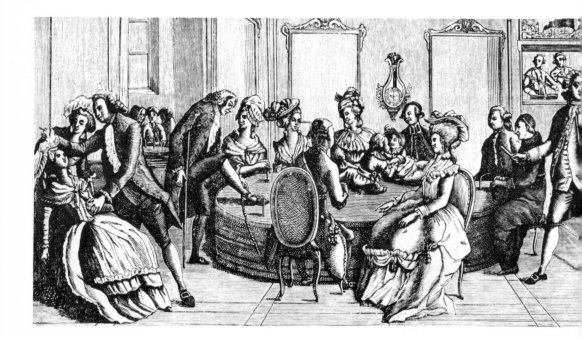

Medical Association gave hypnotism its official blessing, and the Medical and Dental Society for the Study of Hypnosis was formed, which now has over 1000 members in all branches of medicine. In 1958 the American Medical Association investigated the clinical use of hypnosis. Its report warned against the use of hypnosis for entertainment purposes but endorsed the medical use of hypnosis, urging that it be taught in medical schools. It also called for an expansion of research into medical hypnotism.

But patients—and many doctors—continue to consider hypnotism a mysterious entity: they continue to believe in their hearts that the hypnotist is a man with an unusual, if not an unearthly, gift. The ghost of Mesmer is not so easily exorcised however much the hypnotherapist may appear, or want to be, like the dentist or the man next door. Indeed the aura, along with the personality and the prestige of the hypnotherapist, plays a most important role in the result of his treatment. Hypnotherapists, like Mesmer, can list their successes in the many realms of psychosomatic illness, often dramatic ones. But hypnotherapy may be ill-advised. The symptoms may be treated but the cause of the symptoms may still remain.

To such an objection Dr. J. R. Robson, a leading London hypnotherapist, has replied: "Surely the causes of all symptoms, whether treated by drugs or hypnosis, should be investigated prior to commencement of treatment. The influence of psyche over soma is now undisputed, but how many medical men can honestly state that, in every case of insomnia, they have investigated the basic cause before dispensing barbiturates etc. . . . . The danger, if there is any danger, is just as great in direct symptom removal by drugs as by hypnosis. . . ."

Left, a contemporary engraving of *Mesmer's Tub.* Mesmer claimed that the iron hooks on the tubs conducted a beneficial force to the limbs of his patients. The power of suggestion, evident in Mesmer's dramatic "cures"—and in the photo from Tripoli (right) of a man biting into a cactus while in a trance—is the basis of modern medical hypnotic treatment.

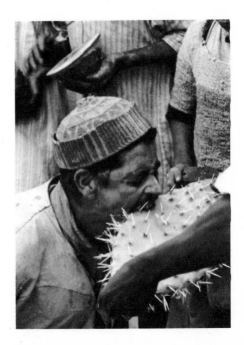

Though hypnotism and hypnotists—medically qualified or not—are regarded by the majority of orthodox doctors with suspicion and hostility, there are few psychiatrists today who would not agree that hypnotherapy can be a useful therapeutic adjunct to psychotherapy in certain carefully selected cases. The warning that Freud gave in 1903 is still very much to the point however: "Hypnosis can conceal," wrote Freud, "the resistances, and for this reason obstruct the physician's insight into the play of the psychic forces. Hypnosis does not do away with the resistances: what it does is to avoid them, and this yields only imperfect information and transitory therapeutic success."

If Anton Mesmer was the father of hypnotism he was also the forebear of those 20th-century "healers" who practice radiesthesia. For radiesthesia is a form of therapy that purports to depend on some kind of mysterious vibration or force akin in some ways, perhaps, to Mesmer's "animal magnetism." The most famous exponent of radiesthesia was Dr. Albert Abrams, who died in 1924 and whose clinic in Sacramento Street, San Francisco, was given the rather 18th-century appellation, "The House of Wonder," by American novelist Upton Sinclair.

Abrams believed, oddly, that the "blood electrons" in a healthy person vibrated at a different rate from those of a sick person; that every disease, like every drug, owned its own vibration frequency. Indeed he believed drugs influenced diseases only when they had the same vibratory rate; but drugs, he felt, had their dangers, and so he invented a machine capable of administering vibrations to a patient at the correct frequency. He called this machine (or black box) an "oscilloclast." Earlier, he had invented another machine, a "dynamizer," which he claimed could diagnose any illness. His technique was to take a sample of dried blood from the patient, and to submit it to his diagnostic machine, which then disclosed the frequency rate of the blood electrons and hey presto, the diagnosis was revealed: tuberculosis, cancer, diabetes, syphilis, or whatever.

This may sound—as it did to many at the time—a crazy, obfuscating kind of poppycock. Nevertheless there were doctors, as well as counterfeit healers, who hired Abrams's machines (at one time Abrams was making $1500 a month from rent). They reported amazing results. Furthermore, Abrams was no mere mountebank, without medical credentials. On the contrary, he had once been professor of pathology at the Cooper Medical College and at Stanford University in California. Earlier in his career he had written substantial medical textbooks, which had been well received by the medical press. As time passed, Abrams and his disciples reported more and more successes, and the popular press in both America and Britain gave him a great deal of publicity. MARVEL OR DELUSION? the headlines read, *It may be that Abrams is a quack, but more probably he is a very great discoverer.* When he died there were many who believed him to be a genius unrecognized by official medical bodies.

Such bodies, though scornful of his theories, were forced by public pressure in the U.S.A. and Great Britain to investigate his machines. In London a painstaking scientific inquiry was set up under the chairmanship of Sir Thomas (later Lord) Horder, the famous physician, whose integrity was beyond question. The committee reported its findings on January 16, 1925. Stringent tests had been conducted, and the committee by and large condemned the machines. Yet they left one loophole: "Stripped of the theatricalities, the chicanery, the quackery, with which Abrams and some of his followers invested their proceedings," Sir Thomas said, "still, nevertheless, there is something unexplained about the machines. On the other hand this finding is in no way a licence for anyone to claim that the box has any curative powers."

Sir Thomas, it seemed, only partly discredited Abrams's machines. Time completed the process. Gradually, it became evident that the dynamizer could err all too often in its diagnoses, that more and more patients were unaffected by the vibrations of Abrams's oscilloclast —and that many of those reported "cured" relapsed. There are some, however, who remain credulous whatever the evidence. Radiesthesia did not end there. Variations of Abrams's machines were developed by later fringe medical practitioners. The Food and Drug Administration in America estimated that as recently as 1954 some 5000 machines of this nature were being used by fringe healers, and in Britain today there are reported to be 1000 radiesthetists.

A discussion of radiesthesia cannot be concluded without a brief mention of Wilhelm Reich—the gifted, indeed brilliant, pupil of Sigmund Freud—who, in later life, took the fringe pathway. Reich came to believe that mind activity was a function of the life force. This in itself was no new postulate. The Hindus, for example, had their "prana," and the Polynesians their "mana." But Reich considered that the source of this life force was a substance called "orgone," blue in color and borne down from the sky by the sun itself. Not for Reich Mesmer's magnetism of the stars but the orgone in the atmosphere.

Wilhelm Reich believed that iron became magnetized when left lying in an "orgone field." To concentrate this life-giving energy (orgone) Reich, like Abrams before him, constructed boxes. These did not contain, as did Abrams's machines, primitive radio equipment.

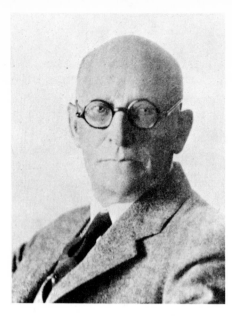

Left, Albert Abrams, the American professor of pathology who was to reject orthodox medicine and develop the practice of radiesthesia. Right, a patient is treated with the "correct" vibration frequency from a portable shortwave "oscilloclast"— a modern variant of the Abrams "black box."

On the contrary, they were simply made of a nonmetallic material and lined with alternate layers of steel wool and glass wool. Reich maintained that his large boxes—large enough to contain a man— drew orgone from the atmosphere, and that once in the box this could transmit its potent health-giving energy. Absurd as this may sound, the power of Reich's personality was such that he convinced many intelligent people that his theories were right, and he did seem to obtain some remarkable results. His co-workers and disciples were often scientifically trained and yet they appear to have been completely dominated by him.

Many odd experiments were carried out by Reich and his assistants. One was outlined by H. W. Heason, in *Frontiers of Understanding*:

"After much careful thought and many preliminary investigations, he [Reich] began a series of experiments in which small quantities of radio-active material were brought into contact with accumulations of this orgone energy. As they proceeded it became apparent that some deadly force was being generated which affected himself and his assistants in a manner similar to radiation sickness. Finally, on the 12th January, 1951, came a climax. A small quantity of radium was placed inside a small box accumulator, which in turn was situated inside the specially constructed laboratory, about 100 yards away. Through the windows of the laboratory they could see the atmosphere become clouded and then a blue luminosity appeared. As they watched, even outside the laboratory the symptoms of sickness began to be felt. Only half an hour had elapsed, but they felt that the experiment must be stopped at once. The radium was immediately removed from the laboratory, but still the effects persisted and *increased*. It seemed that a

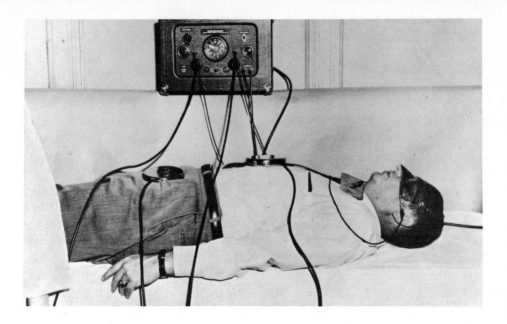

form of 'chain reaction' had been started, and the deadly force continued to spread. Reich's wife and child had to be evacuated from the nearby dwelling house.

"After reaching a peak, the disastrous effects subsided. But for a long time it was impossible to enter the laboratory for more than a few minutes at a time. On February 11th, a month after this crucial experiment, one of Reich's co-workers, a lady doctor, while in the laboratory, had reason to open the door of an old box accumulator, which was being used as a cupboard in which to store glassware. It had not been opened since the time of the experiment. Curious, after removing the glassware, she placed her head in the chamber in order to test for any possible reaction. 'I suddenly felt as if I had been hit with a sledge-hammer,' she remarked afterwards. A violent illness attacked her, with livid discolourations around the mouth and chin and eyes inflamed. So much so that it was only with difficulty that she was kept alive during the first crucial two hours.

"Reich thereon ordered the entire dismantling of the laboratory and all the boxes. Yet for weeks afterwards the effect remained, a strange deadly force that permeated the whole atmosphere in the vicinity.

"From the many tests made by Reich, which are explained in detail in his various books, it would seem that the destructive capacity of radio-active forces coming into contact with the life-giving energy of orgone, sets up a stress, which, while being deleterious to life, is, as it were, a battle of life and death. It is as if two fundamental cosmic forces are at war, and any living things wandering into the centre of the battle, are harmed by the naked strength of the cosmic powers."

Reich had built innumerable orgone accumulators, and other "healers" could hire them. The Federal Food and Drug Administration in the U.S.A. not unnaturally believed that orgone did not exist, and that Reich's boxes were a hoax, and the police eventually seized his books and took over his laboratory. Reich died in prison; but there are still those who believe him to have been a genius, misunderstood and victimized.

One final word about Abrams and Reich. The skeptical will think of them as out-and-out charlatans. If I might venture a personal and of course fallible opinion, I would say that this view is too simple, and indeed wrong. Both Abrams and Reich were brilliant men, but both men, I think, went "mad." Consider for a moment some remarks Abrams made before he died. "The noise of a laugh is masculine," he affirmed seriously, "whereas the sound of a soda water syphon is feminine." He asserted that his machine could register "the scream of a flower when it is torn in half." We may be reminded of the sensitive man's feeling for plants, or the poet's anthropomorphizing of inert objects—of the German poet Rainer Maria Rilke, for instance, who would only with reluctance leave a "lonely" piece of soap in an abandoned hotel room; but these and other bizarre remarks of Abrams go further and would seem to belong within the walls of a mental institution rather than in a scientific laboratory. Moreover, during the last years of his life, Abrams gave all the money he had earned from consultations and all the profits that had accrued from the sale of his boxes to an institution where his method of treatment could be given to the poor and where further research into his brand of radiesthesia could be carried out. Surely a man who, in the 20th century, makes an idol of wires and senseless electrical apparatus and then believes that electrical idol to be all powerful could be termed insane? Many have been certified for less.

As for Wilhelm Reich, there is no doubt that toward the end of his life he developed distinct paranoid tendencies and believed he was being persecuted by communist agents. Obviously genius is no guarantee against insanity. On the other hand, because of their very fanaticism the mad can convince many, can indeed sometimes cure the sane who appear sick in body, can pass on their message to those more than willing, because of their circumstances and personality, to believe in an insane, primitive concept.

Primitive, nonscientific forms of healing will attract those who are sick and who cannot be healed by orthodox doctors committed to scientific methods of treatment. The fringe healer hears over and over the tale of the patient who relates: "Doctors say they cannot do anything for me." Hence the present popularity of acupuncture and faith healing, which are exploited even more than hypnotherapy and radiesthesia—and what after all could be more unscientific than these two forms of treatment?

Acupuncture was first practiced in ancient China. Indeed, a book called *Nei Tsing*, written 2100 years ago and passed down from father to son through the centuries, is said to have recorded 3000 years of acupuncture practice. The Chinese believed that energy flowed in the body along 12 meridians: to the heart, to the liver, to the lungs, and to the other organs of the body. A too feeble flow of energy to the heart, they considered, caused a disorder of the heart; a too feeble flow to the liver, an ailment of the liver; and so on. But they were convinced that by pricking the skin with golden or silver needles at one of some 800 points—according to the meridian, and which organ was disordered—the correct quantity of energy flowing to one or another organ could be restored, and the patient returned to health.

This "magical" theory is of course absurd in the light of modern anatomical knowledge. It has no more validity than the countless other views of health and disease held by healers of other ancient civilizations. But whereas, say, specific Babylonian methods of medical treatment are no longer perpetuated, this does not hold true for acupuncture. In the Far East, and in modern China itself, acupuncture is still widely practiced. A Chinese medical journal printed, in 1959, a report on 46 patients with acute appendicitis who were treated by acupuncture at a Canton medical school. All, it was claimed, recovered without any need of surgical intervention. It is not possible to verify the diagnosis, to say whether the patients would have recovered without treatment, or indeed to verify the figures themselves. But the fact that the Chinese government permits its orthodox doctors to practice acupuncture is indicative of the inadequacies of the medical services in a continent where doctors are all too few and the demands on them enormous. Where there are not enough surgeons to deal with acute appendicitis, sticking "magical" needles into patients may be better than nothing.

The continued existence of acupuncture in a "modern" state like China has sanctioned all kinds of quacks, and even doctors, to practice this form of treatment in Britain, France, and other Western European countries. In the last few years newspapers and popular periodicals have given acupuncture much free publicity; there are journalists too, as well as interested doctors, who have tried to give acupuncture a scientific gloss. All over Britain, for example, there exist acupuncture clinics where men in clinical white coats—resembling the glamorous doctor heroes of television medical romances though often they are not, in fact, doctors—stick needles into hopeful patients. Most of the patients leave the clinic (the decor of which commonly resembles a cross between a lush private nursing home and a Chinese restaurant) with the symptoms they had when they entered. Few leave "cured." All leave with less money in their wallets or handbags.

It is significant that one acupuncture doctor interviewed in the British *Sunday Times* admitted that he prefers to treat "chronic ailments which have defeated Western medicine: for instance, migraines and various other types of headaches; duodenal and stomach ulcers, indigestive disorders; lumbago, fibrositis, sciatica, neuralgia; acne and other skin troubles; asthma, hay fever; high blood pressure; depressions and anxiety states"—all symptoms and ailments known to be related to stress or other psychological disturbance. The doctor would probably obtain the same results if he stuck needles into himself while his patients watched him. On the other hand, the acupuncturist might well respond: "Do orthodox physicians with their placebos, tonics, and vitamins, get better results in some of these chronic, intractable conditions?"

Today, in Western society anyway, one would expect healthy adults to believe more in science than in miracles. Whether or not this be so, the sick, whose desperate symptoms cannot be ameliorated by modern medicines, must be tempted to believe more in miracles than in a science that cannot help them. At times they regress in attitude of mind to dependent childhood—to the time when they owned little critical intelligence and took so many things on "faith"; to the time when they were conditioned by parental simplifications and perhaps by a biblical training; to a time when a belief in miracles was held without question. It is no wonder that those in need of miracles consult those who claim their healing gift to be God-bestowed or those who believe themselves to be instruments of some other supernatural, beneficial power or agent. This agent, such healers claim, might be the spirit of a dead man, or the power and goodness of Jesus Christ himself. In Britain alone approximately 1,000,000 people consult such faith healers each year. Others—over 3,000,000 each year—make the pilgrimage to Lourdes and similar places of "healing" where in longing and in faith a number cry out "I am cured," even when they continue to be blind, or to limp.

Faith healers generally follow the example of Jesus in trying to heal by the laying-on of hands, and by prayer and meditation. Two faith healers who have become internationally renowned in our time —both of them British—are Dorothy Kerin, who worked within the ministry of the Church until she died in 1963, and Harry Edwards,

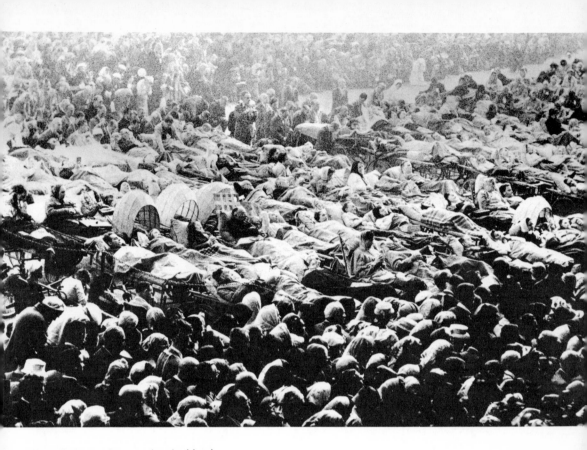

Sick pilgrims wait to receive the blessing in the square at Lourdes, hopeful that a miracle may cure where medical science has obviously failed.

who is still alive and who receives roughly 10,000 letters a week and so has to employ 20 typists to answer his mail.

Dorothy Kerin, even early in her career, was known as "the miracle girl." She suffered several years of invalidism, and when she reached the age of 22 it appeared to her doctors that she was dying from miliary tuberculosis. She had, they believed, peritonitis and meningitis as a result. She became blind, and had sunk into unconsciousness. Then suddenly she opened her eyes, asked for her dressing gown, and told those about her bed that she was quite well. She had seen, she said, a vision: an angel had taken her hand and said, "Dorothy, your sufferings are over. Get up and walk." Let me quote a passage from her own account:

"The Angel again said to me, 'Get up and walk.' They brought the dressing gown. When I had put it on I got out of bed unassisted. Part of the light which emanated from the Angel came to the right side of my bed. I put my hand on it, and it led me out of the room, along a passage and back into my bedroom. Though I had not walked for

175

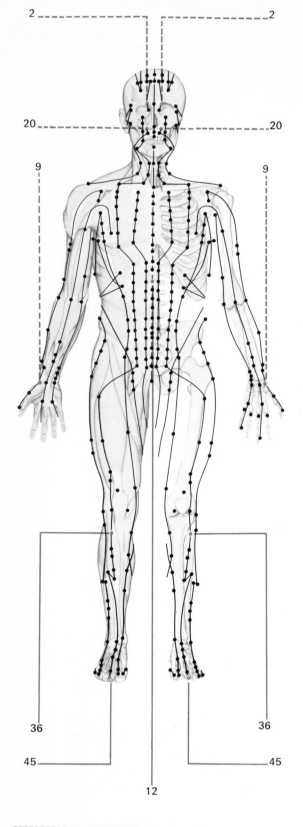

2 - - - - - - - 2

20 - - - - - - 20

9 9

36 36

45 45

12

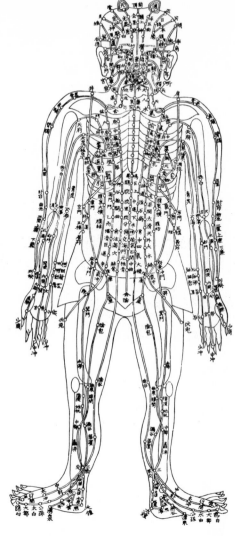

Above, an Ancient Chinese acupuncture chart. Left, the acupuncture points used today by practitioners in the West. (The numbered points are the ones normally selected in the treatment of sinusitis and duodenal ulcer.)

- - - - - - - Points used in Sinus Trouble
———————— Points used in Duodenal Ulcer

Right, an acupuncturist treats a patient for sinusitis. In this case the needles are positioned at the sides of the nose and hands—points that correspond to two of the specific points for sinusitis numbered on the chart.

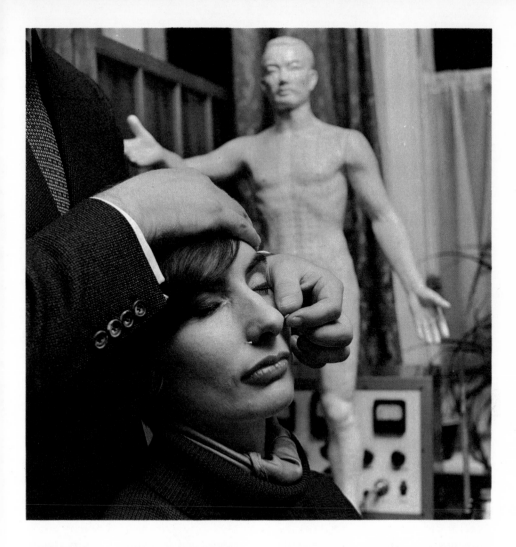

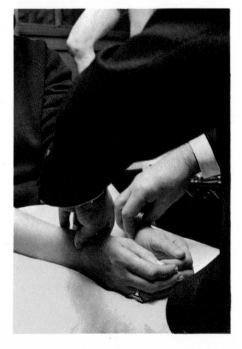

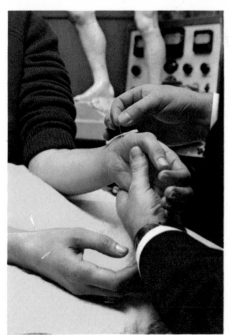

nearly five years, I now walked quite steadily, not the least bit shaky; indeed I felt well and strong and might never have been ill at all."

Her sight had been restored, and 12 hours later the thin, phthisic girl who was Dorothy Kerin had become, according to her account, "quite normal and in a perfect condition. I was quite plump, all my bones being covered with firm, healthy flesh. This in the space of twelve hours! Blessed be God." Her general practitioner, a Dr. Norman, believed she had earlier shown all the gravest symptoms of advanced tuberculosis. He had no theory to account for this miracle cure. He just said: "Had I read of it, I certainly should not have believed it. She is well, how she got better I don't know." Other doctors, of course, had been called in. Also her history had been known before this "miracle," for earlier she had been in various medical establishments: in a sanatorium outside Reading; in St. Bartholomew's Hospital, London; in St. Peter's Home for Incurables at Kilburn. Only a few doctors suggested Dorothy Kerin was an hysteric, for there was the earlier bacteriological report to confirm that there had been active tuberculosis bacteria in her sputum.

One perspicacious journalist, who visited her soon after her recovery, wrote: "Calling at her house I found the young woman sitting on the bed on which she had lain for the past five years. When she speaks her voice, clear and low, is such as would make the fortune of a practicing clairvoyant. Every sentence she uses shows a strong religious temperament. In her own mind she is convinced that she has been miraculously brought back from death's door for a special purpose. What that special purpose is she has not yet discovered." Soon Dorothy Kerin did discover her special purpose. She came to believe that through God she had the gift to heal others. Moreover, this girl, who had lived in a small house in a poor quarter of London, convinced the wealthy and the influential, prominent churchmen and prominent doctors, that this was so. She was taken up by them and, working with them, put her theories into practice: first in The Home of Healing in Ealing, and later in a converted mansion with its own private chapel near Tunbridge Wells in Kent. She had created a legend of her healing powers in her own lifetime. Innumerable sick people had had Dorothy Kerin's hands laid upon them. Many vouched that a current had passed into their bodies, that they had seen Dorothy Kerin's face radiant, that they had been cured by her. "Christ left the power of healing to his disciples," she had said in her dark, hypnotic voice. "The question of whether you believe this power has been passed on to chosen people depends on whether you believe what the Bible tells us." Dorothy Kerin certainly attracted unqualified devotion and love from her disciples and those who worked with her. But it is not uninteresting to note that, as well as a legend, this once poor girl left behind her £180,580 (about $505,000).

Harry Edwards, too, found his vocation through a dramatic incident. His career began when he attended a séance at a spiritualist church. Startled, he heard the medium pass on a message to him from the dead: "Harry Edwards, why don't you use your gift of healing?" Later, he found himself speaking aloud with a voice he did not feel to be his own, as if another intelligence from the spirit world was using his faculties. Harry Edwards went on to become the most famous spirit healer of the 20th century. He believes his spirit guides to be Louis Pasteur and Lord Lister, and, like Dorothy Kerin, holds that his healing power is a divine gift. That people share his faith in his power of healing is evidenced by the enormous crowds that have flocked to places like the Albert Hall and the Royal Festival Hall in London—while Harry Edwards, under spotlights, attempts to exercise his gift. Here is a newspaper report—from *The Sunday Express*—of one such occasion at the Royal Festival Hall in 1956. With Edwards on the platform is a 40-year-old woman crippled with arthritis:

" 'The doctors have pronounced me incurable,' she whispers to Edwards. Her voice continues to carry over the microphones to the 3000 people waiting there. 'Please, Mr. Edwards, heal me. *Please.*' Harry Edwards has his shirt sleeves rolled up. The footlights reveal the beads of perspiration on his brow. Once more he closes his eyes, then says, 'Raise your hands above your head. Place them on the nape of your neck.'

" 'I can't,' says the lady. 'I haven't done that for five years.'

"But her hands are going up. The audience catch their breath. For she has done it, and now she is moving her legs too. It is over. 3000 people have witnessed the apparent cure of a cripple in a matter of two minutes."

Most of Harry Edwards's work is done not on the public platform but at his mansion in Shere, Surrey. There he meditates in the early hours of the morning, to tune in, he maintains, to his spiritual guides so that he can bring about "absent healing" for those many people who write to him. When I interviewed him he told me: "The majority who write to me have been told they are incurable. As a result of my meditations 80 per cent record a measure of improvement, 30 per cent of these have a *complete recovery.*"

I found him to be a bulky white-haired man who chain-smoked, and frankly I was appalled when he told me that among the people he treated were sufferers from conditions like cancer, leukemia, and multiple sclerosis. I recalled how Dr. Yellowlees, an eminent Scots psychiatrist, had warned on a television broadcast: "It ought to be stated that there is a very real danger, a mental danger, to people who occupy themselves with ideas like those of Mr. Edwards. It is pernicious, dangerous for sick people to delay taking modern medical advice while they are seeking spiritual help."

After this broadcast many viewers protested at the vehemence of such an opinion. One woman wrote: "Last night I saw a very fine man judged and condemned. He was brought into the same category as charlatans, liars and witch doctors. This man has helped thousands of people, brought joy into saddened lives by healing many who suffer, and given hope to the hopeless."

There are some who would believe that the practice of osteopathy also derives from a form of faith healing. They would see the manipulations of osteopaths as no more than a forceful "laying-on of hands." The 19th-century originator of osteopathy, Andrew Still, had, it is true, a deep religious conviction. He even went so far as to say that "God is the Father of osteopathy and I am not ashamed of the child of his mind." Still's first patient was a young lady whose nervous symptoms had baffled and defeated the doctors of her native Virginia. All he did was to lift her head, pull her neck, and inform her that she would get better. The lady responded to this "laying-on of hands" and the positive suggestion. And Still found this method to be successful with other patients. He advanced the theory that all diseases resulted from misplaced vertebrae—that these vertebral displacements pressed on the nerves and blood vessels issuing from the spinal column and, in so doing, obstructed the life-force flow. To cure disease it was only necessary to allow the life force to flow unimpeded, which could be done by manipulating the spine or neck.

In Europe today, many people consider osteopaths to be merely bone manipulators and would consult them only for "pains in the back," "a slipped disk," "sciatica," "a stiff neck," and so forth. In the U.S.A. osteopaths are fast losing their separate identity: they are being trained in their schools to adopt more orthodox methods of therapy—and as a result are being recognized by the American Medical Association.

Homeopathy, like osteopathy, is based on a nonscientific principle. It was founded in the 18th century by Samuel Hahnemann, a doctor from Saxony whose guiding principle was "like things are cured by like" (*similia similibus curentur*). By this he meant that if drug X could produce symptoms in a healthy body that resembled the symptoms of disease Y, then drug X taken in minute quantities could *cure* disease Y. This theory allowed homeopaths to prescribe small amounts of belladonna to a patient suffering from scarlet fever—simply because belladonna poisoning can give rise to a clinical picture superficially resembling scarlet fever. All disease, Hahnemann believed, could be treated with drugs producing like effects.

In selecting drugs, moreover, he relied on a theory propounded in the 16th century by the Swiss alchemist and physician Paracelsus, a theory based on the astrological concept that the stars impress the signature of disease upon drugs; this "signature" could be recognized from the color and shape of the plant that yielded the drug. Thus the root of an orchid, which has the shape of a testicle, could be used to cure diseases of the testicle; the black spot in the flower called "eyebright," which resembles the pupil of an eye, could be used in the treatment of eye diseases. Hahnemann also believed that the smaller the dose of the drug used, the greater its effect. In fact, the doses homeopaths gave their patients were too minute to do either harm or good—and they *appeared* to do good, for many patients eventually recover, whatever treatment they are given. As for those who do not, well, as one satirist remarked: "The patients of the homeopaths died of the disease but the patients of orthodox doctors died of the cure."

Homeopathy, it may be thought, based as it is on such a quasi-scientific concept, could hardly last into the 20th century. Yet it

Below, two 20th-century faith healers. Left, Dorothy Kerin, working with an Anglican priest in her chapel in Kent, England. Right, at a public demonstration held in Leeds in 1964, Harry Edwards treats a patient by "laying-on of hands."

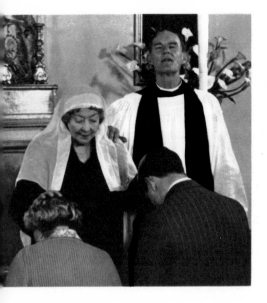
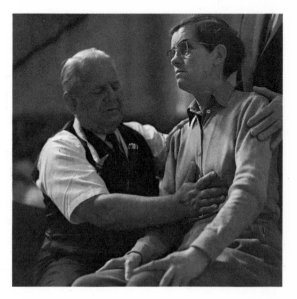

flourishes today—not only in France and Germany, where fringe practices of all kinds find a rich breeding ground, but elsewhere too. In Britain homeopathy is officially recognized and part of the National Health Service. This is because British homeopathic practitioners are medically qualified, and because homeopathy has had long years of aristocratic patronage. In the 19th century, Frederick Foster Harvey Quin, a pupil of Hahnemann, introduced homeopathic medicine into Britain, and he was friendly with the influential Duchess of Devonshire and the Marquis of Anglesey. And in the 20th century homeopathy has found its royal devotees. The late Queen Mary believed in it, and her son George VI also gave homeopathy his blessing. As with the other fringe healers discussed in this chapter, homeopaths have often *seemed* to cure when orthodox doctors failed.

Two questions arise out of this discussion of "fringe healers." First: do these unorthodox men and women really procure permanent cures? Second: if such cures are truly effected, is it because of the methods they use or the result of their own charismatic personalities? At the beginning of the chapter, I stated that about one third of patients suffering from concrete symptoms could be found to have nothing organically wrong with them. In their textbook *Psychosomatic Medicine*, the eminent American doctors Edward Weiss and O. Spurgeon English go much further, maintaining that "between the small number of obviously psychotic persons whom a physician sees and the larger number of patients who are sick solely because of physical disease, are a vast number of sick people who are not 'out of their minds' and yet who do not have any definite bodily disease to account for their illness." They agree that about a third of the patients with chronic illness who consult a physician come into this category. But they continue: "Approximately another third of the patients with chronic illness have symptoms that are *in part dependent upon emotional factors* even though organic findings are present."

These two doctors do not stop there. Justly, they discuss the psychic factor in the final group of disorders that appear to be wholly within the province of organic disease. Many physicians (even those who scoff at psychological medicine) will agree that a surprising number of physical ailments—duodenal ulcer, asthma, migraine, certain kinds of high blood pressure, certain skin conditions, etc.—are emotionally determined. The more one practices medicine, the more one learns that even those diseases with no apparent emotional matrix may have one in reality.

Here are two short case histories from my own medical practice, which I believe substantiate this view:

Case I: *T.S., a young male of 22, suffered his first spontaneous pneumo-thorax (i.e. a collapsed lung) the day after he became engaged in July 1964. Two weeks later he was fully recovered and lived a normal life. But in January 1965 he suffered a second pneumothorax at church when he was best man at his friend's wedding. Again he recovered quickly only to experience a third spon-taneous pneumothorax, this time on the day of his own wedding in April 1965.*

It is surely not necessary to adumbrate the obvious stress factor in this case. Other histories of patients suffering from spontaneous pneumothorax have confirmed my belief that psychogenic factors can frequently operate in the causation of this physical condition.

Case II: *D. J., a male aged 45, had, during the last war, been in a severe air crash. He had avoided boarding an airplane ever since. In 1962, however, he had to fly on behalf of his firm to Finland but was prevented from doing so at the last moment because he suffered from a peri-anal abscess, which finally had to be opened by a surgeon. Since then he remained absolutely fit, journeying when he had to by car, train, and boat. Only recently, this year, when it was necessary for him to travel to the U.S.A. by plane, he developed a second peri-anal abscess. On consulting me he did not relate his infection to his fear of flying. In conversation, however, he said that his forthcoming trip to the U.S.A. was something he did not wish to engage in. "It will be a bore," he said at first. And then later, "Frankly, doctor, the whole thing is a pain in the arse." This is exactly what he suffered from as a result of a staphylococcal infection.*

If, then, it is accepted that even abscesses can be as emotionally determined as many other more obviously functional symptoms, surely the answer to whether "fringe healers" effect cures must be in the affirmative. Aristotle knew that "the mind has the same command over the body as the master over the slave." That Aristotle's wisdom has not percolated through to the average physician after all these centuries is incredible and tragic. As for the fringe healer, whatever method he uses is partly irrelevant. For he has a confidence in his method that an ordinary physician with his "ifs" and "buts" and "maybes" and his many other scientific reservations does not own. The more fanatical the fringe practitioner's faith in the method he uses, the more successful will be his treatment. Nearly 2000 years ago, the great Greek physician Galen wrote: "He cures most in whom most have faith." The emotionally disturbed patient is more likely to have faith in a positive, assertive, optimistic, ignorant healer than in the average doctor, half-educated and beset by any number of scientific doubts and reservations.

Of course, many of the "cures" of fringe healers are all too tem-porary. Their power is basically a suggestive one. Psychiatrists know the limitations of direct-symptom removal by hypnosis. They know that the hypnotist, through suggestion, can frequently "cure" a

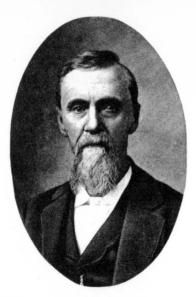

Left, Andrew Still, American originator of osteopathy. Below, an osteopath manipulates the cervical region of his patient's spine to relieve tension of the neck muscles.

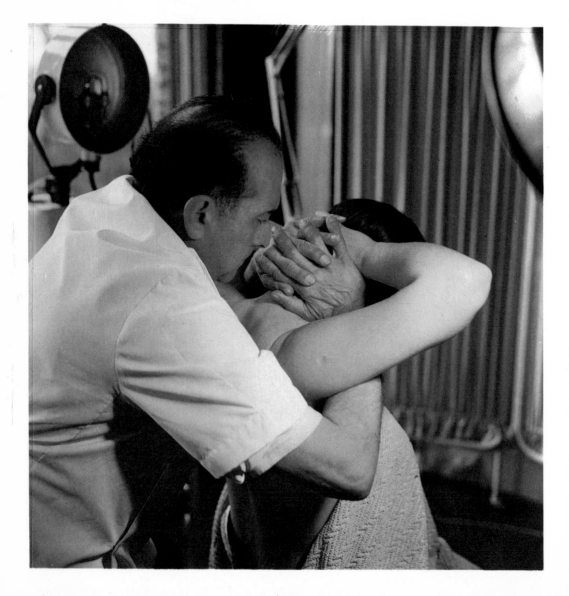

distressing symptom—let us say a paralysed arm resulting from hysteria. They also know that the hysteric may later present his therapist with, perhaps, a vile skin disease. In short, unless the causes of the hysterical symptoms are approached, discerned, and ventilated, one distressing symptom is simply replaced by another—one that can be worse than the original, and even dangerous.

Not all fringe healers' cures are temporary, though. One can begin to understand why this should be only by considering the power of charisma. Max Weber, in *The Theory of Social and Economic Organization*, published in 1947, used the term *charisma* in the sense of an extraordinary magical power and quality possessed by certain persons. From a sociological point of view many leaders—demagogues as well as prophets—dominate others through this power of charisma. A psychoanalyst, Professor D. W. Abse of the University of Virginia, has said recently in a discussion of political rulers that, "for better or worse, charismatic leadership is especially in demand in times of trouble and during emergencies and is then associated with a collective excitement with which masses of people surrender themselves to an heroic leader. The leader dominates by virtue of qualities inaccessible to others and incompatible with the rules of thought and action that govern everyday life."

What is true of the charismatic leader and his followers is also true of the successful fringe healer and his patients. The patient, too, consults his "leader" in times of trouble (illness) or emergency (the knowledge that he has an incurable disease). Masses of people surrender themselves not only to the irrational oratory of a Hitler but also to the showman-like demonstrations of a fringe healer. Just as the political leader dominates his followers, the charismatic healer dominates his bevy of disciples and patients. They, in fact, become "possessed" and the relationship of the patient to the fringe healer may resemble infatuation—and, like falling in love, this surrender can enrich his life.

To understand the power of charisma and surrender let us turn back again to Professor Abse's psychoanalytic view, which emphasizes our early dependence as infants on our parents for survival and growth, not only in body but in terms of the psyche as well. "There is the need for the child to gain a foundation of psychic strength, a foundation which can only be achieved by the evolution of a trustful relationship with the providing parent during the early years of life. At this time grandiose images of the parents are endowed with omnipotence and omniscience, and the child gains strength by identifying with them." In adulthood, too, "for everyone there remains a longing to find again a god-like personage, unlimited in power and wisdom,

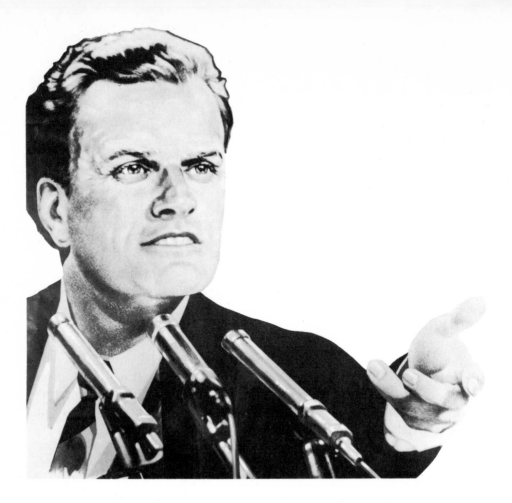

The power of charisma, evident in the mass rallies of American evangelist Billy Graham, is no different in kind from the powers of the successful fringe healer.

and this longing is especially apt to be activated strongly under conditions of frustration. . . ." And one may add, under conditions of illness, suffering, and helplessness too, which are the lot of so many of the fringe healer's clients.

But let us continue with the psychoanalytic view of charismatic leadership—for though this is meant in terms of political leadership it is true also of charismatic healers. "Charismatic leadership approaches more or less closely the model of the rapport of the hypnotist with his subject," writes Professor Abse. "The procedures for inducing hypnosis are basically appeals to *awe* and to *love*. In the first of these, matters of decisive importance are the social and professional prestige of the hypnotist, his imposing behavior and his self-assurance in issuing commands. In the second of these, a mild and friendly attitude, a low monotonous voice, and a restful atmosphere, including perhaps a darkened soundless room and soothing light stroking, are important ingredients. Sandor Ferenczi—Freud's distinguished pupil—discussed the connections of the first method with the child's conception of the firm, infallible, and all-powerful father, whereas the second or maternal method is redolent of scenes in which a mother woos her child to sleep by singing lullabies. The paternal and maternal inductions may be mixed. Appeals to awe and love especially characterize the efforts of charismatic leaders to fascinate their audience and to secure a following."

It may well be that the famous "bedside manner" some doctors instinctively own is based on their ability to be "paternal" and "maternal" to their patients at one and the same time. Charismatic fringe healers certainly exhibit this quality. Dorothy Kerin, for example, had that dark, low voice, that mild and friendly attitude. Moreover she gave commands "like a man" yet her disciples, when interviewed, stressed repeatedly and without prompting, "how feminine Dorothy was." They had a need to say she was a woman, all woman, though why should one doubt it? In the analytic sense, and this is no slur, she expressed the mythic idea that man and woman were, once upon a time, one. Speak to her disciples, read the tracts written by them about her—the language they write is the language of love. As for "awe," well, every famous person is held in awe by some. The public exhibitions, the floodlights, the advertisements, the propaganda, bestow charisma on the subject they are directed at—be he politician, actor, evangelist, or fringe healer.

Indeed, one wonders whether those official medical associations—such as the British Medical Association—that frown on publicity for individual doctors inadvertently prevent some patients from gaining benefit from the orthodox healers who otherwise might be more famous and thus more charismatic. The conditions of love and awe are necessary for the healer—orthodox doctor or quack. That those in the medical profession sometimes instinctively understand this is demonstrated, for example, in the great teaching hospitals.

One only has to listen to the nursing staff talk about this or that consultant (physician or surgeon), Sir Harry This or William That, or go on one of the ward rounds, to understand how the qualities of awe and love operate effectively in this ambience. Yet the medical profession as a whole does not understand that, important as the means of treatment may be, the glamorous aura of those who heal is equally significant. The white cloak of healing may look clinical and antiseptic, but the purple cloak of the magician, of Merlin, of Mesmer, might usefully be hung on the door of every doctor's surgery.

# 6   The Addicts

More and more people are becoming increasingly dependent on drugs. One reason for this is that doctors too frequently prescribe potent preparations for anxiety, depression, and unhappiness, without being able to deal with the root causes of such states of mind. Then again, in affluent societies there has been "the teen-age explosion," which allows adolescents, loaded with money, to look for "kicks" in the way-out coffee bars and jazz clubs. But however many respectable authoritarians consider addicts to be merely young hoodlums, and consequently recommend punitive measures to deal with them, the problem remains primarily a medical, not a police, one. For some of these teen-agers are handicapped by personality disorders and suffer like all others who are afflicted with mental disturbances.

Fortunately, relatively few of the young who dabble in marihuana and the amphetamine barbiturate drugs of the purple heart variety go so far as taking heroin or one of the other dangerous narcotics. And it is the narcotics that continue to be the principal concern of those bodies that have to deal with the problem of drug addiction. The very words "drug addiction," however, are used loosely and have been defined in different ways. The World Health Organization describes addiction as: ". . . a state of periodic or chronic intoxication

An addict's painting externalizes the terrifying hallucinations frequently experienced during the first period of withdrawal from a drug.

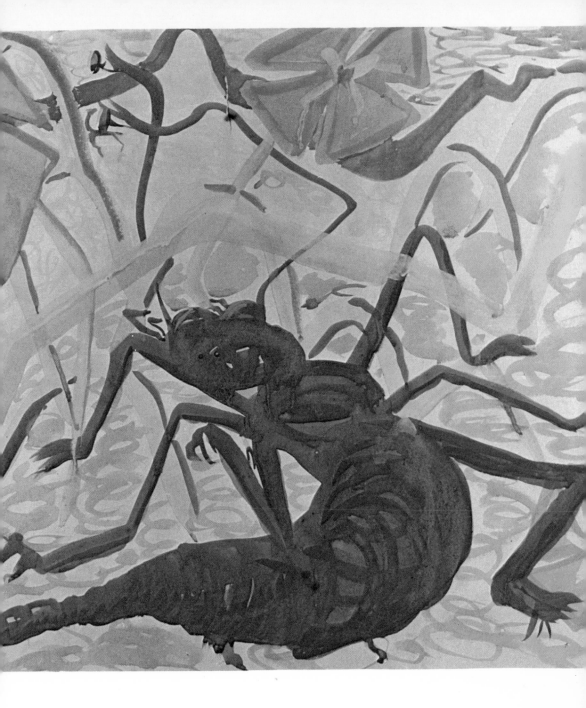

detrimental to the individual and to society, produced by the repeated consumption of a drug (natural or synthetic). Its characteristics include: (1) an overpowering desire or need (compulsion) to continue taking the drug and to obtain it by any means; (2) a tendency to increase the dose; (3) a psychic (psychological) and sometimes a physical dependence on the effects of the drug."

Some may argue with this definition, especially as it makes a value judgment about addiction—"detrimental to the individual and to society." More useful, perhaps, is the strictly medical definition of addiction as proposed by the Departmental Committee on Morphine and Heroin Addiction in Great Britain. This committee defined the addict as "a person, who, not requiring the continued use of a drug for the relief of the symptoms of organic disease, has acquired, as a result of repeated administration, an overpowering desire for its continuance, and in whom withdrawal of the drug leads to definite symptoms of mental or physical distress or disorder." Here attention is focused on the withdrawal symptoms that true addicts experience when deprived of the drugs they depend on. As Edwin M. Schur has pointed out in *Narcotic Addiction in Britain and America*, withdrawal illness is one of the main criteria by which a drug is judged to be addictive or not.

Abstinence from cigarette smoking may be a most difficult and unhappy exercise for some, leading to mental restlessness, inability to concentrate, and depression; but it hardly compares with the acute symptoms of the drug addict's "abstinence syndrome." These include nausea, vomiting, diarrhea, muscular twitching, hot and cold flushes, sexual orgasm, a running nose, involuntary weeping, and heart palpitations. There is also the mental suffering involved. A personal account of one addict's mental state, while deprived of drugs and traveling in an empty boxcar of a freight train, has been reported by L. Guy Brown in his book *Social Pathology*: "I tried everything for relief. I even cried and wailed in my misery. I thought I would go mad. I was on the verge of insanity. I prayed for help, for relief, for death. My clothes must have been wet with sweat. I cursed the habit. If anyone could have seen me they would have thought I was a raving maniac. But no one saw me. I marched back and forth, aching with every step, wondering how I could stand it any longer. I wouldn't stand it again. I prayed that the train would stop so that I might get off and get some dope. I would have done anything to get dope. When I say anything I mean anything. I was in awful shape. It's no use—I can't describe how I felt. It makes me shudder to think about it. . . . There is no use trying to describe what I suffered that night. It was agony, every minute of it."

A New York sheriff lectures high-school students on the effects and dangers of various narcotics.

Despite testimony of this kind the popular view of drug addiction remains, intrinsically, a romantic one. Our innate romanticism conceives of the addict not only as a man apart, as an Outsider—which he undoubtedly is—but as an almost legendary figure. As such, he is dehumanized to become, in fantasy, part tawdry beast and part adventuring angel; part dangerous and part admirable. For he has taken risks, he has become free of respectable restraints, he has sought those forbidden pleasures we do not allow for ourselves, he has engaged in a self-destructive, Dionysian irreverence that we who live in safety, far from Skid Row, can only observe with an ambivalent concern. Perhaps in every fat bourgeois who wears evening dress, a thin ranting Bohemian is trying to struggle out. Again, the drug addict fascinates us in that, like Adam, he has tasted forbidden fruit and is banished from paradise; in reaching for the stars he tempts the gods, and with the inevitability of Greek tragedy, he is punished by the gods. As has been said by Isidor Chein and his colleagues in *Narcotics, Delinquency and Social Policy*: "Prometheus, having illicitly brought the

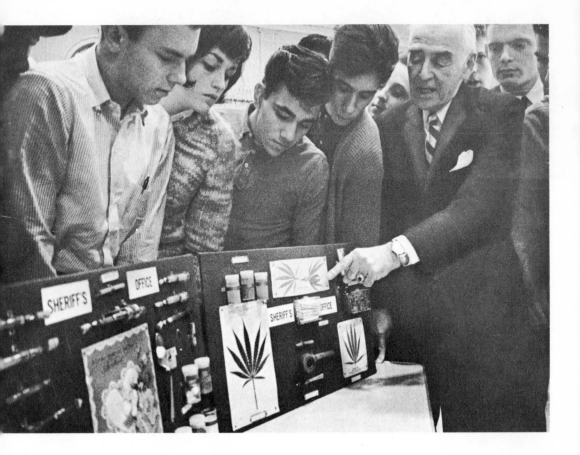

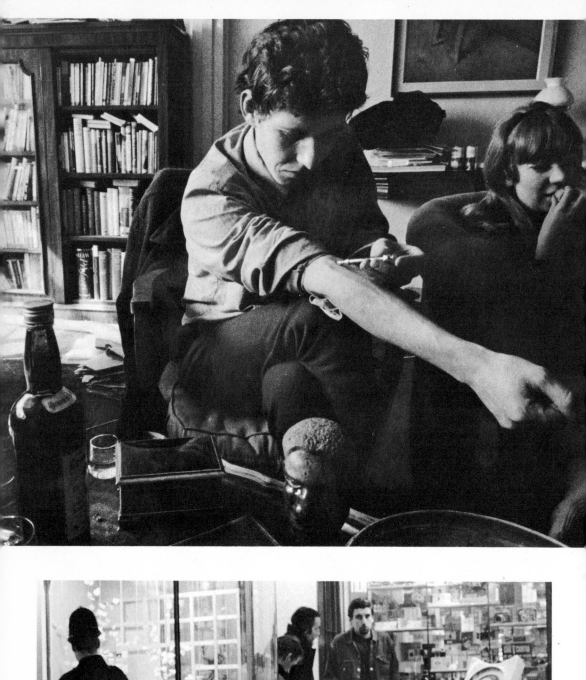

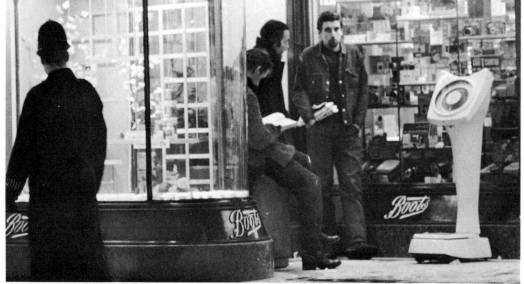

heavenly fire to earth, is condemned to a millennium of being eaten alive; Tantalus, having stolen the ambrosia of the gods, suffers a fate that makes his name a symbol of an exquisite form of torture; Icarus, having soared to forbidden heights, suffers the inevitable consequence of plummeting to the depths; and the addict, having trespassed in heaven, has earned his hell."

Perhaps our romantic attitudes could hardly be otherwise when people are fed so assiduously with the fabrications of commercial mythmaking that propagate the idea of the condemned Outsider as hero. The lives of the alcoholic, or drug-taking, damned artists—the Baudelaires, the Scott Fitzgeralds, the Dylan Thomases—have been told over and over, described with increasing license and exaggeration for the public's delight. Such tormented, neurotic men have been apotheosized into saints by a hundred hacks. True, drug addicts and alcoholics may be gifted: they may be poets or painters or inspired jazzmen. But most own no gift whatsoever, and all are sick, piteous, unhappy, and desperately in need of help. It must be admitted that many of the great writers, such as Baudelaire and Coleridge, have also helped to perpetuate the romantic myth of the drug-taking act.

Samuel Taylor Coleridge paid homage to the escapist and pain-killing properties of opium even as he cursed it. He wrote in his private notebook: "I have never loved evil for its own sake; no! nor ever sought pleasure for its own sake, but only as the means of escaping from pains that coiled around my mental powers as a serpent around the body and wings of an eagle; my sole sensuality was *not* to be in pain." His contemporary, Thomas De Quincey, startled the reading public in 1821 with *Confessions of an English Opium-Eater*, in which he observed: "Opium . . . introduces [into the mental faculties] the most

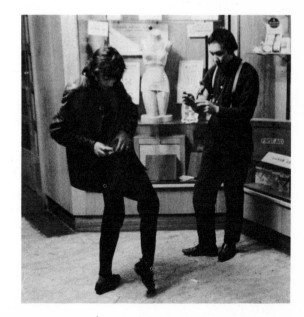

In Britain, addiction is seen more as a medical, than a police, problem. Above left, an addict undergoing gradual withdrawal treatment injects heroin into a vein. Left, addicts outside a London pharmacy wait for midnight, and a new day's ration of prescribed drugs. Right, two addicts stop in the pharmacy's lobby for their first "fix" of the day.

exquisite order, legislation, and harmony.... Oh! just, subtle, and mighty opium!... thou buildest upon the bosom of darkness, out of the phantastic imagery of the brain, cities and temples, beyond the art of Phidias and Praxiteles—beyond the splendour of Babylon and Hekatompylos."

In our own century Jean Cocteau, the French dramatist and artist, wrote (in 1929): "After knowing opium ... it is difficult to take earth seriously. And unless one is a saint it is difficult to live without taking earth seriously." He also maintained: "I owe to opium my perfect hours. It is a pity that instead of perfecting curative techniques, medicine does not try to render opium harmless." Then there was Aldous Huxley who, on taking the hallucinogenic drug peyote—long known to the American Indians—commented: "The flowers in the gardens trembled on the brink of being supernatural.... Later I had returned to that reassuring but profoundly unsatisfactory state known as 'being in one's right mind.'" Similar anti-life, vale-of-tears statements (at least I think that, in their depressive condemnation of normality, they are anti-life) have been made by other literary men who have taken drugs, including of late some of America's Beat poets.

A minority of people, too, feel that the problem of drug addiction is of no great consequence and that, indeed, the junkies are being persecuted by the representatives of a puritanical middle class, who consider drug-taking to be a vicious habit while at the same time hypocritically tolerating alcoholism. They would argue that the majority group-attitude toward such matters merely depends on different social customs and different social adaptations: in the Orient, opium is permitted; in India and Africa, hashish smoking is socially acceptable; in the West, alcohol and tobacco are permitted without question. Indeed, it may be better to be hooked on opium rather than on alcohol. As J. D. Reichard succinctly put it in *Narcotic Drug Addiction*, the alcoholic becomes drunk, returns home, and beats his wife; the heroin addict becomes high, returns home, and his wife beats him. It is generally true, also, that the drug addict suffers less organic deterioration than his alcoholic confrere. Thus D. L. Gerard writes in *Drinking and Intoxication*: "The addict is comfortable and functions well as long as he receives large enough quantities of drugs to stave off his abstinence syndrome. The chronically intoxicated alcoholic, on the other hand, cannot function normally as long as he maintains his intoxicating intake of alcohol."

It is not as simple as that, though. To compare addiction with chronic alcoholism is merely to contrast one circle of Dante's hell with another. The secondary consequences of drug addiction have to be considered. Also, a new drug introduced into a milieu unused to it may cause havoc and general demoralization—as alcohol did with the American Indians. The quality of devastation resulting from drug addiction is told by the American novelist William Burroughs in *The Naked Lunch*. Burroughs had for over 12 years used opium, heroin, morphine, and other narcotics. He observed: "Opium is profane. . . . I had not taken a bath in a year nor changed my clothes or removed them except to stick a needle every hour in the fibrous gray wooden flesh of terminal addiction. I never cleaned or dusted the room. Empty ampule boxes and garbage piled up to the ceiling. I did absolutely nothing. I could look at the end of my shoe for eight hours. I was only roused to action when the hourglass of junk ran out. . . . *I Don't Want To Hear Any More Tired Talk And Junk Con*—the same things said a million times and more and there is no point in saying anything because NOTHING *Ever Happens* in the junk world."

If nothing ever happens in the junk world, if the voluptuous Nirvana of a fix fades so quickly, if narcotic addiction makes a man a social outcast, if the results of narcotic addiction lead to such a miserable debasement of an individual, physically and mentally, it appears paradoxical that the problem of addiction, notwithstanding, is becoming ever more acute in certain areas of the world. Even where heroin traffic does not seem to be increasing—in California, for example—the narcotic pusher reaps new profits from other dangerous drugs. As a governor of California, Edmund G. Brown, confirmed at the White House Conference on Narcotic and Drug Abuse in September 1962: "The decline in heroin sales has been accomplished by a sharp increase in the use of dangerous drugs such as phenobarbital, seconal, nembutal, and benzedrine. In short, the peddlers are turning to a new line of merchandise which is less dangerous for them, but every bit as deadly for their old customers. This is an escape hatch which I intend to close as quickly as possible. [Prison sentences for illegal sales of heroin in California range from six years to life.] I believe we must be as severe on those who spread misery through dangerous drugs as we now are with those who sell heroin."

At present, nobody can say exactly how many true addicts exist in any one place at any one time. Statistics given by different authorities vary widely. In New York it has been estimated that there are from 25,000 to 50,000, but even this varying figure may well be wide of the mark—especially since authorities define addiction in different ways. The only statistical common factor is that day by day, month by month, year by year, the number of those engaging in drug abuse seems to be rapidly increasing.

Drug addiction, however, is not merely a 20th-century phenomenon. Prehistoric man, like his modern counterpart, could not "bear very much reality" and found plants that mitigated his suffering even as they enslaved him. In the Stone Age people had access to plants containing the principal narcotic drugs of addiction—poppies, which are the source of opium, and coca leaves, whose active ingredient is cocaine. Hashish and alcohol, too, were available to our distant ancestors.

Poppies were first actively cultivated some 4000 years ago in the areas around the eastern rim of the Mediterranean, when they were known as "the plants of joy." Homer refers to "nepenthe," which contained opium. Evidently the Greek warriors employed the drug to promote bravery in battle, to assuage their grief for their slain, and as a narcotic for their pleasure. It was also used by the Greeks (as well as by the Egyptians and Persians) medicinally. Galen recommended poppy juice "for it resists poison and venomous bites, cures inveterate headache, vertigo, deafness, epilepsy, apoplexy, dimness of sight, loss of voice, asthma, coughs of all kinds, spitting of blood, tightness of breath, colic, the iliac poison, jaundice, hardness of the spleen, stone, urinary complaints, fevers, dropsies, leprosies, the trouble to which women are subject, melancholy and all pestilence." Opium was recognized as an anesthetic 2300 years ago, yet neglected as a medicine for centuries. The opium poppy spread with Islam into India, and it seems that the Arabs took it with them to China in the ninth century. When it became known again in the West it was rather as a habit-forming narcotic than as a medicinal drug.

Cocaine appears to have been used first by natives of the Andes, who were affected by the drug when they chewed the leaves of the coca plant. They took it as a stimulant when undergoing long marches or hard labor, or during their orgiastic festivals. It was used, also, as an anesthetic when the Andean surgeons performed their remarkable trepanning operations. The ruthless totalitarian Inca state took energetic measures to restrict the use of coca (and chicha alcoholic beer) to prevent its subjects becoming addicted; but to this day coca-chewing remains a serious problem in the Andean geographical areas. For the habit of taking cocaine, like opium, leads to deleterious effects on whole communities and to widespread debauchery.

Cocaine did not come to the West, however, until the early 1880s, when the young Sigmund Freud discovered its medicinal use and suggested to a colleague that it could be used as a local anesthetic for eye surgery. Freud himself took it as a stimulant and enthusiastically recommended it to his fiancée and to his close friends. He lost his enthusiasm for cocaine as a psychic energizer when one of his friends, who had been taking the drug as a cure for morphine addiction, subsequently died. By then, in any case, reports of the powerful addictive properties of cocaine had become widespread.

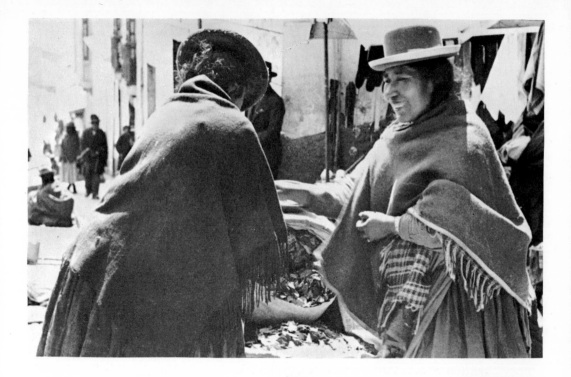

For many centuries cocaine has been the chief drug of addiction in the Andean area, and the coca plant (from which it is obtained) is still sold openly in Bolivia and Peru. Above, a street coca-seller in Bolivia. Below, an addict lies helpless under the influence of the drug.

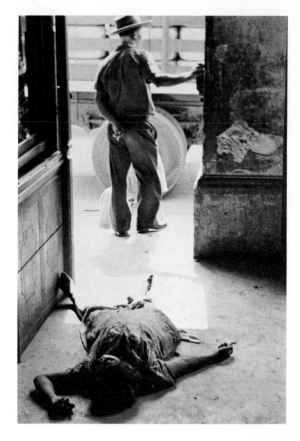

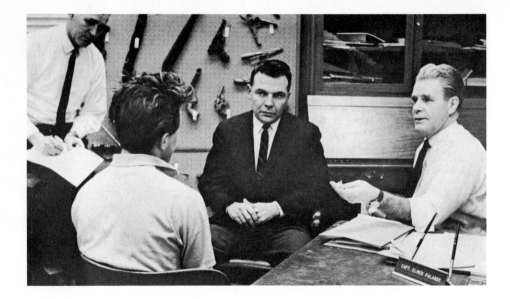

It was in the 19th century also that the alkaloids of opium were isolated. The Germans produced morphine in 1805, and in 1898 the synthetic alkaloid heroin was produced by heating morphine and acetic acid. Heroin was found to be the most addictive of all narcotics, yet at the time of its discovery it was hailed as a miracle drug, "a drug of increased effectiveness with decreased addictive liability." The medical profession dispensed it freely, and in so doing unwittingly increased the number of drug addicts in Europe and the U.S.A.

Early abuse of the narcotics in the U.S.A. resulted also from their inclusion in the different patent medicines popularly consumed. They were even used in soft drinks to ensure that customers would come back for more. The hypodermic syringe became available too, and doctors dispensing morphine during the American Civil War in the 1860s were ignorant of the fact that much smaller doses should be given by this route. Innumerable wounded soldiers were given unnecessarily high doses, and addiction at this time became known as "the army disease." At the beginning of the 20th century, governments all over the world became alerted to the dangers of indiscriminate use of narcotics. In 1906 the Chinese passed an edict prohibiting the cultivation of the opium poppy, and in 1908 public opinion in Britain forced the government to reduce opium exports from India to China. In the same year the U.S.A. prohibited the use of opium in the Philippines other than for purely medical purposes, and in 1912 the first international narcotics convention was held at The Hague. As a result of this convention, control of narcotics became a matter of international law.

Even so, in the U.S.A. it was not until 1914 that Congress passed the Harrison Narcotics Act, which controlled importation, manu-

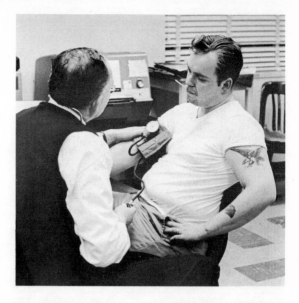

In America, drug addiction is generally linked with crime, and its control is in the hands of special narcotics squads. Left, New Jersey police interrogate a suspected addict; the weapons on display were confiscated from addicts or "pushers." Right, another suspect is given health and coordination tests to establish whether he is actually under the influence of drugs.

facture, and distribution of opium and its derivatives. Alas, no provision was made for those unfortunates who were already addicted, and they were driven underground to seek their drugs illicitly. A new and vicious drug traffic was born and some physicians took advantage of the situation to make fortunes out of the innumerable prescriptions they wrote for their desperate patients. Addicts, dependent then (as today) on narcotics they could not afford to buy in the black market, often had to resort to criminal activities to raise the necessary money. Men became thieves, and women often turned to prostitution.

The average addict in New York today needs $10,000 a year to pay for his drug requirements. An ex-mayor of New York, Robert F. Wagner, maintained in 1962: "The present crime situation in New York City is traceable to a major extent to the insatiable driving need of narcotic addicts for the money to satisfy their habits, regardless of the most heroic police measures to control the thief and mugger." Certainly New York has the biggest police narcotics squad in the whole of the U.S.A.

But large narcotics squads do not, in themselves, solve the problem. Indeed the greater the repressive measures taken against drug addicts, the more threatened they become and the more likely are these social outcasts, with their immature self-destructive urges, to flout authority. It is possible that many of the narcotic psychopaths indulge in anti-social practices simply because of their sense of unbearable guilt, and *unconsciously* crave to be punished. (Men sometimes even commit murder in order to be murdered—i.e. electrocuted, guillotined, or hanged.) Too many authorities, however, do not consider the drug addict as a sick person, which he undoubtedly is, but primarily as a criminal—a socially dangerous person—and as a result argue for

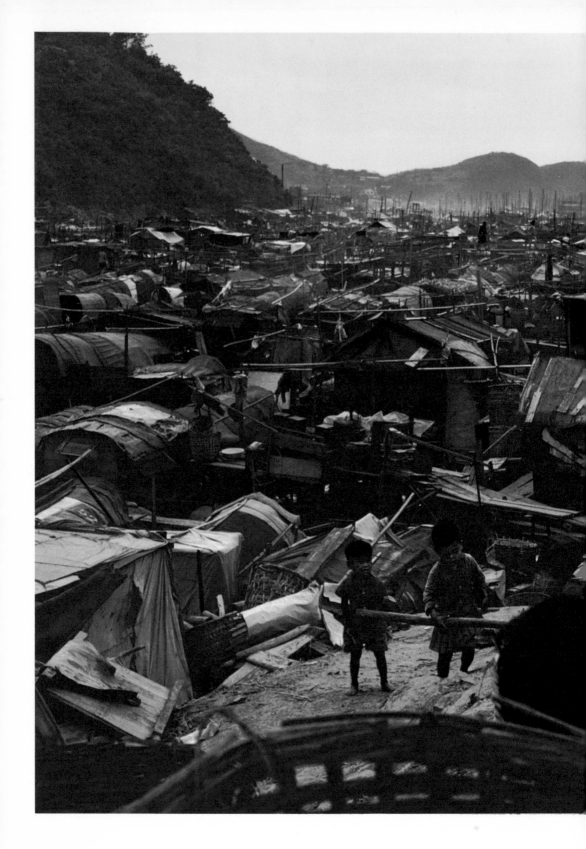

Squatter areas in the hills of Kowloon,
where the majority of Hong Kong's 300,000
addicts and opium traffickers operate.

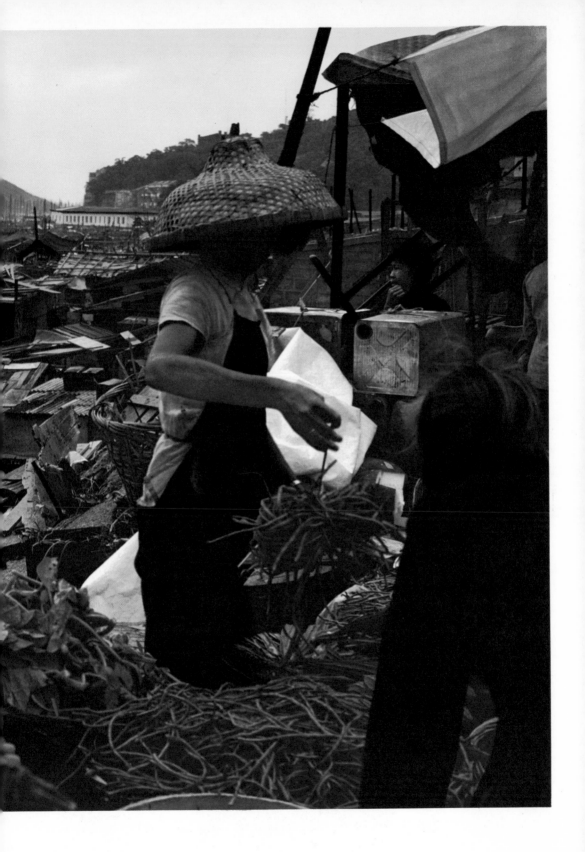

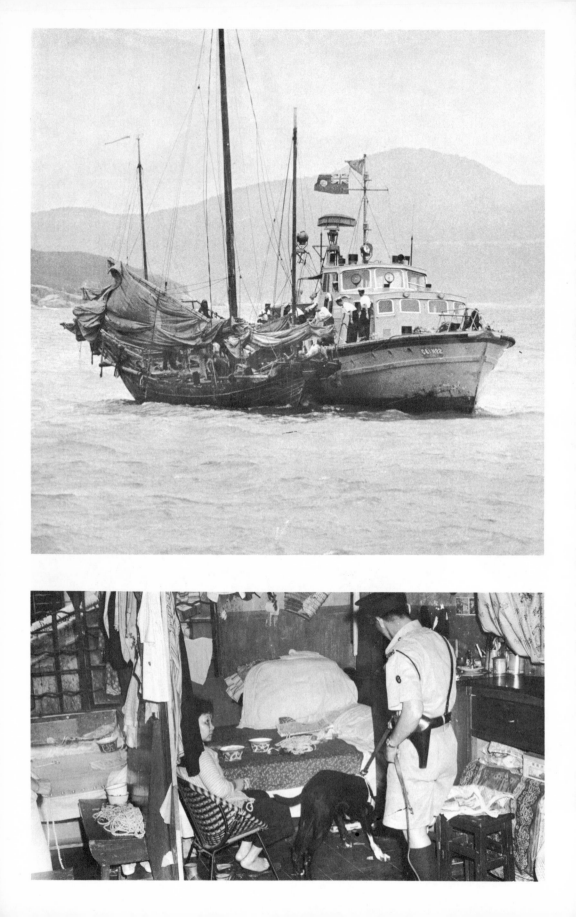

tougher penalties to be enforced against him. Paradoxically, the more effective the activities of narcotics police squads, the scarcer becomes the supply of illicit drugs—and this scarcity leads to rocketing prices on the black market, forcing the addict to involve himself in more serious criminal activities.

I have already indicated that the individual likely to become a drug addict is handicapped by a character disorder. He tends to be immature, inadequate, and unstable. This does not mean there is such a thing as a stereotyped drug-addict personality or one common drug-addict type. In the U.S.A. addicts are likely to be young males brought up in an overcrowded, urban, working-class area. Many are Negroes. In Britain, on the other hand, most reported addicts are over 30 years of age, and women outnumber men. They generally come from middle- or upper-middle-class homes, and there are relatively few narcotic addicts among the colored population. Indeed one quarter of those addicted in Britain are said to be doctors, doctors' wives, nurses, or those who work in the medical auxiliary services.

There are certain features about the drug-addict personality, however, that one can outline in general terms. Most, for example, have sexual difficulties with their marriage partners, and these usually persist even after the addict has given up narcotics. Marie Nyswander writes in *The Drug Addict as a Patient*: "A male addict, having been in prison for two or three years, has no difficulty in answering the question of whether he would rather have a luscious girl or a shot of morphine. Without hesitation he invariably names morphine as his choice."

The adolescent drug addict is often concerned about his sexual inadequacy, or else professes complete disinterest in sex. Many of

Hong Kong's 7000-strong police force (aided by 300 British officers) fights a continual battle to check a growing traffic in opium and heroin. Above left, Hong Kong police board a junk, as it leaves port, to search for contraband drugs. Left, an unsuccessful raid on the home of a suspected trafficker. Elaborate warning systems of lights and bells (right) often foil police raids.

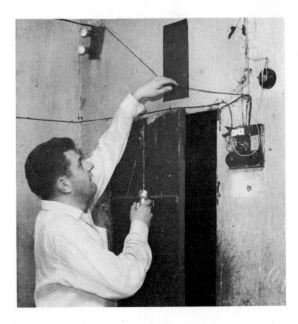

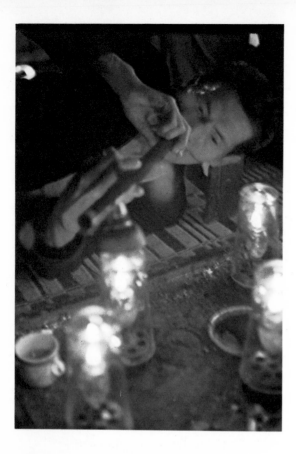

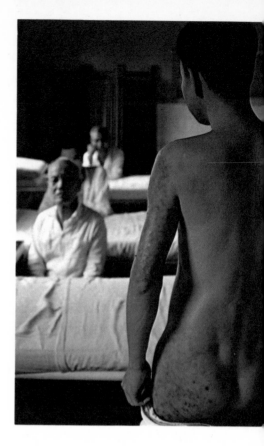

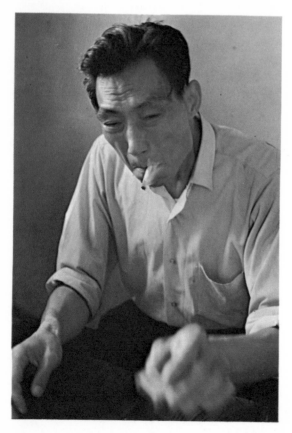

Traditionally, opium and heroin are taken by heating a paste and smoking the fumes through a pipe (above left). The simpler method of inserting pellets of the drug into a cigarette (left) is often preferred— and there are those, too, who take the drug intravenously. As a result their arms and legs become covered with scars from abscesses (above). The photograph (above right) of the inside of an opium den, where the traditional method of smoking prevails, was taken after a raid.

Right, prisoners engaged in occupational therapy at Hong Kong's Tai Lam prison. First offenders (there are about 700, mostly heroin addicts) are given medical therapy during their period of detention.

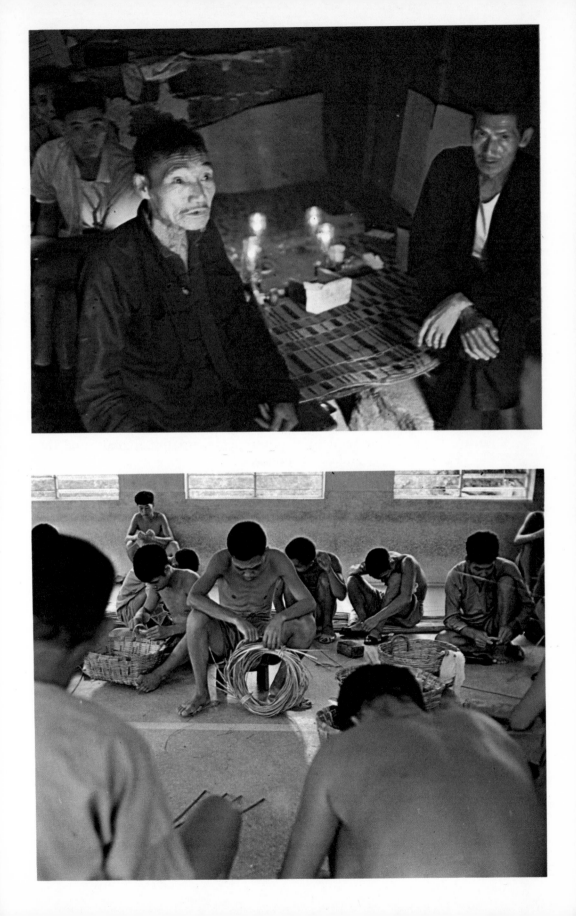

those who do have close girl friends prefer cunnilingus (apposition of the mouth to the vulva) to sexual intercourse. Others have homosexual relationships or exhibit strong latent homosexual leanings, which are expressed, for example, in acute and irrational fear of homosexual assault. As Isidor Chein and his colleagues wrote:

"An extraordinarily high proportion of adolescent addicts can be seen as 'pretty boys.' They would not appear out of place in a musical comedy chorus. They are vain of their appearance. They spend much time preening. They are preoccupied with clothing, which they wish to be of the finest materials and the latest styles. They spend much time before their mirrors experimenting with their hair, moustaches, and goatees.

"None of these preoccupations is alien to adolescent boys; the difference is of degree and not of kind. The degree to which adolescent addicts exhibit these traits and activities suggests the usual traits and activities of adolescent girls. Adolescent addicts do not look, behave, or deport themselves as adolescent boys usually do; they do not try to appear manly, rugged, vigorous, energetic, rough-and-ready. These observations suggest that they have strong feminine identifications, a conclusion to which Zimmering et al., Fort, and the Chicago clinics independently subscribe. A variety of data are offered by those authors illustrating feminine tendencies, interests, occupational goals, and the like. There are occasional exceptions. . . ."

As might be expected, these exceptions protest too much. Their feminine passivity is disguised with overcompensated, Hemingway-like, tough postures. Though the hair on their chests is false, they would describe themselves as dangerous and ruthless toughs. Before becoming addicted many will have been involved with gangs, and engaged in robbery with assault. When discussing these activities they describe them as pleasurable.

Common to many drug addicts is a close and strange relationship with their mothers. After years of addiction, poverty, delinquency, and demoralization, a patient may allow himself to be treated at a hospital. Once over the abstinence syndrome, however, he is frequently restless to return home to a mother who cannot—or so he claims—cope without him. She *needs* him, and these latter years he has caused her so much heartbreak. Often, though, the smothering attraction is mutual. The mother is pleased that her son is so dependent on her. Often she has no husband—the father is dead or has quit the house years ago—and so feels all the more need to be needed. In any case it is generally the favorite son who has become the drug addict: over the years he has developed into her husband surrogate. As Nora Sayre reported in *The New Statesman* of May 7, 1965:

"Recently, the Lower East Side Narcotics Center completed a two year study on male drug addicts in their twenties which revealed that few of the mothers wanted their sons cured. Often these women directly sabotaged the programme. One flushed her son's withdrawal medication down the lavatory. Another who had requested treatment for her son developed her yearly ear-complaint so that he couldn't leave her on the day he was to enter the hospital. A 'prize-addict', near to recovery, visited his mother just before taking university entrance examinations; she gave him three dollars for a haircut. But a haircut costs 1.50 dollars, whereas three dollars buys a bag of heroin."

The study also showed that the addicts' mothers "prefer their sons on heroin rather than barbiturates since heroin is quieter." Also heroin might have the advantage—from the possessive mother's point of view—of extinguishing her dear son's sexuality, so neutralizing her deep fear of real-life rivals. As for the son, the very taking of heroin may provide him—though he will be generally unaware of it—with a symbolic incestuous gratification. Isidor Chein and his colleagues report that there are "those patients who tell us quite directly that the syringe and needle ('the works' as they are called in the argot) are like a breast; when he is high, he feels that he is together with his mother, long ago, warm, comfortable, happy, at peace; when he injects the opiate solution, he mixes the solution with his blood and bounces the blood-opiate mixture back and forth from syringe to vein, and, as he does this, he has fantasies about intercourse."

There are many who consider such psychoanalytical interpretations of drug addiction to be farfetched or even downright nonsense. Too many doctors, alas, think in this dismissive way. Even now, in the second half of the 20th century, doctors who have never read Freud jeer at his teachings; but how, except through analytical interpretation, can the addict's loving description of a fix be understood? Consider novelist Alexander Trocchi's account of a fix and his attitude toward it in the following passage from *Cain's Book*:

"When one presses the bulb of the eye-dropper and watches the pale, blood-streaked liquid disappear through the nozzle and into the needle and the vein it is not, not only, a question of feeling good. It's not only a question of kicks. The ritual itself, the powder in the spoon, the little ball of cotton, the matches applied, the bubbling liquid drawn up through the cotton filter into the eye-dropper, the tie round the arm to make a vein stand out, the fix often slow because a man will stand there with the needle in the vein and allow the level in the eye-dropper to waver up and down, up and down, up and down, until

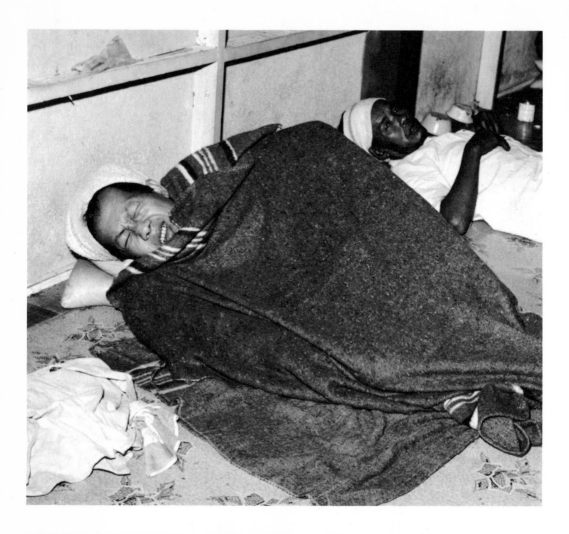

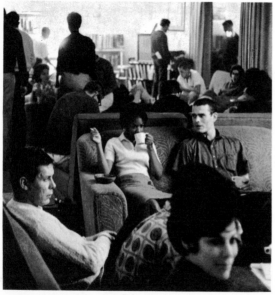

Above, an opium addict going through the first stages of withdrawal at a new cure center in Bangkok that can house up to 3500 addicts. Although the temperature is in the 90s, the man has huddled under blankets for extra warmth.

Left and right, two views of Synanon, the revolutionary home for drug addicts established at Santa Monica, California, in 1958. There are now six Synanon communities in America, housing more than 500 ex-addicts between them. Synanon, a nonprofit-making corporation, works entirely on the principle of self-help (employing no psychiatrists or doctors) and accepts only those with a genuine desire to be cured.

there is more blood than heroin in the dropper—all this is not for nothing: it is born of a respect for the whole chemistry of alienation. When a man fixes he is turned on almost instantaneously . . . you can speak of a flash, a tinily murmured orgasm in the bloodstream, in the central nervous system."

Not only doctors, of course, are dismissive of psychological interpretations of drug addiction. Many articulate addicts or ex-addicts not unnaturally resent being thought of as stunted personalities, and would naïvely attribute drug addiction to external physical causes. William Burroughs wrote in *The New Statesman* of March 4, 1966: "Addiction is an illness of exposure. By and large, those become addicts who have access to junk. In Iran where opium was sold openly in shops they had three million addicts. There is no more a pre-addict personality than there is a pre-malarial personality despite all the hogwash of psychiatry to the contrary."

Believing that psychiatry is so much hogwash, it is not surprising that Burroughs, like many doctors, feels aggressive toward psychotherapeutic methods of treatment. He writes: "I feel that any form of so-called psycho-therapy is strongly contraindicated for addicts. Addicts should not be led to dwell on or relive the addict experience since this conduces to relapse. The question 'Why did you start using narcotics in the first place?' should never be asked. It is quite as irrelevant to treatment as it would be to ask a malarial patient why he went to a malarial area."

Some may be impressed by William Burroughs's arguments. He speaks, after all, with the authority of an ex-addict, and one, moreover, who has been cured by apparently physical means—by administration of apomorphine (a drug made by boiling morphine with hydrochloric

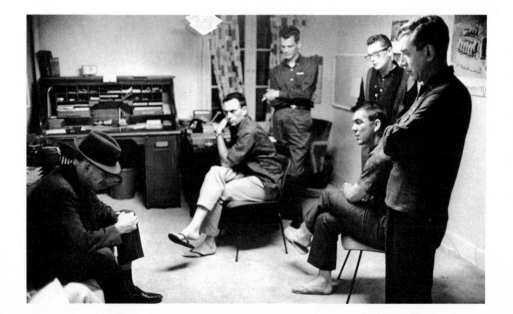

acid and whose action, physiologically, is quite different from the narcotic). There are also arguments to show that a man becomes physically—not merely psychologically—dependent on narcotics as a result of an altered metabolism. Dr. Abraham Wikler, who works at the Addiction Research Center in Lexington, Kentucky, reported at the White House Conference of 1962: "Investigations in our laboratories have yielded evidence that rats previously addicted to high daily dose levels of morphine continue to show deviations from normal rats in several respects for over 60 days following drug withdrawal. In man, also, residua of 'physical dependence' may persist for as long as 6 months after drug withdrawal."

Dr. Wikler's findings do not reduce addiction to the metabolic illness Burroughs would have us believe in, but they do confirm that there exist two components of drug addiction: the primary one is those psychological tensions that drive a man to find relief by taking narcotics (Nirvana for an addict who is "high" is not a place of active pleasure but one of no pain, no tension, no anxiety, and no distress); the secondary one is the physical dependence that follows on altered cellular metabolism. Many addicts who, like Burroughs, have been treated with apomorphine or other drugs, have (unlike Burroughs) relapsed because their psychological tensions remained and were relieved only by taking narcotics. Burroughs evidently managed by an act of will and a changed personal mental climate to overcome these tensions without resorting to the prop of narcotic drugs.

Alas, to argue that an addict needs supportive psychotherapy does not in itself solve any problems. (Most addicts take a long time to accept even simple counseling.) Israel has had a relatively enlightened policy toward its drug addicts, and at an institution at Bat Yam therapeutic activities have been directed toward physical weaning followed by brief psychotherapy and group sessions; but the final results have been disappointing. At first the Bat Yam doctors believed they had achieved a 20 per cent stable cure—a most favorable result when comparison is made with figures from other parts of the world. After 18 months the Israeli doctors still thought they had permanently cured 15 per cent of their patients. Now after 5 years they have had to admit that those who did not relapse constituted only 2–3 per cent.

Doctor Z. W. Jermulowicz, director of the Bat Yam Institute, finally concluded: "Our entire experience has taught us that the principal stress must be laid on the prevention of drug addiction since psychological weaning of drug addicts depends on so many factors that its chances of success are hardly favourable." This is a defeatist and most depressing conclusion. For prevention of drug addiction can be achieved only by preventing *all* drugs from reaching the potential addict, which seems an impossibility. In the U.S.A., for instance, vigorous and competent narcotics police squads have so far failed to wipe out the vice rings and drug pushers. Nor are they likely to succeed in the future. At least 100,000 "hard" addicts are supplied with heroin by international criminal agents, despite the harsh penalties that threaten them. There is always a back door in the night, a secret passageway, and in the shadows the narcotics are passed from hand to hand even as the sirens of the police cars fade on the air like the sound of hunting horns.

Since illegal traffic in narcotics cannot be stopped by the police authorities, the problem can be engaged in only three other ways. First, society can allow the addict to stay narcotized to his heart's content through unrestricted doctors' prescriptions. (Some doctors believe that in extreme cases the addict can be helped only by being allowed to remain chronically narcotized. They feel that, like a patient suffering from incurable cancer, he is entitled to such treatment.) Second, society can persecute the addict, hunt him down like a dangerous wild beast, and compulsorily outlaw him to prisons or special centers. Third, society can provide clinics where a favorable and compassionate ambience prevails; where the addict can receive his maintenance dose of narcotics; where he can feel that he is wanted and deserving of attention; where weaning can take place; where group and individual psychotherapy is encouraged (and for a much longer period than at Israel's Bat Yam); and where social workers, doctors, psychologists, and psychiatrists can work together with all the financial assistance they need. The alternatives are clear. None can hope to be fundamentally successful. The second alternative, though, is inhumane, and one to which a civilized society cannot be committed.

It seems likely that the British system for dealing with drug addicts will be altered in the near future and that treatment centers will be set up. If so it is to be hoped that they will have the amenities suggested above and that a permissive atmosphere will dominate. British psychiatry, frankly, is as a whole so organically orientated that the experts who will presumably staff such treatment centers may do more harm than good. The Brain Committee, which was convened to consider whether, in the light of recent experiences, the prescribing of addictive drugs by doctors needed revising, urged in 1965 the ending of independent doctors treating addicts in their consulting rooms. The Committee was alarmed by the addiction problem in Britain—which, though small, has been increasing with great pace in recent years—and recommended the setting-up of prescribing and treatment centers. The British policy of permissiveness under which

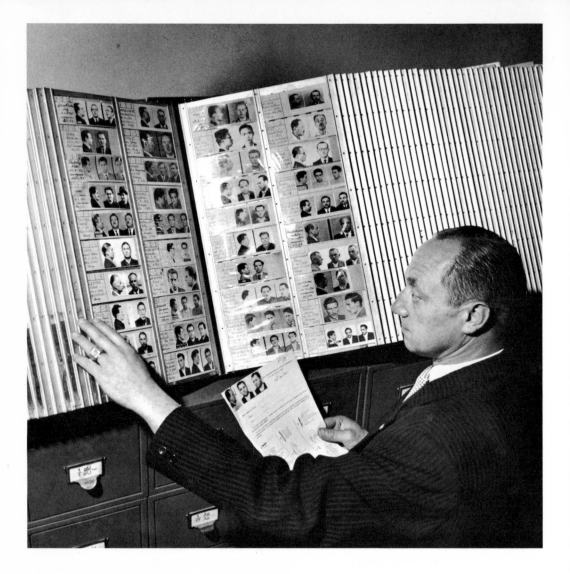

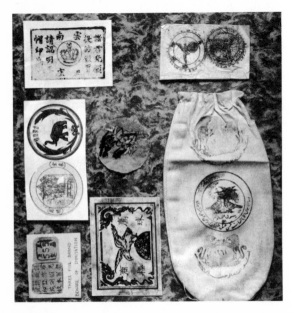

At the Interpol headquarters in Paris, detailed files are kept on all suspected traffickers (above). Despite Interpol's vigilance, the quantity of narcotics seized each year represents only some 10 per cent of the total traffic. Left, examples of the coded grading labels used by clandestine laboratories that produce heroin and morphine from illicit supplies of opium. Right, some favorite hiding places—these objects were seized by the Washington D.C. narcotics squad.

heroin could be obtained free on a National Health prescription signed by any doctor, had until recently been very successful. But some half a dozen "junkie doctors" in London have been overprescribing narcotics: one of them prescribed as much as 15 per cent of the total consumption of heroin in Britain during 1962. The Brain Committee, citing such examples of overprescription, reported: "We heard of other instances of prescriptions for considerable, if less spectacular, quantities of dangerous drugs over a long period of time. Supplies on such a scale can easily provide a surplus that will attract new recruits to the ranks of the addicts."

In Britain at present, there is certainly no significant traffic in dangerous drugs—stolen or smuggled. Because of permissive prescribing the black market price of narcotics has been kept down and illegal trafficking, by and large, has not been "worth the candle." Whether or not this state of affairs will continue depends, I imagine, on the permissiveness of those doctors who will prescribe in the new centers. A London "junkie doctor" had a point when he said, in an interview with the *Sunday Times*: "Restricting the supply won't help a bit in treating these people. It's hard enough as it is: junkies are often rather pleased when they manage to evoke authoritarian and disciplinarian responses."

The taking of narcotic drugs is not the only problem. Fashions in taking non-narcotic drugs—marihuana, purple hearts (amphetamines)—come and go in the metropolitan cities of the world. The aimless and restless young, anarchic students, and show-biz personalities become natural prey to the vendors of Drugs for Kicks. Often those taking them are misinformed about the properties of the drug in question. Thus hashish, derived from Indian hemp or cannabis (a

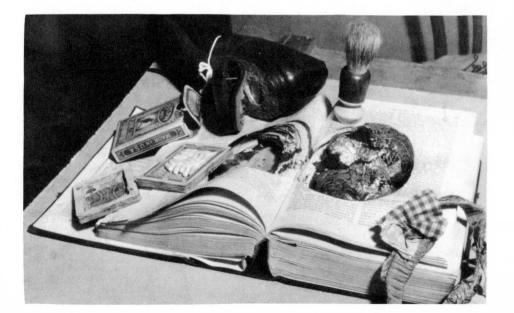

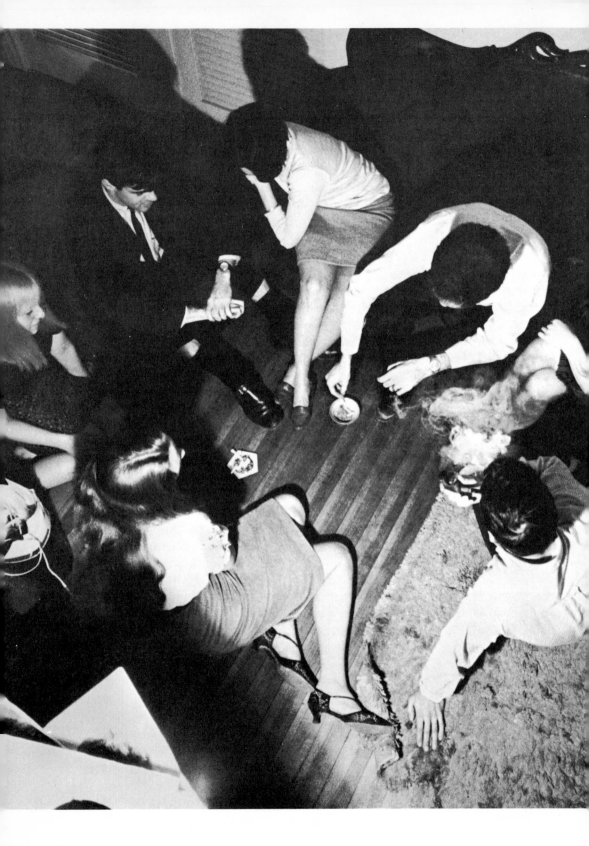

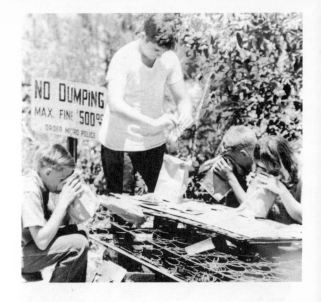

Drugs for kicks. Left, Harvard students at a marijuana party held in a Cambridge, Massachusetts, apartment. The *New York Times* has estimated that between one fifth and one half of Harvard students try marijuana at some time during their stay at Cambridge. Estimates for other American colleges are equally alarming.

Right, a glue-sniffing session held on an abandoned road south of Miami. The photograph was taken with a telephoto lens shortly before the boys' arrest by Miami Beach police.

weaker form is known as marihuana), has a reputation for being an aphrodisiac. The drug does tend to dissolve inhibitions, and for this reason it has been taken by uncertain teen-agers at petting parties. Alcohol, too, may increase the desire, only to reduce the performance. Actually, the initiate inhaling the smoke of burning cannabis (a reefer) can sometimes improve his sexual performance, achieve a more formidable erection—but often he fails to experience a rewarding orgasm. Continual use of hashish in fact leads to sexual inertia. As the 19th-century French poet Théophile Gautier wrote: "A hashish addict would not lift a finger for the most beautiful maiden in Verona." Indeed, at one time Eastern monks took hashish in order to subdue their sexual appetites.

Some notable jazz musicians have been known to smoke reefers in order to be "sent" and so improve their musical performance. Their musical ability, however, will generally deteriorate under such conditions. Hashish merely impairs the critical intelligence. In this respect it is like Benzedrine, which not uncommonly is taken by nervous students about to embark on their examinations. Answering the papers they feel they have done magnificently, whereas in fact they are likely to have written so much nonsense and accordingly fail. Their critical sense awry, they have deceived themselves.

These drugs, however, usually do no more harm than alcohol. Few become addicted in the true sense of the word, though abuse of these drugs, as with alcohol, can lead to catastrophe. Some elderly heroes of young intellectuals write dramatically of the pleasures of taking such offbeat drugs. The hallucinogenic variety—mescaline, psilocybe, and particularly the more powerful LSD—have all had their famous advocates. Thus the poet Robert Graves enthusiastically commended

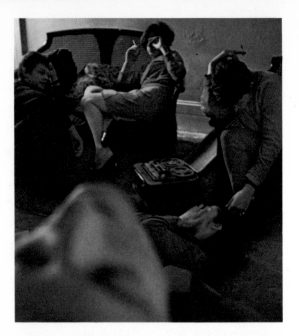

Though the indiscriminate use of LSD can lead to serious mental breakdown and disorder, the drug's "hip" image still draws young people to this kind of LSD party.

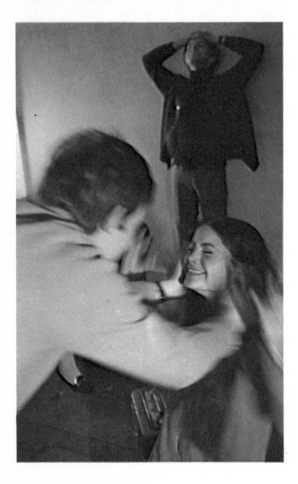

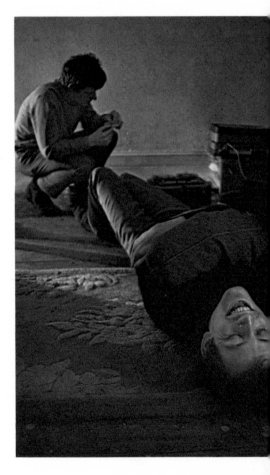

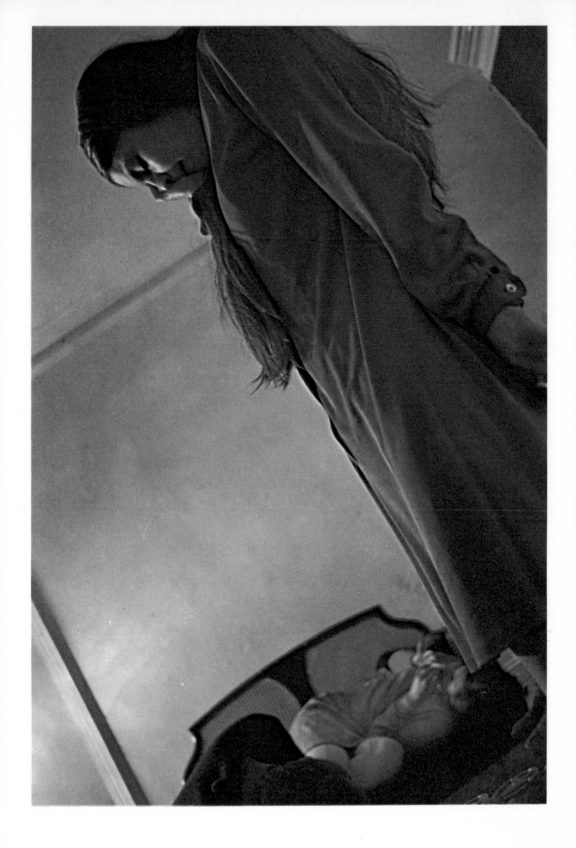

psilocybe: "Any use of hallucinogenic drugs, except for medical purposes, goes against civilised conscience; perhaps because, in this Christian world, only visions won by prayer and piety are ascribed to God, rather than the Devil. Because of my Protestant conditioning, I would never take cocaine, heroin, hashish, or marihuana, even experimentally; but the Mexican mushroom [psilocybe] does not belong to this range of drugs, nor is it habit-forming. So far from stupefying the senses, it quickens them. An experimentalist's mind will stay conscious throughout—indeed supraconscious. This peculiar virtue, of enhancing reality, turns the Greek command 'know thyself!' into a practical precept; psilocybe illuminates the mind, re-educates sight and hearing."

Such claims for psilocybe are romantic and exaggerated. In the same article, *A Journey to Paradise*, Robert Graves describes a session in which he took the drug:

"I reached for a notebook and wrote: *9 p.m. Visions of . . .* but got no further: things were happening too fast. Besides, the pen felt strange in my hand, and its scratch on paper sounded offensively loud. After a while I remember saying, 'I have seen enough treasure for a lifetime. Is there no human beauty in Paradise?' At once the diadems, tiaras, necklaces, crosses, and sceptres vanished, as the demons had done. Instead, a row of lovely, live, naked caryatids appeared, lined along the wall, as if supporting the dome. Their faces were shrouded. Yet I hesitated to indulge in erotic fancies, lest the caryatids turned into filthy, deformed devilkins like the ones in Flemish pictures of St. Anthony's Temptations. Blushing, I dismissed them, too, and emerged from the tunnel into daylight.

"Around me lay a mountain-top Eden, with its jewel-bright trees, its flowers, and its pellucid streams. And I experienced not only the bliss of innocence, but also 'the knowledge of good and evil'. . . .

"Indeed, my mind suddenly became so agile and unfettered that I felt capable of solving any problem in the world; it was as if I had immediate access to all knowledge everywhere. But the sensation of wisdom sufficed—why should I trouble to exploit it? . . .

"An unseen voice began singing. I rejoiced that it was a woman's. . . .

"I fell wholly under her spell, and presently enjoyed the curious experience of *seeing* sound. The song-notes became intricate links of a round golden chain that coiled and looped in serpentine fashion among jade-green bushes: the only serpent I saw in Eden. . . .

"Each song was followed by a pause, and always I waited in a lover's agony for her to begin again. Once she seemed to sing off key. Perhaps this was quarter-tone music; I saw one edge of the golden chain formed by the sound spread out into a spectrum, and laughed for pleasure. Towards the end came a quick, breathless, cheerful song of creation and growth. The notes fell to earth but rose once more in green shoots which soared swiftly up, putting on branches, leaves, flowers, until it dominated the sky.

"My spirit followed after into the clear blue air, gazing down on cornfields, fields of poppies, and the spires of a heavenly city. . . .

"At last the music came to an end. The visions were fading now. My corporeal self sighed, stretched luxuriously, and looked around. Most of the company had left the room. . . .

"At two o'clock in the morning we said goodbye. By eight I was on my way to Idlewild, headed for Europe: profoundly refreshed and, in Wordsworth's phrase, trailing clouds of glory—wisps of celestial memory which persisted nearly a month."

I must say that I have had more interesting dreams than that, and certainly less Wordsworthian ones, without the assistance of any hallucinogenic drug. I imagine others also have had equally pleasurable night visions in the most exciting technicolor. To eat cheese at night, however, is obviously much more mundane than taking psilocybe or mescaline to break down the doors of perception.

Another "star" glamorous to the young—Cary Grant—sings the praises of LSD: "I take it as a short cut to the subconscious. You don't become addicted to it. Once it has shown you the way to meditation and the subconscious you can cut it out. I began using it because I wanted to find out more about myself. It has given me a stauncher belief in God. People ask why I don't try religion. I wish I could but I wasn't brought up to it. This is my short route to the kind of thing experienced by the religious mystic."

But, as I have indicated in an earlier chapter, the indiscriminate use of LSD is a grave matter. It is a most powerful chemical agent, capable of inducing permanent mental changes and leading to nervous breakdown and suicide. Nevertheless there is a flourishing black market in LSD, particularly on college campuses in the U.S.A. It seems that LSD has largely replaced barbiturates and pep pills in those circles that think it smart to be "hung" on one of the non-narcotic drugs. It has been estimated that as many as 10,000 students at the University of California have taken LSD at least once. No wonder sensational incidents are reported in the popular press following the taking of LSD. Thus, one American student took the drug at a secluded beach and, believing that he could walk on water, was found floating in the Pacific. Again, as a jet airliner took off from Los Angeles one of the 120 passengers suddenly went berserk and tried to break into the pilot's compartment; later it required four policemen to subdue him. He had taken LSD. Finally, let me conclude this short catalog by quoting a recent report from an evening newspaper. The headlines read: MAN KILLED UNDER LSD INFLUENCE SAY POLICE. Then followed: "New York, Tuesday—A man has been charged here with the murder of his mother-in-law while under the influence of LSD, the hallucinatory drug. Police claim that when they went to 30 year old Stephen Kessler's home he was just coming round from the effects of the drug. He asked them: 'Did I kill my wife? Did I rape anybody? What have I done?' What he did, they said, was to go to the home of his wife's parents in Brooklyn, where she had returned, and stabbed her 57 year old mother. Police quoted Kessler as saying: 'Man, I've been flying for three days on LSD. I'm high. I'm really high."

No doubt LSD will soon be replaced as the in-drug by another—it is to be hoped by a less dangerous one. Meanwhile it behoves the heroes of the young to be responsible and cautionary about the effects of any particular drug, be they film stars, pop singers, or poets. It seems some people need very little encouragement to try any drug for the hell of it, and certain people become "addicted" to anything. On January 22, 1966, *The British Medical Journal* reported the case of a young motor mechanic who accidentally drank some gasoline while siphoning a tank. Subsequently this 17-year-old—who, by the way, was of superior intelligence—took a liter of gasoline a week for a period of almost three years. He either drank it straight, or soaked a wad in it and inhaled the fumes, to become oblivious of everything else. It only needs some folk hero to write articles on how he was a teen-age gasoline inhaler to set the campuses alight in more senses than one. I hastily add here that the young mechanic was eventually admitted to hospital suffering from peripheral neuritis. The gasoline had so affected his nerves that he suffered from "floppy feet" and could not move his legs easily. He also began to experience progressive weakness of both arms. At hospital he was cured of his "addiction" but it took some eight months before his neuritis finally cleared up and he was free of all symptoms.

To drink gasoline may seem to most of us ridiculous: to gulp down alcohol, sublime. Certainly alcohol (in the West anyway) is consumed year in, year out—a habit independent of fashionable whims. Yet alcohol is a drug, and like almost all drugs will act as a poison when taken in excess, or over a long period. In Britain it is the fourth largest cause of premature death. In the U.S.A. alcoholism is next only to heart disease and cancer in disease incidence. In Czechoslovakia two per cent of the total population are alcoholics. (Czechoslovakia is one of the few Iron Curtain countries where figures on alcoholism have been published.) The prevalence of alcoholism in Europe and the Americas

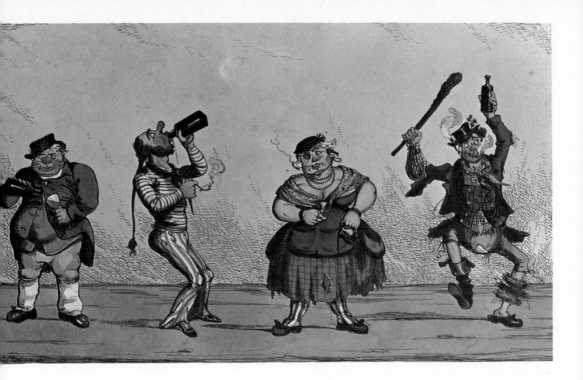

Above, an early-19th-century caricature, *The Comforts of Life*, showing (from left to right) Brandy, Rum, Gin, Whisky.

Below a shared moment of oblivion for two Harlem drunks—under one roof for the night at a home for vagrants.

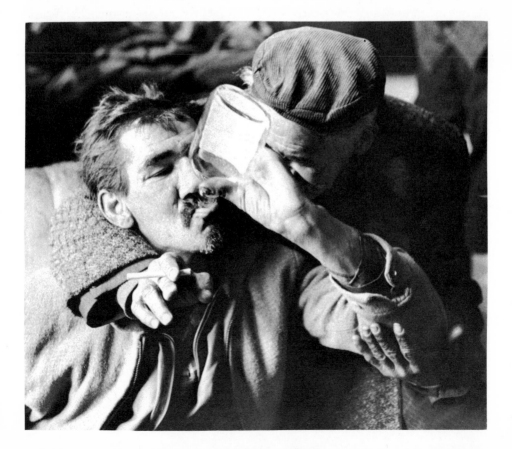

is altogether more marked than narcotic addiction. The following comparative statistical table of adult alcoholics per 100,000 people in various countries as given by Robert E. Popham *et al.* in 1958 is instructive:

|  | Alcoholics per 100,000 popn. (20 years and over) | Year |
|---|---|---|
| France | 5200 | 1945 |
| U.S.A. | 4360 | 1955 |
| Chile | 2960 | 1950 |
| Sweden | 2580 | 1946 |
| Switzerland | 2100 | 1953 |
| Denmark | 1950 | 1948 |
| Canada | 1890 | 1956 |
| Norway | 1560 | 1947 |
| Finland | 1430 | 1947 |
| Australia | 1340 | 1947 |
| England and Wales | 1100 | 1948 |
| Italy | 700 | 1954 |

Though these estimates have been made at different dates, Popham's table does reveal the gravity of the problem. The numbers of those addicted to narcotics seem trivial in comparison. In West Germany there are only 4374 *known* narcotic addicts (618 of whom are doctors); in Italy a few hundred; in Switzerland and France about 100 each.

Despite the great disparity between the numbers dependent on alcohol in the West and those addicted to narcotics, the press search-lights seem to be directed almost exclusively on the latter. The public tends to think of a drinker as a hearty he-man and the drunkard as a boring sot, quite without the fascination of a narcotics addict. Perhaps this is simply because alcoholics are numerically so commonplace.

At one time, however, writers waxed ecstatic about alcohol rather as Aldous Huxley and Robert Graves have in their descriptions of the hallucinogens. Thus the Roman poet Horace (65–8 B.C.) wrote: "What wonders does not wine! It discloses secrets; ratifies and confirms our hopes; thrusts the coward forth to battle; eases the anxious mind of its burden; instructs in art. Whom has not a cheerful glass made eloquent; whom not quite free and easy from pinching poverty." Nowadays, more people are likely to curse the excesses of alcohol than sing its praises. For when a person becomes dependent on that liquid drug, misery and unhappiness follow behind him like a shadow. Karl Menninger has defined alcoholic addiction as "a form of self-destruction used to avert a greater self-destruction, deriving from elements of aggressiveness excited by thwarting, ungratified eroticism, and the feeling of a need for punishment from a sense of guilt relative to the aggressiveness." This definition, of course, implies that alcohol dependence is basically a result of the alcoholic's personality disturbances. (The American Medical Association defines alcoholism more simply as ". . . a disease which is characterized by compulsive drinking of alcohol in some form. It is an addiction to alcohol. The drinking of alcohol produces continuing or repeated problems in the patient's life.")

The personality of the chronic alcoholic tends to exhibit certain traits. He or she is an individual who may be sexually fixated, to a large degree, at the oral stage, and who is likely to own unconscious doubts regarding his or her sexual identity. It is not for nothing that alcohol has been described flippantly as "the adult's mother's milk." In 1942, H. Duchêne and his colleagues showed how statistically significant numbers of male alcoholics were married to women older than themselves.

Freud maintained that alcoholism can be a substitute for repressed homosexuality—an opinion that appals many alcoholics whose unconscious fear of their own latent homosexuality often drives them to condemn homosexuals with a particular venom. It is surely true that men like to drink together, and "legitimate" emotional bonds do form between such male drinkers. A non-drinker among such a group becomes suspect—he is not "one of the boys"; after all, he may even prefer to play with one of the girls! Karl Abraham, a pupil of Freud, believed that the alcoholic's homosexual tendencies derived from the time when, as an infant, he was frustrated by a withdrawn mother and so became over-identified with his father. Abraham also related alcoholism to those fetishes where precoital play of a curious kind becomes more pleasurable and significant than the actual sexual act itself, the forepleasure of the alcoholic being obtained at his fixated oral level.

The analytical approach may be disputed by some and resented by many, but all will surely agree with Menninger's concept of alcoholism as a form of chronic suicide. For, apart from the alcoholic's original character defects, alcohol itself leads to secondary personality changes. Further, alcohol dependence poisons the body, organ by organ. It leads to chronic gastritis, and ulceration may occur that could require surgery; it leads to cirrhosis of the liver, which eventually can be a cause of death; it leads to kidney and heart damage, which may finally result in kidney or heart failure; and it leads to death of the brain cells, along with poisoning of the peripheral nervous system. In

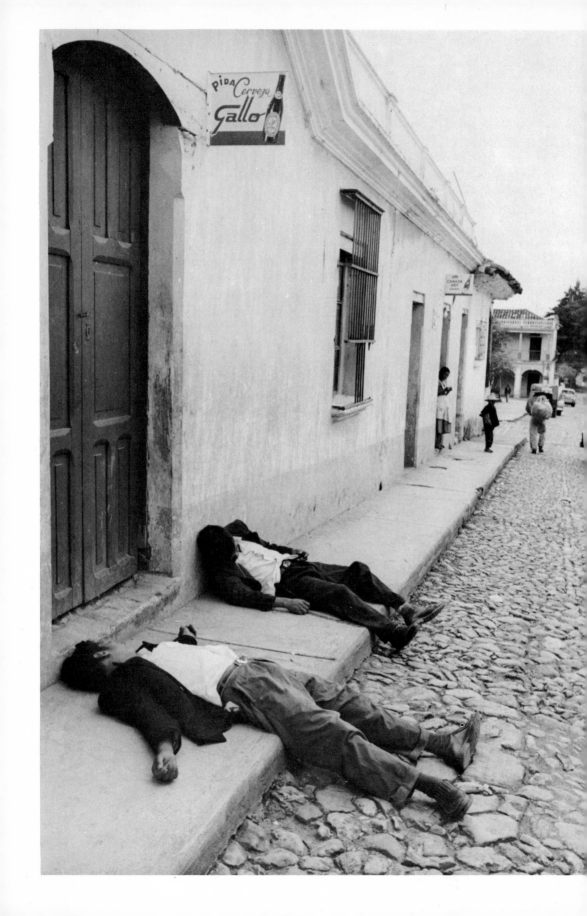

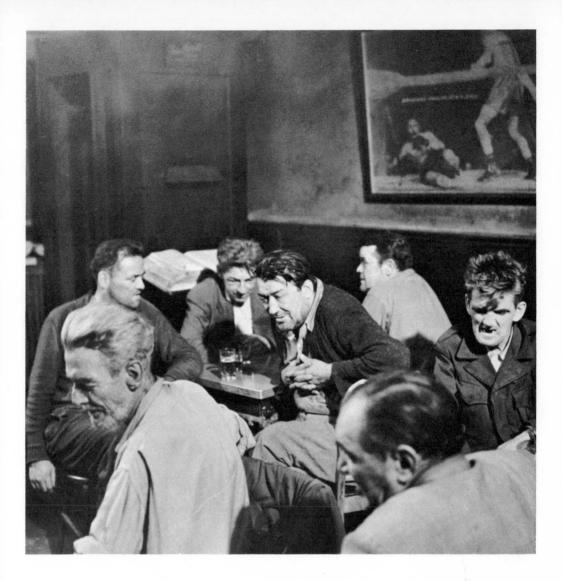

Left, afternoon scene in a Mexican street. Above, a bar on the notorious Bowery in Lower New York City, formerly the haunt of the city's derelicts and alcoholics.

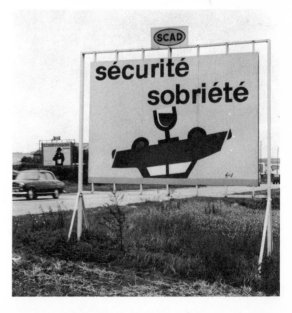

Right, a roadside poster put out by the French government in its campaign to curb drinking—especially wine-drinking.

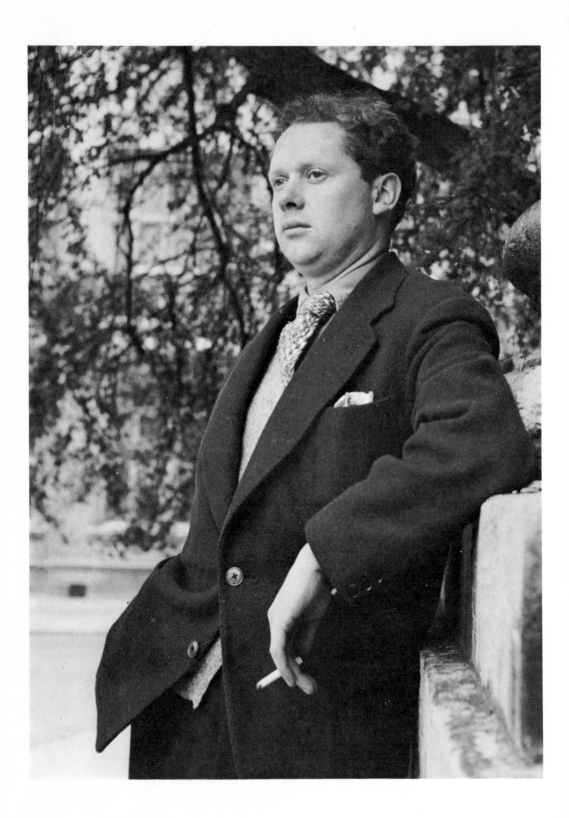

short, the common remark that this or that person "is drinking himself to death" has an all too real basis. One thinks of the sad death of the poet Dylan Thomas after his performance of *Under Milk Wood* at the Poetry Center in New York in 1953. Constantine Fitzgibbon writes, in *The Life of Dylan Thomas*:

"In New York Liz Reitell took charge of him, and immediately the rehearsals of the new and, as death willed, final version of *Under Milk Wood* began. The strain on Dylan was too great. Drink no longer helped, and he was in a state of near collapse. Liz Reitell arranged that her doctor give him an injection of ACTH (a cortisone-type drug) which briefly pulled him together and enabled him to go on at the Poetry Center. This was then a comparatively new drug, the effects of which were not fully understood. The doctor did warn Dylan against drinking after this injection, but it must have been obvious that Dylan would go on drinking. The combination of alcohol and ACTH can be, I am told, poisonous. He was also taking sleeping pills. It has been said that certain of his friends were giving him pep pills as well. Nevertheless, as John Malcolm Brinnin's account in *Dylan Thomas in America* shows, he struggled on. He managed to do the Milk Wood performance, and one reading, and then, on November 3rd, he collapsed.

"At 2 a.m. on November 4th he struggled from his bed and despite Liz Reitell's protests insisted that he must go out and have a drink. She did not go with him. After an hour and a half, according to her account, he returned and said laconically: 'I've had eighteen straight whiskies. I think that's the record.' This characteristic remark was certainly untrue. Within a matter of weeks his friend Ruthven Todd and Stuart Thomas, a Swansea lawyer, checked on those ninety minutes. He had had perhaps four or five whiskies; eighteen would have killed him outright. But even this was enough to undo him.

"Next morning the doctor was summoned again, and another injection of ACTH administered. (One of the noxious qualities of this drug is that it may make the patient highly liable to any sort of infection. It does decrease strain, however, which is presumably why it was administered.) That afternoon when he had awoken from a troubled sleep, he developed delirium tremens. Again the doctor was summoned. Yet another injection was given, which Brinnin describes simply as a sedative: I am told—though not by the doctor in question, for he does not reply to questions on this subject—that it was morphine. Within a matter of hours Dylan was transferred to St. Vincent's Hospital in a coma and an urgent message was sent to Caitlin [Thomas's wife] to come to the hospital immediately. He never recovered consciousness, and died on November 9th. (The doctor does

The poet Dylan Thomas, photographed at Laugharne, South Wales (where he is now buried), seven years before his death.

not appear to have been summoned at once and the hospital authorities were thus initially in ignorance of the various injections that had been previously administered.) The terminal cause of death was pneumonia, which he contracted while in coma. According to his autopsy the cause of his death was: 'Insult to the brain', a phrase equally meaningless in British and in American medical parlance.

"He was brought back to Wales, and his body lies buried in Laugharne."

Apart from the individual tragedies consequent on alcoholism, this disease also has wide social implications. An estimated 10 per cent of all suicide attempts each year result from chronic alcoholism, and although it is impossible to give the figures of automobile accidents attributable to drinking, these too must constitute a high percentage. In Britain, 25 per cent of family separations are due to alcoholism. In the U.S.A. drunkenness represents more than 40 per cent of all police arrests.

The problem is complicated by the fact that it is not easy to persuade an alcoholic to undergo treatment—at least not until he "hits bottom." Often he will deny he is ill, and lacking insight will become defiantly aggressive. Only four per cent of alcoholics are likely to recover without treatment. So despite the difficulties, it is imperative for the doctor to convince his patient that he is an alcoholic. Only then can he refer him to a special clinic (if there is one available), to a psychotherapist (recently some have reported an encouraging cure rate with the use of LSD), or to a body such as Alcoholics Anonymous (AA claims that the sobriety rate of its members exceeds 50 per cent). Too many general physicians, though—whether American, Russian, or European—think of alcoholics as criminal delinquents rather than as patients desperately ill. Generally they will think of referring them for treatment only if they are suffering from such physical complications of the disease as polyneuritis or delirium tremens. They do not, or will not, think of Skid Row as an open-air sick ward without nurses and without doctors. Too many nations, East and West of the Curtain, have barely repressed punitive attitudes toward their alcoholics. Sadly their doctors for the most part share the prejudice and indifference of the general population and the governmental representatives. Just as the alcoholic involuntarily fails his family, his friends, his employers, and himself, too often his doctor, because of wrong moral attitudes, ultimately fails him.

One cannot conclude a chapter entitled *The Addicts* without some brief reference to tobacco smoking. For, though some would not classify smoking as an addiction, it is, all the same, more habit-

A Russian anti-smoking poster links cigarette smoking, illness (cancer in particular), and death.

forming than drinking alcohol. Tobacco can take such a hold of a person that the relationship of the smoker to his cigarettes compared with that of a drug addict to narcotics is a quantitative rather than a qualitative one. In 1952, L. M. Johnston reported in *The Lancet* that the cravings of chronic smokers can be satisfied by injections of nicotine. Apart from any psychological factors involved, then, it would seem that smokers become pharmacologically dependent on their tobacco consumption.

The degree of dependence on cigarette smoking in Western communities can be gauged by the attitude of semistarving nations in World War II and the priority of their needs between food and tobacco. As Dr. C. Van Proosdy points out in his book *Smoking*: "By plundering food and vehicles in '44–'45, the Germans in occupied Holland brought complete starvation and want to Dutch cities; [nevertheless] there were many among the holders of allotments who preferred to grow tobacco for their own use rather than vegetables and other foodstuffs. Even in concentration camps, where a crust of bread

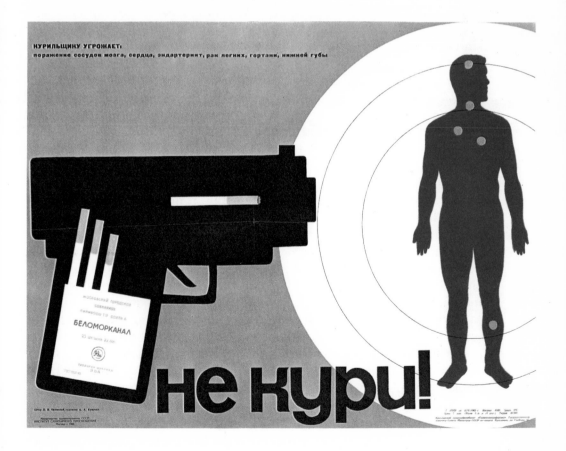

might have decided between life and death, food was repeatedly exchanged for cigarettes."

Dr. Van Proosdy, like others, also speaks of the use of tobacco "as offering a means of partial escape from reality." Now I happen to be a chronic cigarette smoker myself and this judgment does not tally with my own experience. On the contrary, as long as I have access to cigarettes I can face up to reality. If I feel a need to smoke and there are no cigarettes at hand, my craving preoccupies consciousness to such an extent that "reality" is partially blotted out. I agree with one opinion expressed at a conference at Birmingham University in 1958: "An addict has to smoke before he is up to what he recognises as his best mental efficiency." Those who do not smoke cannot understand the smoker's weak dependence on tobacco. With Ben Jonson they feel: "Ods me, I marvel what pleasure or felicity they have in taking their roguish tobacco. It is good for nothing but to choke a man, and fill him full of smoke and embers." Perhaps only by thinking of tobacco smoking as an addiction rather than as a bad habit can nonsmokers begin to understand the difficulties confronting any person trying to give up his "vice."

It has been suggested that those who smoke may have a different kind of personality from those who do not. Some psychoanalysts have discussed the unconscious drives that turn a person into a heavy smoker. As long ago as 1921, A. Starke wrote in *The International Journal of Psychoanalysis* that the pleasure of smoking was an oral one, and he stressed the connection between smoking and the smoker's early deprivation of the maternal breast. Later, other analysts commented on the compulsive characteristics of the smoker, and his unconscious desire to set things alight. That smoking gratifies some basic oral need seems to be borne out by the fact that as many as one third of ex-smokers gain weight. It seems that they find it necessary to eat more—to put things into their mouth; but sometimes the gain in weight is only a transitory phenomenon.

Nowadays more and more people are trying to give up smoking. For though tobacco was introduced to Europe in the 16th century, only recently has scientific evidence been put forward to implicate smoking in the etiology of serious diseases. Multiple statistical surveys carried out in several countries reveal that more lung cancer patients smoke than do not. Prospective studies have indicated that the death rate from lung cancer increases steeply with an increased consumption of cigarettes. It seems that substances other than nicotine in cigarette smoke—the polynuclear hydrocarbons and some radioactive isotopes of polonium—are carcinogenic. Arsenic, too, has been identified in tobacco smoke, but to a lesser extent since tobacco plantations reduced the quantity of arsenical insecticides they were using. Tar condensed from tobacco smoke has been applied to the skin of mice, and skin cancer has resulted. On the other hand, despite intensive experimentation, animals made to inhale tobacco smoke continually have not produced any lung cancers.

The chronic smoker may also receive some slight solace from one or two other paradoxical facts. Lung cancer occurs in only a minority of smokers. Again, the death rate from lung cancer in some countries—for instance in the U.S.A., Japan, and White South Africa—does not correspond with the degree of cigarette consumption of these respective populations. Finally, the question of inhaling cigarette smoke and its relationship to lung cancer seems odd. A recent French survey showed that inhaling seemed to increase the liability of light smokers to lung cancer but not so evidently that of heavy smokers.

It would appear, then, that smoking is not the only causal factor in lung cancer. H. J. Eysenck has put forward the hypothesis that persons constitutionally predisposed to smoke are also constitutionally predisposed to develop cancer. In his book *Smoking, Health and Personality* Dr. Eysenck presents evidence to show that those who are extroverted are more likely both to smoke cigarettes and to suffer lung cancer than those endowed with an introverted temperament.

In the 16th century, tobacco was considered to be a cure-all. Its leaves were applied to wounds and its smoke was blown up the rectum. Nowadays, it is known that cigarette smokers are more likely to suffer not only from lung cancer but also from various other diseases. These include chronic bronchitis and coronary heart disease. Since, statistically, it seems that over the next 10 years the chance of a 35-year-old cigarette smoker dying is 1 in 23 compared with the non-smoker's 1 in 90, clearly it is a doctor's duty to recommend that his patients give up smoking. If I light a cigarette myself, even as I conclude this chapter, I can only say to the smoker, without flippancy, "Don't do as I do: do as I tell you."

# 7 Drugs Have Made Us Old

Thanks to the success of vaccines, antibiotics, and other drugs (together with the social advances in hygiene and housing, etc.), more people are now living out their potential life span than was the case even a decade or so ago. In Great Britain alone, the proportion of people over the age of 70 has increased from 1 in 36 in 1891 to 1 in 15 in 1955 and 1 in 13 in 1964; by 1975 the proportion is expected to be as high as 1 in 7. In the United States the proportion has increased in the last 10 years from 1 in 19 to 1 in 16. Civilized communities are becoming old; and with the probability of more revolutionary drugs being discovered soon to combat the present "incurable" diseases, such societies are liable to become even more aged.

But, accidents and drugs aside, what is the possible life span of any one human being? The world champion of *authenticated* longevity is still Pierre Joubert of Quebec, who died at the age of 113 years 124 days in 1814, and whose records were officially investigated by the Canadian government in 1870. There have been many other pretenders to the title, however. In the first century A.D. the Roman scholar Pliny recorded that in the city of Parma there were two individuals of 130 years of age and three of 120. Asclepiades, a Greek physician who practiced in Rome in the second century A.D., is

A 16th-century conception of *The Fountain of Youth,* by the German painter Lucas Cranach. While the secret of eternal youth remains elusive, more and more people are living out their potential life span—a problem that now challenges scientists and sociologists in a very real way.

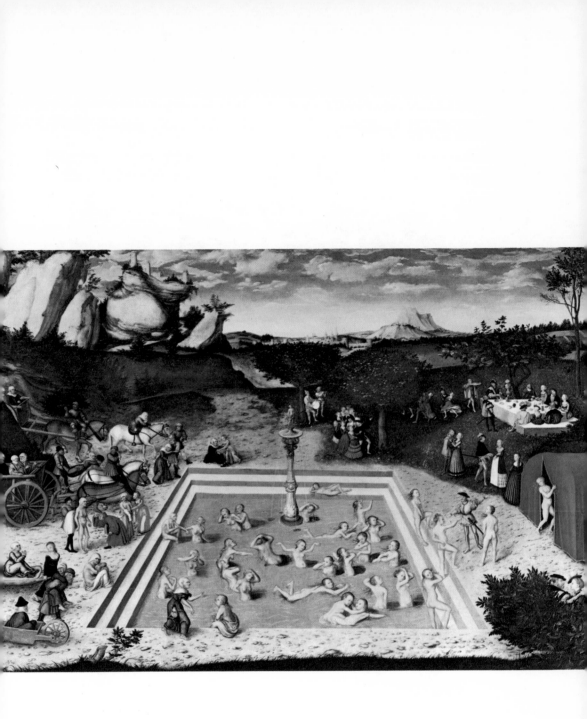

233

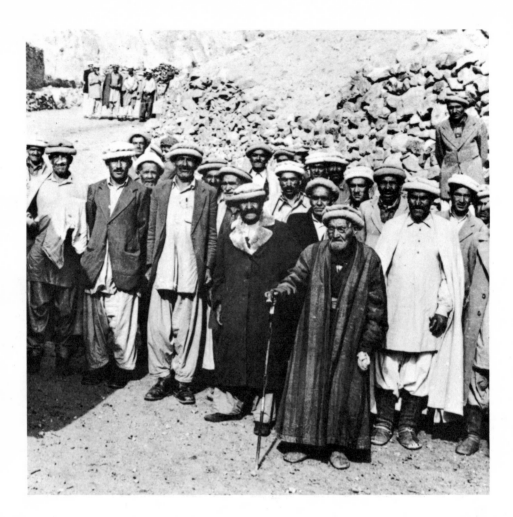

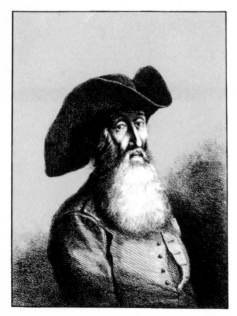

Above, some of the aged inhabitants of Hunza (in northwest Kashmir) photographed at the end of a five-mile walk; the man in the foreground claims to be 118 years old. The clue to the exceptionally long, disease-free lives of these people is supposed to lie in the very rich mineral content of the local water they drink. Left, a contemporary portrait of Henry Jenkins, the Yorkshire fisherman who died in 1670—allegedly at the age of 169. The conflicting stories and birth dates produced by Jenkins during his lifetime leave little doubt that he was a fraud.

Right, a graph comparing recent life expectancy figures in various countries with the corresponding figures of about 30 years earlier. The upper (lighter) lines represent the figures for men; the lower ones, the figures for women.

reputed to have reached 150 before being killed by a fall down some stairs. And what of the Cretan prophet and diviner Epimenides who, according to the historian Theopompus, lived to 157?

"In Bengal there was once upon a time a certain peasant who reached the age of 335," records John Henry Cohausen, an 18th-century German writer. Indeed, in his book *Hermippus Redivivus, or The Sage's Triumph over Old Age and the Grave*, Cohausen lists a number of candidates for the old age stakes. There was "one Marcus Apponius, who was 150. Vincent Coquelin, a Clergyman, died at Paris in 1664, at 112. Lawrence Hutland lived in the Orkneys to 170. James Sands, an Englishman, towards the latter End of the last Century, died at 140, and his wife at 120. . . ." More recently (in November 1965) the British writer Noel Barber described on BBC radio a visit to the state of Hunza, on the northwest frontier of Kashmir—supposedly the original Shangri-La of James Hilton's famous novel *Lost Horizon*. "Here," he said, "every man has his patch of ground on which he tends sheep or cattle—and grows two or three crops a year of fruit and vegetables—not for a short life span of three score years and ten, but often for 100 years or more. . . . I talked to one man of 118 who had just returned from a five-mile walk. I went to the christening of a newborn son while his father of eighty-nine stood by chuckling."

Whatever the claims of the Methuselahs from past or present centuries the fact remains—in the "developed" countries anyway—that while more and more people join the aged legions, the *potential* life span of human kind remains basically the biblical three score years and ten: it has not itself been greatly raised by the discovery of modern "miracle" drugs—though the average *life expectancy* has. This increase in life expectancy, of course, is in part due to the *decrease*

| Selected Countries | Period | Life Expectation at Birth (Years) |
|---|---|---|
| England and Wales | 1930-32 | 58.74 |
| | 1960-62 | 62.88 / 68.0 / 74.0 |
| France | 1933-38 | 55.9 / 61.6 |
| | 1962 | 67.96 / 74.5 |
| India | 1921-30 | 26.91 / 26.56 |
| | 1957-58 | 45.23 / 46.57 |
| Italy | 1930-32 | 53.76 / 56.0 |
| | 1954-57 | 65.7 / 70.0 |
| Japan | 1926-30 | 44.82 / 46.54 |
| | 1962 | 66.23 / 71.16 |
| New Zealand | 1934-38 | 65.46 / 68.45 |
| | 1955-57 | 68.2 / 73.0 |
| United States of America | 1939-41 | 61.6 / 65.89 |
| | 1962 | 66.8 / 73.4 |

in infant mortality, which has been dramatic. In the United States, for example, the infant mortality per 1000 live births in 1961 was 25.3, compared with 74 per 1000 in the years 1921–25. This compares strikingly with the corresponding figure for India, which in 1961 was still 83.1 per 1000 live births.

It would seem, then, that revolutionary thinking is required to deal with the increasing problem of aging communities. The plight of old, solitary people is no longer an idiosyncratic one. It is not chance that, of late, the social problems of the old have been aired increasingly in films, television plays, and novels. In an Italian film like *Umberto D.*, which depicts the isolation of an old man, or an American television play like *Holiday Song* by Paddy Chayevsky, which outlines the alienation of an old person from his family, or a novel like *Memento Mori* by the British writer Muriel Spark, which exhibits the proximity of death for a group of octogenarians, the problems of the aged are more graphically brought home to society at large than by thousands of statistical tables.

The training of medical students the world over, though, is not attuned to the present problems—medical or social—of the aged in the community. The needs for a different education are all the more pressing since increasing infirmity is to be expected with the advent of old age, and general practitioners will have to deal with larger and larger numbers of the aged. Obviously, the health of the elderly is more delicate than that of the young; nor is illness in the elderly so easily recognizable—it is often confused with the basic aging process. Few medical phenomena are more striking than the apparent rejuvenation of an old patient after successful therapy of a previously unrecognized ailment.

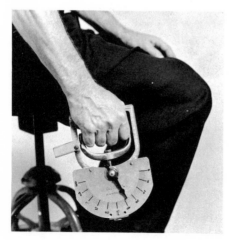
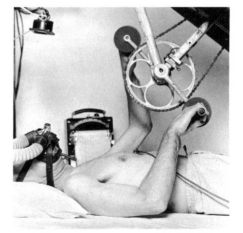

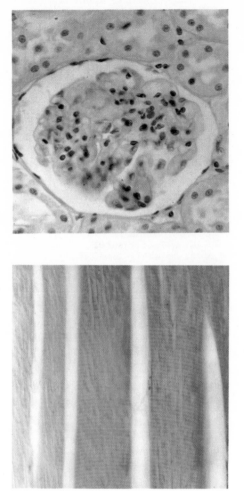

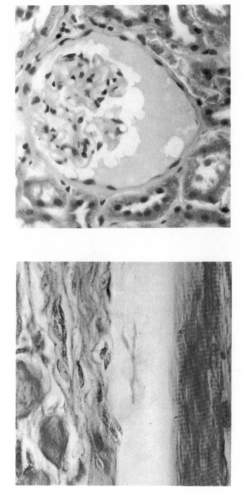

In 1958 the gerontology branch of the Baltimore City Hospital, in the U.S.A., initiated a 20-year study on 400 men of various ages. Such attempts to chart the aging process scientifically are a relatively new aspect of 20th-century medicine. Two of the experiments to test working ability are shown on the left-hand page. Far left, the function of various muscles is isolated and observed in a test of grip strength. Left, a subject breathes into a face mask (to record oxygen consumption) while turning the crank of an ergonometer.

The four microphotographs above show the effects of aging on the kidney and leg muscles of the rat. Top left, a section through the kidney of a normal adult rat; top right, the atrophied kidney of a senile rat. The kidney's reduced efficiency with age affects the blood flow and processing of body wastes. Lower left, a section through the leg muscles of a normal adult rat, as compared with those of a senile rat (lower right). The deterioration of muscle fibers and their replacement by connective tissue largely accounts for the physical weakness of the aged.

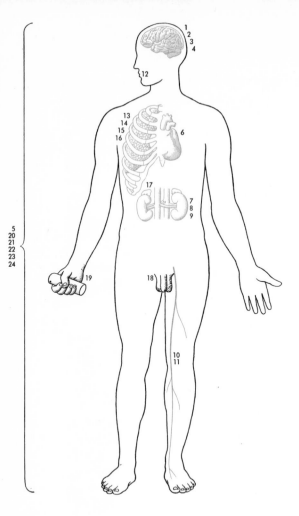

1 Brain weight 56%
2 Memory loss
3 Slower speed of response
4 Blood flow to brain 80%
5 Spread of return to equilibrium
of blood acidity 17%
6 Cardiac output (at rest) 70%
7 Number of glomeruli in kidney 56%
8 Filtration rate of kidney 69%
9 Kidney plasma flow 50%
10 Number of nerve trunk fibres 63%
11 Nerve conduction velocity 90%
12 Number of taste buds 36%
13 Maximum oxygen uptake
(during exercise) 40%
14 Maximum ventilation volume
(during exercise) 53%
15 Maximum breathing capacity
(voluntary) 43%
16 Vital capacity of lungs 56%
17 Less adrenal activity
18 Less gonadal activity
19 Hand grip 55%
20 Maximum work rate 70%
21 Maximum work rate
for short burst 40%
22 Basal metabolic rate 84%
23 Body water content 82%
24 Body weight for males 88%

Left, a diagram indicates the decline in
efficiency of various parts of the human
body in the average 75-year-old man: the
percentages in the key (above) indicate
the approximate degree of function or
tissue remaining, taking 100 per cent
as the norm for a 30-year-old man. The
graphs (below) compare percentage decline
with age in nine different physiological
functions—again taking 100 per cent as
the norm at the age of 30.

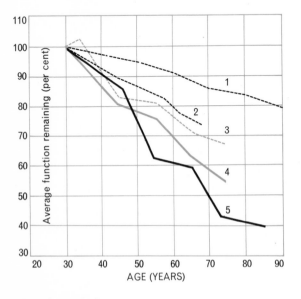

1 Basal metabolic rate
2 Maximum work rate
3 Cardiac output (at rest)
4 Vital capacity of lungs
5 Maximum breathing capacity (voluntary)

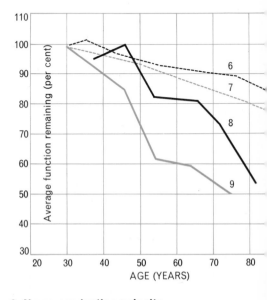

6 Nerve conduction velocity
7 Body water content
8 Filtration rate of kidney
9 Kidney plasma flow

The physical process of aging is complicated and varied, and not always measurable. But certain physical processes, discomforts, and conditions *are* common to old age, and these can be observed. There is, for example, a tendency for bones to become decalcified, and for calcium to be deposited in arteries, in scar tissues, and elsewhere. Atrophy of cells often occurs because of a decreasing blood supply to the tissues. Blood pressure rises as age advances. Old people are likely to experience a degree of deafness or poor sight. Arthritis, painful feet, bronchitis, and urinary disorders are also common afflictions. And it is interesting to observe that the physical deficiencies of the aging process are apparent earlier in men than in women.

Apart from physical illness, mental disturbances—depression, loss of memory, disorientation, apathy, etc.—are common in the elderly. These disturbances may result from a combination of organic, pyschological, and environmental factors. They cannot be treated successfully by drugs alone. True, the introduction of tranquilizers and sedatives helps in the management of the elderly; as a result many can be treated at home instead of in hospital. Yet old people do not show a common response to such drugs. And doctors do not always seem aware that there are special dangers in the administration of tranquilizers to the elderly: basal pneumonia is only one of the many complications that may follow a spell in bed induced by tranquilizers.

But for even the wisest and most sensitive doctor to carry out his duties effectively, the aid of an efficient domiciliary service of nurses, home helps, and night attendants is essential—as is the total co-operation of local authorities, who can help not only in the matter of housing but also by promoting group activities among the old, perhaps through voluntary services, to combat their natural feelings of isolation. Too many of us—relations, friends, neighbors—do not want the increased responsibility of supporting old people in our midst. Yet if old people are deprived of the sense of being useful and wanted they lose their self-esteem. This leads to rapid mental deterioration. And since many young and middle-aged people do find an older person living with them an intolerable burden, resentment builds up until they secretly wish grandmother or grandfather be put away. Perhaps Baudelaire only exaggerated a little when he wrote: "When a man takes to his bed, nearly all his friends have a secret desire to see him die: some to prove that his health is inferior to their own, others in the disinterested hope of being able to study a death agony."

A vigorous poet like Robert Browning could write, romantically, at the age of 52, "Grow old along with me! The best is yet to be." More realistically the American, Robert Frost, experiencing the trials of old age itself, wrote:

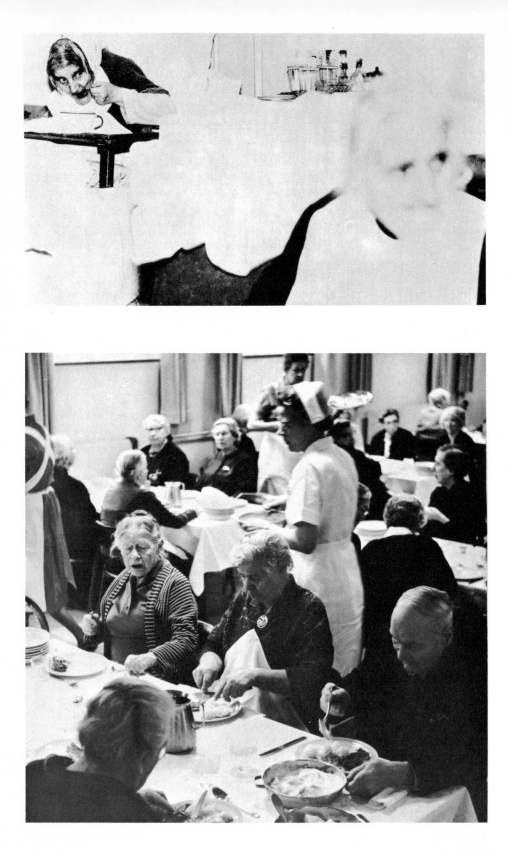

Above left, two women in the ward of an old people's home in Italy. Many old people come to dread the physical and financial dependency that may compel them to accept whatever help they can get from social welfare services. By accommodating both sexes within the one institution, the Danish state-run home for the aged (below left) is following a relatively enlightened policy.

Right, a Chinese family (from Taipei, Formosa) pays formal respects to the grandmother on her birthday. Reverence for age is deeply rooted in the oriental tradition, though the social upheavals of this century now threaten the old people's status. With the modern emphasis on youth and the small family unit, the old can no longer be assured of an honored place in a large integrated household.

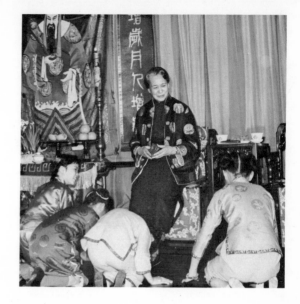

> No memory of having starred
> Atones for later disregard,
> Or keeps the end from being hard.
>
> Better to go down dignified
> With boughten friendship at your side
> Than none at all! Provide, provide!

The young and the middle-aged only half understand the problems of the old. They even forget that the libido does not necessarily disappear with age. The Kinsey Report, published in the United States in 1948, surprised many people with its revelation that the incidence of impotence rises from 0.1 per cent of the population at the age of 20 to only 27 per cent at 70 years of age. Yet many old people's homes still segregate husband from wife—as if cohabitation in old age was either unnecessary or repugnant.

It seems that just as we have a resistance to recognizing sexuality in children, so also we consciously reject the sexuality of our grandparents. We even need to make a joke of the matter—*literally*. For innumerable stories are in currency that, in allowing us to laugh at the sexual ability of the old, in fact protect us from thinking about the matter seriously. Here is but one of this genre of "jokes."

Joe Smith, aged 80, rings up his insurance broker. "Tom," he says, "if I give your insurance company £1000 tomorrow, will they give me £5000 in 10 years' time providing I'm alive?"

Tom feels he must consult on this matter. And after the statisticians have been at work the insurance company concludes it is on to a good thing. So Tom rings back to tell the old man that it's a deal. "But

241

first," Tom says, "you'll have to have the routine medical checkup with our insurance doctor. Will next Thursday be a good time for you?"

"Can't next Thursday," says old Joe Smith. "You see I'm playing football then."

Surprised, Tom stutters, "Football? Well, what about the following Thursday?"

"Oh, can't then either," replies Joe. "You see my grandfather is getting married."

"Getting married!" gasps Tom. "What does he want to do that for?"

"He doesn't *want* to," Joe says. "He's *got* to."

Old age, though, is no joking matter. The fear of impotence, of senility, is only too real. No wonder that since the first man turned gray the human race has longed for a rejuvenating agent. If drugs have made us old, it has been thought—and indeed is still thought—that one day there will be a drug or agent capable of revitalizing our lethargic cells, our flagging tissues, our vigor. Maybe doctors will even find a Faust-pill to make us young again. But our ancestors, too, had dreams of eternal youth and the substance of these dreams can be seen still in the neglected yellowing pages of documents by philosophers, alchemists, and "scientists" of different civilizations.

Often this search for a rejuvenating agent has been linked with the idea of maintaining sexual potency. In China and India 3000 years ago, for example, the elders and priests would consume the sexual organs of wild animals in an attempt to hold back the ravages of old age. In Old Testament times it was believed that the proximity of young women could revitalize the aged. Thus we have the story of King David and Abishag: "Now King David was old and stricken in years; and they covered him with clothes, but he gat no heat.

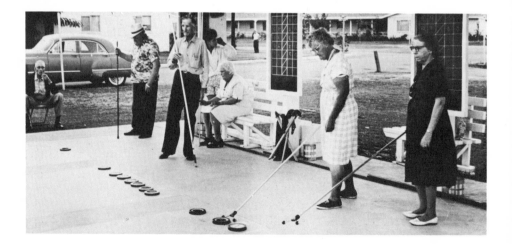

Wherefore his servants said unto him, Let there be sought for my lord the king a young virgin: and let her stand before the king . . . and let her lie in thy bosom, that my lord the king may get heat. So they sought for a fair damsel throughout all the coasts of Israel, and found Abishag a Shunammite, and brought her to the king. And the damsel was very fair, and cherished the king, and ministered to him: but the king knew her not." (I KINGS I: 1–4)

Later in history this "therapy" was still being advocated. The English Franciscan philosopher Roger Bacon, who resigned his Chair at Paris University in 1247 to devote himself to experimental medicine, believed young girls could rejuvenate the wizened old. Four hundred years later Hermann Boerhaave, the famous Dutch physician, recommended a deviation from this long-established practice. He placed two healthy youths, one on either side of an aged ailing burgomaster—with what result no one knows!

Not all rejuvenators equated longevity with sexuality. Gold had always been held in esteem as a magical rejuvenating agent. After all, alchemy in ancient China was harnessed not only to the idea of changing base metals into gold but also to the idea of finding the secret of immortality. The European alchemists, too, believed in the healing powers of gold. And in medieval Germany, medicines like the "Red Dragon" and the "Swan," which had gold as an ingredient, were supposed to act as rejuvenators. The 17th-century French physician P. J. Faber declared in his *Myrothecium Spagiricum* that gold, properly used, would retard old age by strengthening the inborn heat (*calor nativum*) and by renewing the innate moisture (*humidum radicale*).

The use of blood drawn from young persons or animals to revitalize old people has a long history too. There is the medieval legend of

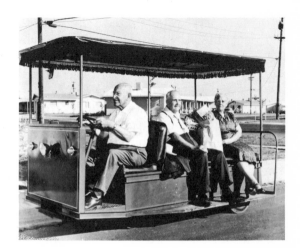

Two views of America's largest Senior Citizens' Village (for the over 62s) in Fresno, California. The last 20 years has seen the creation of many such communities in the United States. They provide a home and all the attractions of a year-round holiday camp for those who choose to spend their years of retirement in voluntary exile from a society from which they feel alienated. Only people in reasonably good health and able to care for themselves, however, are accepted in these villages.

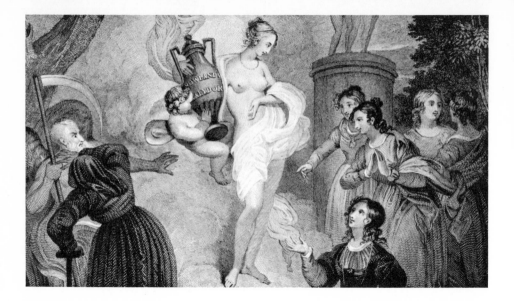

Artephus, a 12th-century alchemist, who boasted of having lived for 1000 years by distilling a spirit from boys' blood and inhaling the fumes. In those days people believed that witches, anxious to extend their lives, attacked children and drank their blood. Pope Innocent VIII (1432–92) when 60 years of age was reported to have had a transfusion from three young boys who, according to the 19th-century Italian historian Rodocanachi, were paid one ducat each for their blood. Shortly after, the Florentine savant and physician Marsilio Ficino gave detailed advice on how aged people could be rejuvenated with blood taken from the young. He advised the aged to drink their blood "in the manner of leeches" from freshly opened veins. He did recommend, though, that they should imbibe the blood only from volunteers.

Sex, gold, blood—what else? Well, the flesh of vipers was consumed in the Middle Ages, for people believed that by shedding their skins vipers rejuvenated themselves. There were some, though, who obviously could not stomach vipers' flesh neat; so a rejuvenating cure was devised whereby patients lived for weeks on a diet of chickens that had themselves been fed solely on minced viper. Only the rich of the time could afford such "cures," however.

All this may seem strange, even ridiculous, to modern readers, but our century too has produced its own extraordinary remedies—from homely advice on the value of eating yogurt to the rejuvenating potency of ultraviolet light. A choice example appears in *Life-shortening habits and Rejuvenation* by the Czechoslovak physician Arnold Lorand who wrote (in 1922) that "the rejuvenating effects of arsenic have already been known for a long time." Many people took Lorand seriously when he listed as the 10 chief life-shortening habits: alcohol,

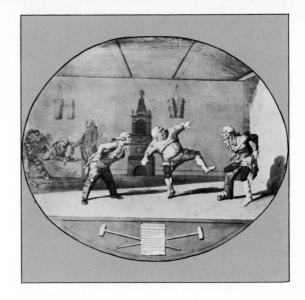

Left, in a 19th-century advertisement Venus and Cupid temptingly display a jar of "Rowland's Kalydor," a potion designed to ward off the ravages of Time. Right the *Ballet Arthritique,* an aquatint published by Paul Sandby in 1783 to satirize the current popularity of quack rejuvenatory potions of all kinds.

overeating, tobacco, sexual indiscretion, uncleanliness, ambition, avarice, anger, vanity, and avoidance of parenthood.

True modern experimental gerontology began in Paris with the great neurologist and physiologist, Charles Brown-Séquard (1817–94). Early in his career he came to believe that internal secretions of different organs might be useful in the treatment of different ailments. He even suggested that if semen was injected into the bloodstream of old men they might show signs of rejuvenation. But it was not until 1889 that Professor Brown-Séquard began his real rejuvenating experiments. He was then 72 years of age. In the late May of that year he adventurously injected into himself the ground-up testicles of dogs and guinea pigs. Over a period of two weeks he gave himself six subcutaneous injections, and the results were such as to convince the old professor that he had at last solved the question of rejuvenation.

On June 1, 1889, he reported the details of his experiments to the *Société de Biologie*:

"I was 72 years old on the 8th of last April. My general vigour, which was considerable, has diminished notably and gradually during the last ten or twelve years. Before the experiments, which now occupy me, I had to sit down after standing for an hour in the laboratory. After three or four hours, and sometimes after only two hours of experimental work at the laboratory, although I sat down, I was left exhausted. On returning home by carriage about six o'clock in the evening, after some hours passed thus in the laboratory, I was for many years so tired that I had to go to bed almost as soon as I had taken a hasty meal. Sometimes the exhaustion was such that despite the need to sleep and a drowsiness which prevented me even from reading the papers, I could go to sleep only after many hours.

"Today and since the second day, and above all the third day after the first injection, all that has changed and I have regained at least all the force which I possessed a number of years ago. Experimental work at the laboratory tires me little now. I can, to the great astonishment of my assistant, remain standing for hours together without feeling the need of sitting down. There are some days when after three and a quarter hours of work standing, I have been able, contrary to my habits for twenty years, to work at the preparation of a memoir for more than an hour and a half after dinner. All my friends know what an immense change that implies for me.

"I can also now without difficulty, and even without thinking about it, go up and down stairs almost running, a thing which I always did before the age of sixty. By using the dynamometer, I have established that there has been an incontestable increase in the force of my limbs. For my forearm, in particular, I find that the average of trials since the first two injections is greater by 6–7 kilograms than the average before the injections."

This was no pronouncement of a quack. Brown-Séquard's reputation was worldwide. He was known as a scientist of integrity. No wonder, then, that during the next six months as many as 12,000 doctors injected testicular extracts into their patients. Of course there were many who poured ridicule on his ideas of revitalization of "nervous energy," which he believed triggered off the rejuvenating mechanisms. In Britain and America particularly, there were those who found the idea of injecting the seminal fluid of animals into human beings "disgusting." One American doctor wrote: "The idea is as old as stupidity, wicked as superstition, cruel as savagery: it is false in its premises, false in its logic, false in its conclusions." Those conversant with modern psychoanalytic theory can account for the over-reactive, charged abuse of such statements.

On the other hand, the 12,000 reputable doctors who had followed Brown-Séquard's recommendation began to report amazing successes. Some, it seemed, had found it to work not only as a rejuvenator but also as a wonder drug in the treatment of such varied conditions as paralysis agitans, gout, goiter, and cancer. Brown-Séquard himself was doubtful whether testicular injections could cure so many of these ailments. But he did believe that the injections could bolster up "the nervous force" of individuals and that this in itself would help the body to fight many diseases.

Brown-Séquard had believed in his nervous force theory for over 40 years. In 1851 one of his patients, a 21-year-old woman, had regularly on each Sunday morning at 8 A.M. climbed onto the rail of her bed. There she stayed, on tiptoe, her body rigid, her head thrown

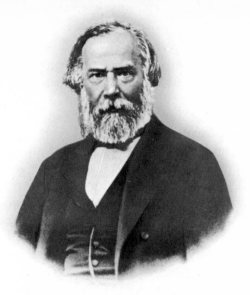

Dr. Charles Brown-Séquard, the distinguished French physician whose pioneer experiments in rejuvenation won wide acclaim in the 1890s.

back, her eyes glaring, for 12 hours, praying all the time. Only when the bell of the nearby church of St. Sulpice struck eight times in the evening would the young lady move down from the rail on her bed. Once, while the girl stood in her hysterical, catatonic trance, Brown-Séquard gave her a strong electric shock; but his patient stayed motionless as before, erect and still praying. A policeman watching this episode thought the current must be too weak, so Brown-Séquard gave him the same electric shock. The policeman literally jumped into the air, screaming with pain. Brown-Séquard believed that only the girl's nervous force—the force in her mind—could control her body in the way it did; that is to say, the patient's symptoms confirmed his views on the power of nervous over bodily functions. This, after all, is not such a bizarre idea, given 20th-century knowledge. Anyway, it seemed to Brown-Séquard, in 1889, that testicular extracts revitalized the nervous force, making the body young again.

It must have been his own power of suggestion and autosuggestion, though, that augmented the nervous force we all indeed have; for after a time the suggestive power of testicular therapy faded. The ill patients who had seemed to benefit became just as ill again; the old men became just as aged. And when Brown-Séquard died in 1894, the injections he had advocated became irrevocably discredited.

Yet, in passing, one would like to pay tribute to the extraordinary man who was Charles Brown-Séquard. He remained a scientist in the best sense of that word to his last days. Even when dying with a right-sided hemorrhage of the brain, Brown-Séquard continued to give a detailed account of his own symptoms, correctly diagnosing his illness, and stating his bleak prognosis—as if observing another patient. The next day he was dead.

Two other pioneer scientists were to carry on Brown-Séquard's work in rejuvenation at this point in time. They were Eugen Steinach (1861–1944) and Serge Voronoff (1866–1951). In the Biological Institute of Vienna, Professor Steinach began his experiments the very year Brown-Séquard died. At first he transplanted ovaries from young female albino rats and guinea pigs into castrated males of the species. This was not the first time successful transplants had been effected. In 1770 the great British surgeon John Hunter had transplanted testicles from one dog to another, and the transplanted tissues had survived for a time in their new host. The German biologist Professor A. A. Berthold of Göttingen had carried out similar experiments in 1849, with encouraging results. But Steinach went altogether further. After his experiments he noted that the castrated male rats and guinea pigs—because they now had grafted ovaries in them—began to look and behave as females. When he removed the ovaries from female rats and grafted testicles onto them, they in turn began to assume male characteristics.

It was now only a short step for him to consider grafting the testicles of young male rats onto the old males of the species, and young ovaries into aged female rats. After several weeks, the aged animals on which Steinach had operated began to manifest signs of "rejuvenation." Professor Steinach, who published the results of these experiments in 1910, did not then take the logical step of trying to rejuvenate elderly humans by similar methods. This was left to the Russian surgeon, Serge Voronoff.

Steinach, a research biologist, thought there might be a simpler method of producing rejuvenation. He knew that certain vital testicular cells—the so-called interstitial cells of Leydig—degenerated in aged animals. If these cells were "vitalized," he felt, the animal should show the same signs of rejuvenation that had followed the more radical grafting experiments.

Steinach believed he could revitalize these decaying, interstitial testicular cells by increasing their blood supply—in this way bringing them more oxygen and nutrition. He thought he could do this by simply tying off the sperm ducts, through which seminal fluid normally leaves the testicles. As long before as 1852, the celebrated French physiologist Claude Bernard had discovered that tying off the sperm ducts caused more blood to flow into the testicles.

So on male senile rats of 28 months old, Steinach performed the operation of tying off one sperm duct in each animal—leaving the duct of the other testicle alone, so that, if rejuvenation did take place, the rat would still be able to breed. Prior to the operation the old rats shared all the usual outward signs and symptoms associated with senility. They lay about listlessly, their eyes were dull, they no longer cleaned themselves, and their skins showed bald patches. They even ignored the pieces of fat bacon—a favorite food—that were offered to them on a stick. Their sex instincts, too, had completely vanished. They had no interest in female rats and they retreated from young male rats, showing none of the pugnaciousness they would have displayed had they not been senile.

A few weeks after Steinach's operation amazing changes occurred in the rats. New hair grew on the skins, the bald patches vanishing. They became agile, ate with relish, fought young rats, and experienced what Professor Steinach called "a sexual paroxysm." For the once senile rats now exhibited insatiable desire for the females of the species and showed every indication of alarming sexual vigor and potency. These rejuvenated rats apparently did not care whether or not the females they pursued were in their mating period—as young rats almost invariably do. And not only were these hitherto senile rats youthful again; their life span appeared to increase also. In one rat the rejuvenation effect lasted some eight months. That the Leydig interstitial cells of the testicle were responsible for these extraordinary developments was shown by microscopic examination of sections from the testicle, and it was seen that these cells had now grown larger and had increased in number.

Various surgeons—among them the Viennese surgeons Professor R. Lichtenstern and Dr. K. Doppler—tried to carry out these operative procedures, or refinements of them, in human beings. Professor Lichtenstern published the results of a number of his cases. Some of his patients maintained that after the operation they felt much younger—and their symptoms of shortness of breath and dizziness had subjectively improved. In one case, a man aged 72 with marked arteriosclerosis, sexual desire returned after an absence of many years, and his ability to take advantage of it happily returned too. In the cases reported, hair grew more richly and abundantly after the operation and memory seemed to improve.

Steinach's methods, then, did seem to work at least *temporarily* in selected cases in that there was some increase in the output of sexual hormones and a revival of sexual activity. But no true rejuvenation occurred, for senility is not only allied to degeneration of the interstitial cells of Leydig. There is, as we have seen, deterioration of many other tissues of the body. Besides, in September 1920, Professor Payr of Leipzig and Professor Kummel of Hamburg warned doctors of the dangers of the Steinach procedures. Payr pointed out that severe shock had resulted from cutting the sperm ducts and Kummel reported several deaths following the operation. So, because of the disappointing

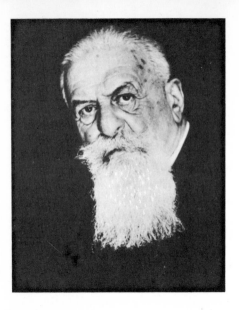

The great Viennese biologist Eugen
Steinach, who believed that degeneration
of the human body could be arrested by
revitalizing the interstitial cells.

results and because of the dangers, the operation gradually fell into
disrepute. Once again, it seemed, doctors had based their hopes on
unjustifiable analogies between laboratory animals and man.

Professor Serge Voronoff, a Russian surgeon living in Paris, began
his grafting operations on human beings in 1920. He knew of Steinach's
work and had read the published results of his experiments. But
Voronoff had already begun to think of testicular grafting in 1898,
when he visited Egypt where he examined many eunuchs. After that
experience he felt that testicular activity was related not only to
sexuality and the secondary sexual characteristics of the male—the
growth of hair on the face, the narrower pelvis, the deeper voice, and
so on—but also to more general body functions. "My observation of
eunuchs now led me to infer that the internal secretion of the testicle,"
he wrote, "also influences the development of the bones of the leg and
cranium: that it either destroys adipose tissue or prevents its development: that it combats sclerosis, stimulates the intelligence, maintains
courage, and prolongs life."

On his return to Paris, Voronoff began experimenting, like Steinach,
with animals. In 1908 he obtained some senile rams whose wool was
thin with bald patches. These rams were so old they could hardly
stand, and their limbs trembled. Voronoff grafted portions of testicles
from young rams into their scrotums, and observed them subsequently
from month to month. After a time their appetites returned; they had
a new thick growth of wool and their general condition improved
enormously. "My old rams became young in their gait, bellicose and
aggressive, and these changes were progressive. The miserable old
beasts became full of vitality," Voronoff declared.

Voronoff, it must be remembered, was a surgeon, and he wished to go further than Steinach had. He wanted to graft young testicles into old men, hoping that what had happened in animals would also occur in man. Of course he was faced with an insoluble difficulty. Young men were hardly likely to sacrifice their healthy testicles to prove Voronoff right or wrong.

Professor Voronoff thought for a long time about this difficulty. Perhaps testicles could be taken from people sentenced to death? Or perhaps young men could be persuaded to part with one testicle if they were assured that physical health and sexual activity would in no way be impaired by such a sacrifice? In the end he realized that such ideas were impracticable. Instead, he began to concentrate on the idea of grafting testicles from apes into man—for anthropoid apes were closely related to the genus *Homo*. It was necessary, anyway, he felt, to try out such an operation. He recalled a dictum of Claude Bernard, that great scientist and colleague of Brown-Séquard: "the presentiment of truth justifies experiment." In fact, his first graft from ape to man was performed on June 12, 1920.

Encouraged by the results, he managed to obtain more and more apes, and more willing patients. He was haunted by the idea that so many of the great deeds of life, so much great creative activity, had been carried out during the time when the sexual glands were most active. He thought of creative geniuses like Goethe, who retained their reproductive ability until the end. Indeed, Goethe at 74 was still enthusiastically in love with a 19-year-old girl. Even on his death bed, Goethe, 83 years old, expiring, said: "Look at this lovely woman's head, with black curls, in a black background . . . ."and then, after a pause, continued, "Light, more light!" Voronoff believed Goethe was asking for more light so as to see that lovely woman's head better. He saw a moral in this.

Between June 12, 1920, and October 15, 1923, Voronoff performed 51 testicular grafting operations from ape to man. The operations, which had to be done with great speed on the anesthetized man and ape, were carried out simultaneously. Man and ape were placed on separate tables in the same operating theatre. The operation on the ape was carried out by Voronoff's assistant while Voronoff performed the graft into the man's scrotum. Among those operated upon were seven medical men: three Frenchmen, two Englishmen, one Italian, and one Spaniard.

Voronoff maintained that physical and mental restoration often resulted from his operations. Here is but one "successful" case history as given by Voronoff himself. It concerns a 74-year-old Englishman—a chronic alcoholic incidentally—who, when seen by Voronoff, had all the appearances of an old man: he was obese, bent, and walked with a stick; his memory was bad, his intelligence sluggish; he had been sexually impotent for 12 years.

"He was operated upon on February 2, 1921, at the Maison de Santé, Rue Montaigne, Dr. Didry assisting," wrote Voronoff. "He was grafted with the right testicle of a Cynocephalus (Papion).

"There were no sequelae to operation and the wounds healed by first intention.

"The patient left Paris twelve days after his operation and I did not see him again until eight months later. My clinical assistant, Dr. Didry, and I were literally stupefied when Mr. E. L. appeared. He had lost half his obesity, his manner was jovial, his movements active, his eyes clear and twinkling with amusement at our astonishment. His superfluous fat had disappeared, his muscles had become firm, he held himself erect and conveyed the impression of a man in perfect health. He bent his head and revealed to our astonished eyes a growth of white down, where formerly there had been a bald expanse.

"He came to see us from Switzerland, where he had been climbing and taking part in the various sports so favoured by Englishmen. The man was literally fifteen to twenty years younger. His whole condition, physical, mental and sexual, had undergone a radical change. The grafting had transformed a senile, impotent, pitiful old being into a vigorous man, in full possession of all his faculties.

"Since then I have heard from him nearly every month and the news is more and more reassuring. Some months ago he sent me photographs showing him fencing, weight-lifting, and running upstairs, four steps at a time.

"I examined him again recently, twenty months after operation, and I found that the beneficent change which had taken place in the entire organism was not only maintained but was definitely progressive. His manner then was youthful, his carriage upright, and his walk springy. What surprised me most was to discover that his bald head was covered with hairs 3 centimetres in length. This objective sign is very interesting. Taken in conjunction with the restored intellectual faculty, the improved intestinal function, the muscular tonicity, and the sexual recovery, it completes the clinical picture of the generalized effect upon the organism of the testicular hormone, as provided artificially by the graft.

"I saw Mr. E. L. for the last time on July 28, 1923, in London. Not only had he retained all the benefits of his graft, but his general condition then, two and a half years after operation, was better even than when I had seen him previously.

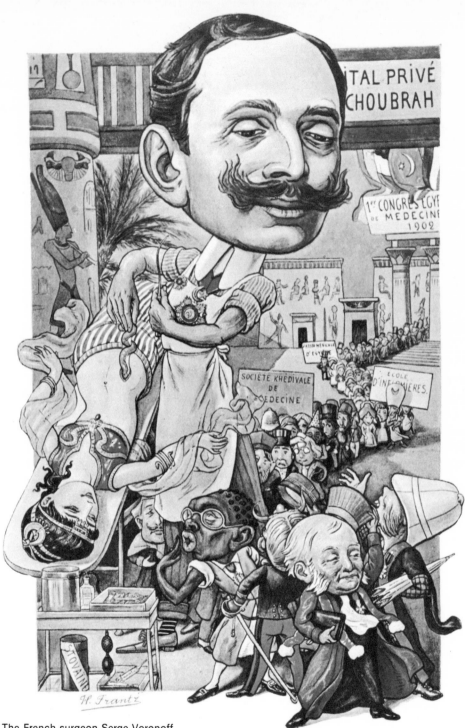

The French surgeon Serge Voronoff,
caricatured at the International Congress
on Tropical Disease held in Cairo in
1902. During his years in Egypt, Voronoff
began to consider the possible rejuvenatory
effects of testicular transplants.

"He told me of yet another symptom of improved muscular tonicity, as presented by an organ of peculiar sensibility, namely, the eye. Long-sighted, like the majority of old people, he had been unable to read without glasses. But when I saw him he was able to read without glasses for two or three hours at a time, a thing which formerly had been quite impossible.

"On September 4th, 1923, I heard of his death during an attack of delirium tremens. His intemperance was confirmed, and, unfortunately, the graft had no effect in this direction."

Voronoff continued with these grafting operations but there were sometimes sequelae arising out of his extensive surgery and he had many failures. Moreover, the beneficial effects that sometimes resulted faded too often and too soon. By 1939 even Voronoff was less dogmatic about his wonderful rejuvenating operations in man. Rather he emphasized the success attendant upon his animal experiments. He reminded the world of a ram he had operated upon that lived to the age of 20. This was equivalent, in terms of human life, to the age of 160. The ram was an old ram indeed, for it maintained its vigor until the last six days of its life, and the ewe with which it had cohabited during its later years produced five lambs only a few months before the patriarch ram died.

"The case of this ram," Voronoff bravely declared, "indicates to us the course to be pursued, the ideal to be attained: the prolongation of the length of life and the shortening of the period of old age. . . ."

Today Voronoff is dead, Steinach is dead, Brown-Séquard is dead, but the human condition has not changed. There are still those who seek out the latest rejuvenating wizard. There are still doctors alive who claim, by their methods, to restore successfully golden youth to the old, not like Faust in exchange for their souls, but for dollars, pounds, francs, or other coinage.

Many rich and famous people in the West—and many neither rich nor famous—have visited a discreet clinic near the Swiss lakeside town of Vevey. The man in charge of the *Clinique Générale La Prairie* is 83-year-old Professor Paul Niehans, who believes that injections of fresh young embryo cells taken from a newly-killed animal fetus can revitalize the failing tissues of aging human beings. He claims that fresh embryo animal heart cells can revitalize a failing human heart, that fresh fetal liver cells can stimulate a worn-out human liver, that fetal brain cells can reactivate the brain, that embryo bone marrow cells can be efficacious in certain blood diseases that result from a damaged bone marrow, and so on.

He considers that these fetal cells can not only help to stay the years but can also be used beneficially in the treatment of certain radiation diseases and other maladies. He even suggests that the brain power of retarded children can be improved by his therapy. No wonder official medical bodies remain skeptical of his claims. The American Medical Association has announced: "There is insufficient explanation of the Niehans treatment and the exact physiological action in the body." The Board of Physicians of the Federal German Republic, like a number of other orthodox bodies, has stoutly rejected fresh-cell therapy.

The reason for the hostile position of orthodox doctors is not only that fresh-cell therapy is based on an insufficient scientific foundation; there is also the publicity-seeking and self-advertising associated with some of the fetal-cell practitioners. There has been, too, a commercial exploitation of the alleged cell therapy successes. Above all, orthodox medical bodies are concerned about the danger of disease transmissions and the risks of unpredictable allergic reactions if living animal fetal cells are injected into the human body.

Yet many of Niehans's disciples—doctors won over to his position in Germany, Japan, Spain, and elsewhere—continue to carry out his therapy and have contributed papers to medical symposiums on its efficacy. It is claimed that treatment of blood disease caused by roentgen irradiations has led to some positive results. Thus Dr. Mathé and Dr. Salmon, two French doctors, treated Yugoslav nuclear scientists with fresh fetal marrow cells following an accident at Wintra, in Yugoslavia, on August 15, 1958.

Perhaps the most remarkable claims for the Niehans cell therapy have come from Dr. H. Feldmann at the University of Geneva, after treating 37 mongoloid, retarded children. He gave them a series of injections—as explained in his paper "The Value of Cell Therapy for Cases of Retarded Development." "We are aware," he writes, "of the fears entertained by the medical profession, more accustomed to classical types of treatment, concerning this new type of therapy, and we must confess that many paediatricians have disparaged this method stating that the greatest prudence and a sharp critical sense are essential for the interpretation of possible progress in mongolian children. . . ."

He goes on to report: "We were extremely surprised to see that it was precisely with actual mongolians and retarded mongoloids that we had the best results. . . . After three weeks—sometimes five—the child suddenly shows a marked progress not only from the point of view of intellectual and social behaviour, but also physically. . . . Their facial expression, previously inane, expressionless, sometimes brutish or comical, became more lively, and the child acquired the possibility of becoming more readily integrated into groups of normal children

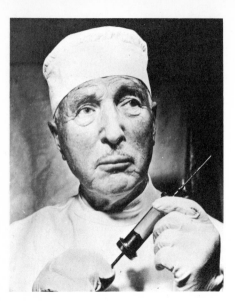

Left, Professor Niehans, head of the Swiss *Clinique Général La Prairie.* Below, Niehans demonstrates the extraction of embryo cells from a sheep for injection into the human body.

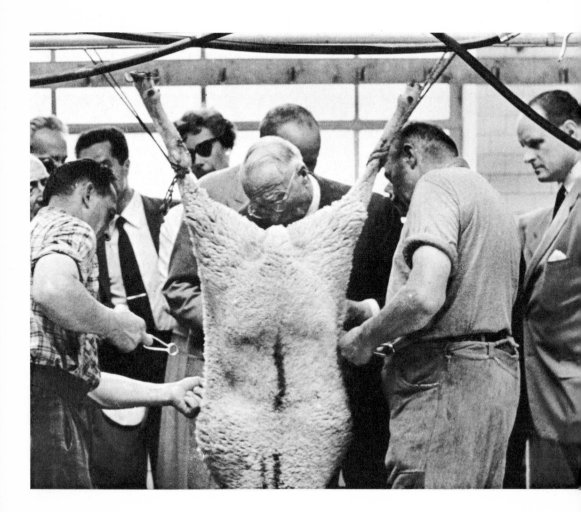

and no longer felt rejected, as before. . . . One important fact should be noted: the younger the mongolian, the more effective the treatment. The most interesting results were obtained with children under 5 years of age."

Other Niehans disciples testify to other extraordinary gains in other conditions. Thus Professor H. G. Rietschel of Herford, Germany, reports on the old-age condition of arteriosclerosis. Arteriosclerosis, he maintains, is an indication for Niehans's fresh-cell therapy. "In 21 cases with arteriosclerosis and endarteric vascular involvements of the lower limbs, the patients were able, four weeks later, to walk three times as much as before." And he asserts, "old age diseases can definitely be improved by the action of cell therapy."

Doctors may raise their eyebrows at such extravagant claims—and they may note how small a number of patients is used in these clinical "trials." But whether they sneer or not, patients still trek to Vevey to see Professor Niehans himself. Among those said to have been treated by Professor Niehans's fresh-cell therapy are the German statesman Konrad Adenauer, the British writer Somerset Maugham, the Arab potentate King Ibn Saud, and the French painter Georges Braque. Pope Pius XII, too, was treated by Professor Niehans; indeed, it was through his association with the pope, when the latter was seriously ill in 1954, that Niehans became world-famous.

I, myself, went to interview Professor Niehans in April 1964. I was not impressed by his conversation. Many of his remarks, scientifically speaking, were bizarre or just did not make sense; but I was taken aback by his own vigor. He did not seem to be a man over 80 and he maintained that his youthfulness was due to the fact that he had treated himself with fresh embryo cells.

But there are still no convincing controlled experiments on fresh-cell therapy, no convincing statistics. Skeptical doctors are hardly likely to be swayed merely by Niehans's disciples or Niehans's rhetoric. "The Creator," Niehans has said, "has placed a magnificent power in the fresh cell—and if one thousand injections do not guarantee one thousand cures, we can nevertheless help and ameliorate certain conditions at present incurable in a number of patients." He does talk with a kind of religious fervor and it is hard not to recall, when talking to him, that this great-nephew of Kaiser Wilhelm II was a doctor of theology before he studied medicine and became a surgeon.

Perhaps it is significant that a number of Niehans's famous patients subsequently trailed to see another professor, thought by some to hold the passport to Shangri-la—a woman, Professor Ana Aslan, who works in Bucharest. Certainly Adenauer and Ibn Saud, despite their political orientations, were recently reported to have been treated by

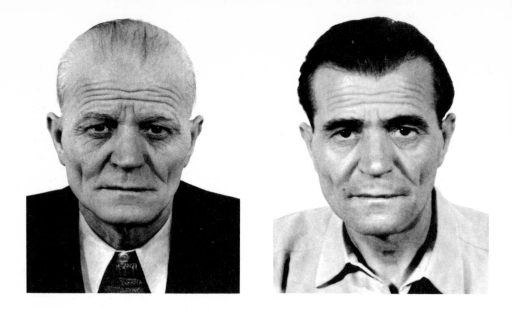

this 57-year-old lady doctor of a communist country; and Mao Tse-tung and Nikita Kruschev, too, have apparently been treated by her. Communists of different complexions, just like "western deca-dents," it would seem, grow old and yearn for youth. And just as inveterate neurotic patients will go from doctor to doctor for relief of their symptoms, those morbidly hungry for the green and palmy days will journey from one "rejuvenator" to another, however dubious this man's theories or that man's claims.

What is the drug that Professor Aslan uses and that, she claims, can reverse hardening of the arteries, improve the impaired hearing of premature senility, loosen old arthritic joints, make wrinkled skin smooth again, and repigment the white hair of the aged? This magic, regenerative drug is basically nothing more than procaine.

Now procaine is essentially a local anesthetic, and countless people the world over have experienced injections of it before minor opera-tions or prior to having a tooth cavity filled by a dentist. However, for many years it has been known that procaine may have functions other than that of a local anesthetic. In 1944 Michael Good, a British doctor, used procaine in the treatment of certain rheumatic disorders with some mildly encouraging results. Originally, too, Professor Aslan gave injections of procaine to sufferers from rheumatism. She noted to her surprise that the patients' general condition improved: many seemed more active in mind and body. This improvement, she felt, could not be accounted for by the local relief of rheumatic pain. Moreover, other concurrent ailments (asthma and skin conditions, for example) sometimes cleared up magically as well.

She induced rheumatism artificially in rats and treated these animals with procaine. These and other animal experiments appeared

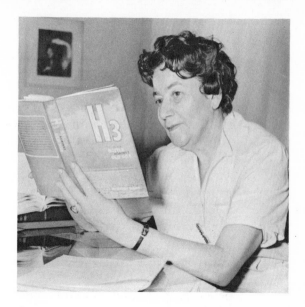

Left, "before and after" photographs from the Bucharest Institute of Geriatrics: a 52-year-old subject exhibits a dramatic growth of dark hair and loss of age lines, allegedly as a result of injections with H3. Right, Professor Ana Aslan, director of the Bucharest Institute.

to confirm her earlier findings, especially when she increased the acid content of her procaine solution. She began to believe she was witnessing "a biological rejuvenation" in these animals, as well as in her older patients. Professor Aslan, convinced that she had discovered new possibilities for the old drug procaine, now called her acid solution of the local anesthetic "H3."

When in Bucharest recently, I asked Professor Aslan whether she thought the renaming of procaine merely obscured matters. "For aren't H3 and procaine intrinsically the same thing?"

"We have potassium in our solution," Professor Aslan replied. "This potentiates the action of procaine. With procaine solution such as you use in England I would only expect to get a 25 per cent success. With H3 I obtain a 60 per cent success."

In 1959, Professor Aslan had been officially invited to Britain to address a meeting of skeptical doctors. The invitation came from Lord Amulree, president of the Medical Society for the Care of the Elderly. At that London meeting she presented her clinical reports to the startled British doctors. With lantern slides she demonstrated how her patients had looked before and after she had given them H3. The orthodox medical response was summed up by a leader in the *British Medical Journal* at the time: "A study of the clinical reports makes sad reading for the clinician trained in scientific method. There is an almost complete absence of controls, and blind trials were never used. At the Apothecaries' Hall last week, Professor Aslan created a most favourable personal impression as a woman gifted with humour, charm, enthusiasm, and boundless therapeutic optimism. The word 'statistical' was heard frequently but no worthwhile statistics were shown. The audience heard little but a series of medical anecdotes."

After Professor Aslan returned to Romania some British doctors carried out trials with procaine injections on geriatric patients. These trials were a total failure. But when I interviewed Dr. Aslan at the Institute of Geriatrics in Bucharest, of which she is head, she maintained that the British doctors had not carried out real trials. "First they selected desperate cases," she insisted, "whose life expectancy was no longer than one year. Second, they did not use the correct method. They only gave two injections a week instead of three. Third, they did not treat the patients for a long enough period. Fourth, they did not give H3—they gave procaine injections. So that is why they had poor results."

In her clinic she introduced me to many of her old patients. A number of them were apparently over 100. One in particular I shall never forget; after shaking hands with him my fingers were white, crushed. That he had a strong handshake was indisputable. That he was vigorous could not be denied. That he had a sense of humor was evident. But whether all this was a result of H3 I do not know. Professor Aslan pointed to another old person who had black hair. "You have heard of people going white," she said, "but have you before known a white-haired man go black?"

Certainly more encouraging preliminary reports on the efficacy of H3 have been published recently in the U.S.A. as a result of work done at the Chicago Medical School and at the St. Peter State Hospital in Minnesota. And an Italian medical journal reported recently: "In 1960 our investigations were resumed, this time with the Romanian compound. We found that the drug had beneficial effects in arthritis, in general disorders of pre-senility, in resistance to stress, etc. No miracles—but a whole series of positive results which would justify the use of H3 in old age therapy and the furtherance of its study."

There are many doctors, too, who are impressed by the fact that Professor Aslan has the Romanian government's backing. But not too much should be made of this. H3 is exported now in quite large quantities; and Westerners go to Professor Aslan's clinic in Bucharest for treatment. They bring with them valuable foreign currency. It may be that the Romanian government is more interested in the economic benefits of H3 than in the medical ones. In any case the claims of Professor Aslan are too much founded on personal testimony, on unacceptable photographs, on inadequately controlled blind trials. Dr. Alex Comfort, a leading British gerontologist, recently summed up the orthodox Western viewpoint in his book *The Process of Aging*: "Dr. Aslan's recent experiments with procaine injections probably produce some physiological effects but certainly do not produce rejuvenation." He admits that "such procedures might have their uses, but as a palliative only."

It would seem, then, that there is as yet no drug that indisputably slows down the aging process. This is no cause for pessimism, however. Research into old age is being carried out more and more extensively each year. In 1960 the U.S. Department of Health alone spent $12,400,000 on such research and some cautious gerontologists believe they will discover means for retaining vigor within a score of years. Experiments on animals have already yielded much information on longevity. Thus rats, which normally die at the age of three, have been kept young throughout their life history by purely dietary means—in fact by feeding them a diet deficient in calories. More, the life span of Wistar rats has been *increased* by simply fasting them every third day: the longevity of these rats has been increased by 20 per cent, that of female rats by 15 per cent. Similar results have been obtained with mice. So perhaps Seneca, the Roman philosopher and tutor of Nero, had a point when he said: "More people are killed through their stomachs than by the sword."

Another laboratory fact worth noting is that if a female rat is incarcerated with aging male rats the condition of the latter seems to improve and as a result they tend to live longer. But before hopes rise too high it should be added that King Solomon, despite his "thousand wives," did not reach the biblical span of three score years and ten.

Of course the conception longevity and sexuality are linked is not new! When Brown-Séquard injected himself with testicular extracts, when Steinach tried to stimulate growth of the testicular cells, when Voronoff transplanted chimpanzee testicles into a man, these early modern gerontologists were only acting out the fundamental age-old equation of sexual vigor=longevity. It is not, alas, as simple as that. We have learned that sex hormones do not halt the aging process in man: eunuchs live as long as the rest of us. Indeed, it has been demonstrated in the laboratory that if sex hormones are given to a castrated male animal, its life span may be shortened.

If, one day, a drug is found that can indisputably extend our life span, it may be that yet another drug will be needed to bolster our "will to live." There is something in the vague philosophical idea that we die only when we are ready for death. And from the standpoint of modern analytically orientated psychiatry everyone has a suicide potential, varying from very low to very high. In his book *Man Against Himself*, Karl Menninger emphasizes the concept of "partial suicide." We all know people who, as we say, are drinking themselves to death. Certainly many people bring about psychological and

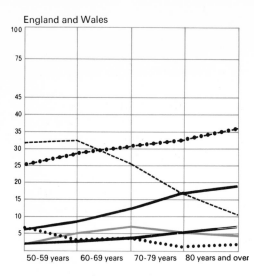

England and Wales

| | | | |
|---|---|---|---|
| •–•–•–•–•–•–•–• | Heart diseases |
| --------------- | Malignant neoplasms |
| ▬▬▬▬▬▬▬ | Vascular lesions |
| •••••••••••• | All accidents |
| ═══════ | Pneumonia |
| ▬▬▬▬▬▬▬ | Bronchitis |

50-59 years    60-69 years    70-79 years    80 years and over

physiological alterations within themselves that result in premature demise. Thus the will to live can in itself actually change bodily function, and affect the span of life.

This will to live, judging from suicide statistics, is most frail in the elderly. One has only to remember the physical discomfort, the incapacity, the loneliness, the feelings of futility, that the aged endure, to understand the association of suicide with old age. Recent investigations of mental illness after the age of 60, moreover, have clearly shown the importance of depressive illness and suicidal acts in that age group—suicide, incidentally, resulting not only from taking overdoses of sleeping pills or other poisons, but more commonly from dramatic acts such as drowning, hanging, or shooting.

If one remembers that once every minute in the U.S.A. someone is killing himself or trying to kill himself, and that the suicide rate is likely to increase with aging populations, the enormity of the problem can be encompassed. Recently, old people who had attempted to commit suicide were investigated in Scotland. The given reasons in more than 50 per cent of the cases were loneliness, the sense of being unwanted, the feeling of being a burden on other people—in short, social isolation.

Then, again, it is common for old people "just to give up the ghost" simply because their lives have become meaningless. Changes in their life situation often hasten their death. An old man dies—then very soon his aged widow "goes out like a light," though until her husband's final illness she was full of vigor. When old people move, through force of circumstance, to another town, so that they are devoid of their old friends, cut off from old avenues of entertainment and interest, it is astonishing how quickly they deteriorate.

France

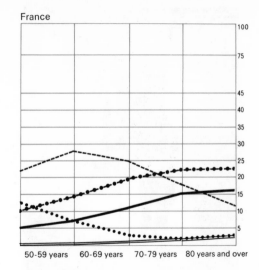

50-59 years    60-69 years    70-79 years    80 years and over

Graphs based on recent WHO figures for six countries show how the over 50s are affected by six major causes of death: the horizontal lines represent the percentage of deaths from all causes attributed to the particular diseases. Thus in America, 40 per cent of all deaths at the age of 70 are caused by heart disease, which contrasts strikingly with the corresponding figure of 10 per cent given for Japan.

Italy

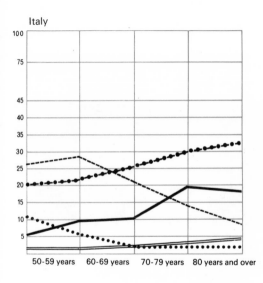

50-59 years    60-69 years    70-79 years    80 years and over

Japan

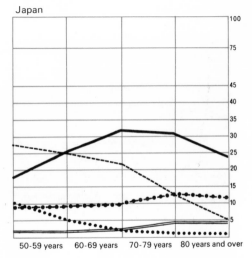

50-59 years    60-69 years    70-79 years    80 years and over

Netherlands

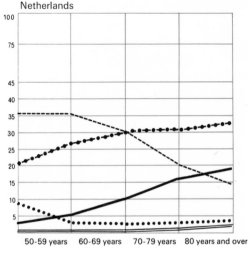

50-59 years    60-69 years    70-79 years    80 years and over

United States of America

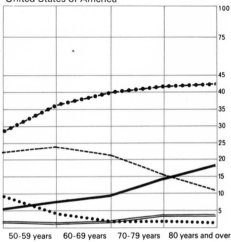

50-59 years    60-69 years    70-79 years    80 years and over

263

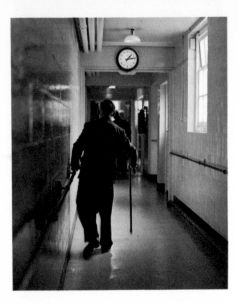

Patients at work and exercise in the geriatric department of the pioneer Chesterton Hospital, Britain. Organized activities of this kind are a positive attempt to engage patients' interest and keep their minds and bodies alert.

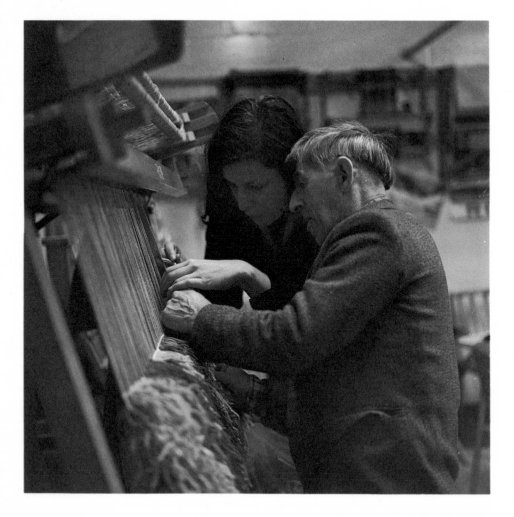

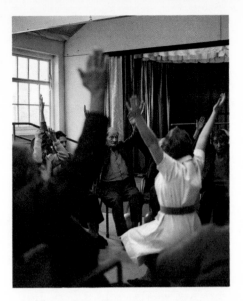

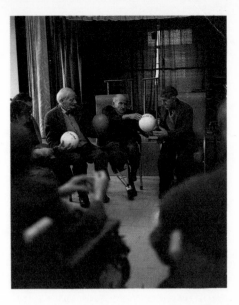

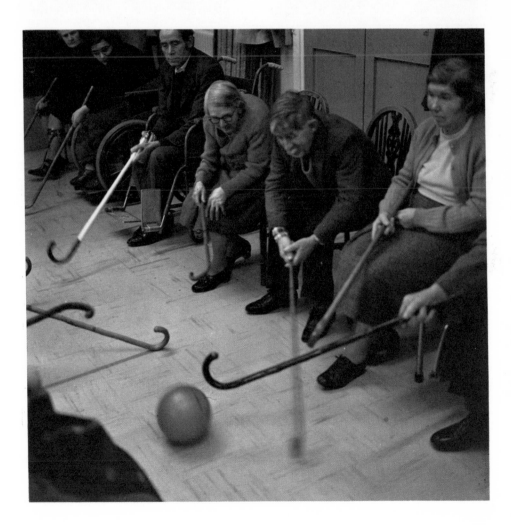

265

As long ago as 1897 the French sociologist Emile Durkheim, in his study *Le Suicide*, postulated the concept of *anomic* suicide—that is to say, suicide that results when new adaptations are required as a result of life changes. Where the actual suicide figures rise one can be sure that the "partial suicide" potential or the "will to live" for many other people is also altered.

Durkheim has shown how the suicide rate increases in times of financial stress—as for example after the famous crash on the Paris Bourse during the winter of 1882. But he also shows how with sudden prosperity the changes in life situation also increase the suicide rate. Durkheim gives as an example the conquest of Rome by Victor Emmanuel in 1870, which caused a wave of prosperity in the country: trade boomed, salaries rose, the material comfort of the workers improved, the price of bread fell, and private wealth multiplied. But together with this collective gain in prosperity between 1871–77, the suicide rate increased by 36 per cent.

It is evident that where the social regulation of the individual is altered he is vulnerable to mental disturbance, and the "will to live" may then be altogether less vigorous. Professor D. Wilfred Abse has written: "The speed and intensity of the changes in 20th-century society have no precedent in recorded history. Technological advances, increases in population, large scale immigration and resettlement, the vast expansion of education and communication, the widespread trend towards urbanization, are all new factors which readily give rise to *anomic* conditions on account of their sheer velocity." Obviously the gerontologist cannot work alone, cannot hope to increase our life span with drugs unless the factors that control our psychological will to live are also understood and accounted for.

Meanwhile certain basic problems, like the care of the aged sick, remain half neglected—though there are welcome signs of change. The Scandinavian countries, in particular, adopt an enlightened policy toward the aged. Sweden already has more than 1400 old-age homes accommodating 50,000 pensioners, and 20,000 places in hospitals and nursing homes reserved for the chronically sick—most of whom are old people. There is a special housing allowance for the old, a rapidly expanding home-help service, small but modern pensioners' flats. The story is much the same in Norway. In Britain there are now 100 geriatric units, with hospitals like the Chesterton in Cambridge carrying out exciting rehabilitation work in the geriatric departments. America, too, is beginning to come to grips with the gargantuan problem of its aged community.

But there is still a long way to go. Even the fundamental question of euthanasia, presumably because it is so unpalatable, is put on one side—yet too many patients on the point of death are kept alive needlessly because the doctor cannot face the religious, ethical, and social problem he is faced with. The whole psychological approach of modern medicine, naturally, is to cure. In our modern hospitals, the medical drive is to make people well again. But comes the hour when surgeon and physician are helpless: we may put an animal out of its misery but the law and the doctor's own education often inhibit him from being truly human at the last.

Too often large doses of narcotics are withheld for this reason. Too often radical surgery is desperately attempted when it is best to leave well alone. Too frequently "miracle drugs" and antibiotics are given right to the end when it would be more merciful to withhold them. If drugs have made us old, if new drugs will in the years to come make us yet older and at the same time vigorous, if King Solomon's dictum that there is "a time to be born and a time to die" can be disproved, so drugs must be allowed to help us when we do eventually draw our last breaths. For "after the first death there is no other."

# 8 The Cost of Drugs

In the chapter entitled "The Fringe Healers," I discussed briefly how manufacturers of specious proprietary medicines advertised their products in popular media and how they made handsome profits from their sale. Doctors disapprove of such proprietary patent medicines not least because, on occasions, their use may be dangerous. A man with piles, gulled by advertisements into trying out one or another patent ointment, postpones seeing his doctor when his condition may be secondary to a serious disease requiring immediate medical attention; another with a cough may take a useless patent expectorant mixture when his symptom is the result of tuberculosis or cancer, which could become more widespread because of such delay; a woman with a headache may (though rarely) be suffering from a kidney ailment or even a brain tumor—and so forth. In short, self-medication follows on self-diagnosis: there has been no clinical examination to elucidate the cause of the particular symptom. No doctor can be happy about that kind of situation.

Moreover, the taking of such medicines is so widespread a habit that catastrophe must follow more frequently than proprietary patent firms are likely to admit. A recent survey conducted on a council housing estate in London revealed that two out of every three people

A doctor's receptionist throws out a week's accumulation of pharmaceutical circulars, pamphlets, and free drug samples.

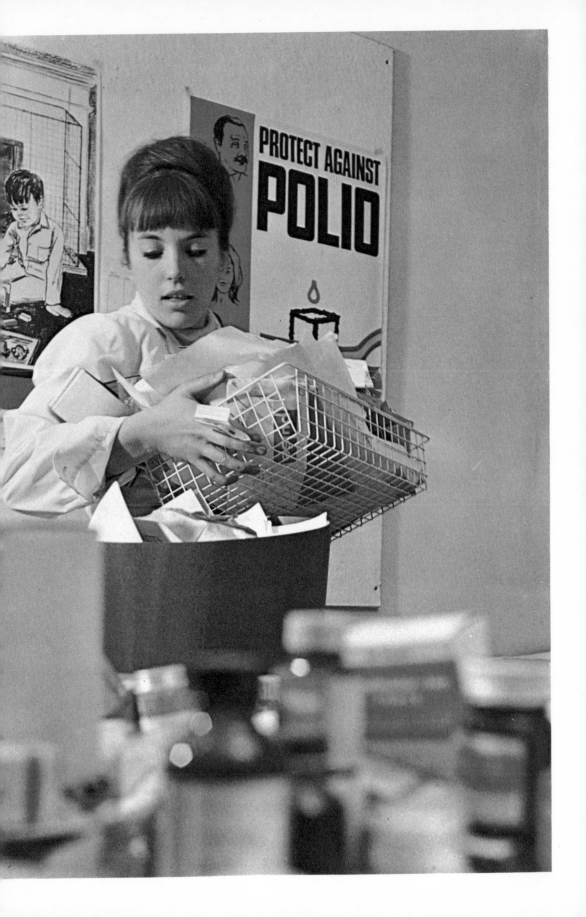

took a patent medicine over a period of one month. For every person who took a laxative on doctor's orders, 16 bought nonprescribed laxatives over the pharmacist's counter. Worse, 90 per cent of the children who had been given laxatives were not even constipated in the first place. The misguided mothers gave them to their young "just in case."

No wonder, then, that many doctors disapprove of the firms that sell patent medicines. In some cases, however, the companies manufacturing these patent remedies also make those drugs the doctor himself prescribes. Some firms even market a product under two different names—one for the public and one for the medical profession. That manufacturers usually have different factories to produce the mild patent medicines on the one hand, and the more powerful prescription drugs on the other, is hardly relevant. Either way, the drug manufacturer is in business to make money—the more the better. The manufacturers use the same techniques to sell their medicines as do soap firms promoting detergents. And if their advertising copy seems more sophisticated when directed at the doctor rather than at the man in the street, it is simply because they feel they will get better results this way.

Sometimes the advertising copy doctors receive is different only in degree from that seen on television or in newspapers. Here are but two examples from the many advertisements sent to British doctors daily—the first from British Schering Ltd., advertising their "Orasecron" pregnancy test; the second from William R. Warner and Co., advertising "Peritrate" for heart anginal attacks:

"Tomorrow she will ask you . . . dreaming . . . hoping. . . . There comes a breathless time when a woman wonders, decides no, wonders again—and finally asks you for confirmation or denial of pregnancy. So many prosaic things for her to consider. Should she buy that new summer dress?—When will she have to stop work?—How much do cots, prams, baby clothes cost?—What about the nursery? She needs to know the truth as quickly and certainly as possible. . . ."

"Angina has always been a great favourite with writers and actors, perhaps because it is at once dramatic, serious but not necessarily lethal, and has to do with the heart. It must be an aristocratic kind of thing to have angina, for Mr. Evelyn Waugh's Lord Marchmain, also mysterious and romantic, had it too, though he died of it only at 73. . . . And finally in one of her films Miss Bette Davis, who could always give a really nasty look better than the next, took the part of a woman who gives one to her husband, as, suffering an anginal attack, he struggles towards the relieving medicines she has placed beyond his reach. . . . What exactly would Miss Davis do if faced with a

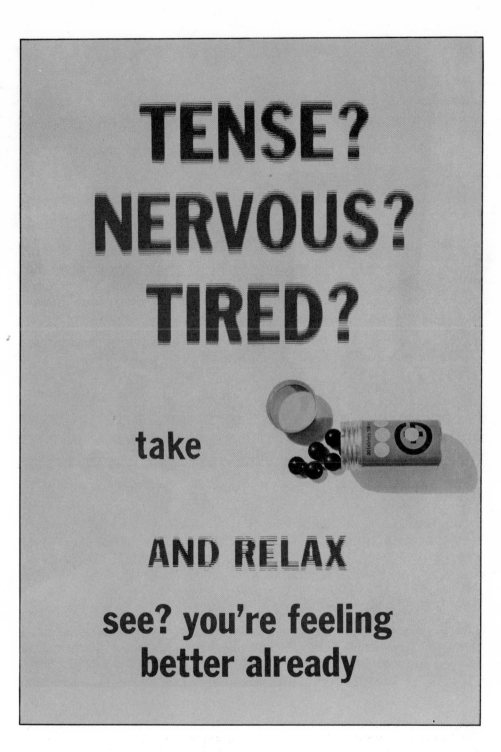

A parody of one kind of technique used
in pharmaceutical advertising. An actual
sensation of physical stress is produced
by the blurred type; the contrast of
the clear-cut lettering at the bottom
then suggests relief.

271

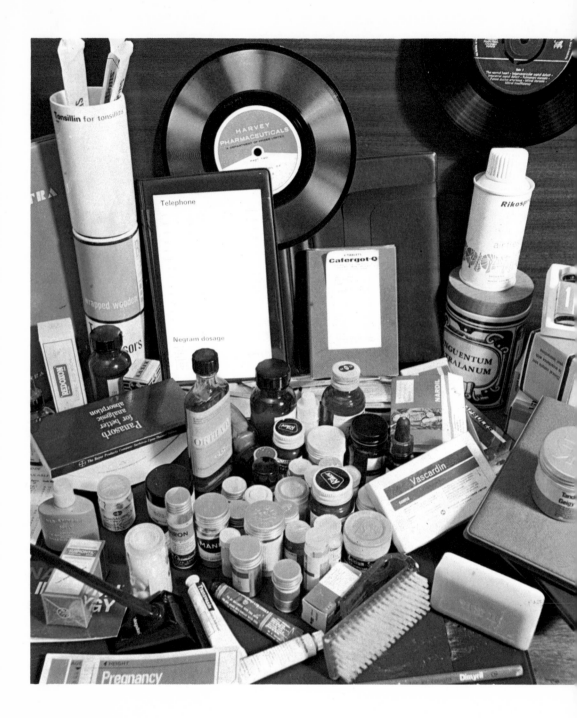

Many drug companies have adopted the sales technique of offering the doctor free gifts in addition to the usual drug samples and handouts. The selection here (from firms in several countries) includes items of general use—soap, a ball-point pen, calendars, a nail brush—all bearing the trademark of the donating company.

husband on Peritrate SA, with its effects sustained for twelve hours?"

In any one year a British doctor receives about one hundredweight of advertisements through his letter box. The Association of the British Pharmaceutical Industry has revealed that on sales of £67 million worth of drugs (about $187 million), trade advertising costs have amounted to £6½ million (about $18 million), of which roughly half is spent on sending out drug representatives (detail men) to doctors' surgeries. The drug firms do not pay out these large sums for nothing. They are aware that their two-pronged promotion attack of postal advertising and personal visiting by their representatives is amply rewarded. The general physicians, it seems, obtain about 30 per cent of their information about drugs in this way. The specialists, for their part, are more influenced by advertisements in the orthodox medical press; but the advertisements sent to doctors highlight the good points of a new drug and tend to minimize the bad ones. All business salesmen are likely to follow this procedure, but whereas vacuum cleaners that go wrong may irritate the housewife, drugs that misbehave may kill her. Thus one would expect pharmaceutical firms to show a greater awareness of their responsibilities than other kinds of commercial enterprises. Too often, alas, they do not seem to do so.

To assess the value of any new drug the general practitioner is largely dependent on the information given him by the representatives of the pharmaceutical companies. Many doctors welcome the regular calls made on them by representatives for this reason. But judging from the "situations vacant" columns for prospective medical representatives only 13 per cent of the "ethical" companies require applicants to have had a pharmaceutical training. When a new product is launched the company representatives are given a full account of its pharmacology and clinical indications; but sometimes, because their training is inadequate, they themselves cannot fully grasp the implications of the information. When the representative later leads the doctor on to trying a drug out, it seems too often a case of the blind leading the blind. The representative, committed to selling the new drug, is inevitably biased in its favor, and so even if he happens to be particularly well-informed the system becomes suspect.

One ex-medical representative or detail man, Ted Whitehead, wrote in *The New Statesman* of June 12, 1964, about his experiences as a drug peddler. "Inevitably," Mr. Whitehead said, "the detailman makes certain that he gets across the favourable details of his products and hopes that there will be time at the end for describing such negative points as precautions, contraindications and undesirable side effects. In fact he will probably avoid describing these at all and satisfy his conscience, if he must, by saying that such points are fully detailed in the literature provided—at the same time plonking his file of folders on the doctor's desk. He then goes whistling on his way. . . ."

It is evident that an expert, uncommitted advisory service for doctors is needed. Such a service could analyze the merits of similar drugs put out by competing manufacturers and, in this way, guide the doctor. It is likely that such an independent service will come into being in various countries sooner or later. Already, in New Zealand, the Ministry of Health employs doctors who provide the general practitioners with all the growing information about drugs, new and old, and who assist them in rational prescribing.

As I have already said, specialists are influenced to a greater degree than general practitioners by advertisements in the orthodox medical press. Even these, though, contain misleading information. A pharmaceutical company may advertise the same product differently in several medical journals. For example, Niamid, an antidepressant, was advertised in two American medical journals. In one, the manufacturer warned: "Niamid has not been reported to cause jaundice. However, in patients with a history of liver disease, the possibility of hepatic reactions should be kept in mind." In the other, the doctor was not warned but reassured: "A high degree of safety already

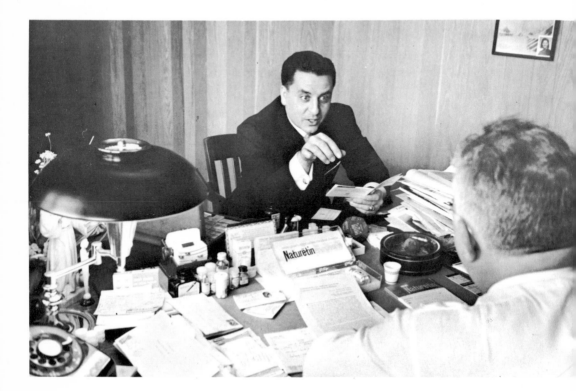

An American detail man briefs a doctor on the advantages of his company's new product —in this case, a drug for dropsy.

274

proved in several thousand patients. Niamid has not been reported to cause jaundice or glandular symptoms." It should be borne in mind that these two advertisements were published during the same month. The patient with liver damage who needed an antidepressant could only hope that the consultant he had been referred to was one who remained uninfluenced by advertisements in the medical press or, at least, had read the more admonitory copy.

Professor O. L. Wade of the Department of Therapeutics and Pharmacology at Queen's University, Belfast, with a colleague, examined the advertisements in the *British Medical Journal* of October 20, 1962. There were 44 advertisements in all and the investigators concluded that 26 of them made excessive claims, while in seven, serious side effects were not even mentioned. As Professor Wade said at the Second International Pharmacological Meeting, held in Prague in August 1963: "Almost every drug has some undesirable effect. My own teaching to my students is that no drug should ever be used unless there is good reason for its use, and when a drug is used the benefit that the patient stands to derive must outweigh the harm which may result from its use. This philosophy is not shared by those who advertise drugs. Many drug manufacturers are prepared to market and advertise drugs before controlled clinical trials have proved their merit or before extensive use has given reliable evidence of the incidence of side effects. The fact that modern drug advertising leads to the use of ineffective and sometimes dangerous remedies and to the misuse of many effective drugs is a criticism not only of the pharmaceutical industry but of our own profession and of the teaching in our medical schools. But it is impossible to examine current advertisements without realizing that some sections of the pharmaceutical industry manifest a cynical determination to benefit commercially from our professional ignorance. What worries me is that this has serious consequences for patients."

In Britain, a committee headed by Lord Sainsbury was set up in 1965 to investigate the relationship of the pharmaceutical industry to the British National Health Service. The Council of the British Medical Association, in submitting evidence to the Sainsbury committee, opined that advertising in medical journals is "not only an effective means of sales promotion but is also an important source of information to the medical profession." Since the B.M.A. publishes (among other journals) the *British Medical Journal*, it is not surprising that the Council continued: "The medical scrutiny given to advertisement copy by medically qualified staff is a protection against false and misleading claims." Judging from the above analysis by Professor O. L. Wade of advertisements in one issue of the *British Medical*

*Journal*, it would seem that the council's faith in medical editorial censorship is misplaced. In any case, it is lamentable that professional journals, especially those of the highest grade, should be financially dependent on advertising revenue. The evidence given on this issue by the B.M.A. Council does not appear to be disinterested. Indeed, its memorandum seems to me to be generally timid or complacent—even, on occasions, contradictory and hypocritical.

It is hard to know whether the Council is being sanguine or cynical when it states: "The influence of the pharmaceutical houses in disseminating information . . . is significant and contributes to the continuing education of the medical practitioner. The doctor's critical faculties which have been developed during his medical education aid him in analysing the wide variety of therapeutic information provided by the industry. Such information may be presented as straight advertising material, as explanatory literature, or as lectures and films and the Council is confident that the medical profession is discriminating in its use of this information." The Council has no reason to be confident; the medical profession is all too susceptible to the sophisticated propaganda of the pharmaceutical sales departments. The sales departments are confident that this is so—and hence spend the enormous sums available to them for promotion. They know—even if the Council does not—that a doctor's previous education cannot help him in assessing critically the value and dangers of any new drug marketed. What the medical profession needs is some objective and disinterested guidance, and the Council of the British Medical Association should say so without equivocation.

The Council does not even condemn the entertainment given by the pharmaceutical houses to medical groups. Such entertainment is often lavish and expressly undertaken to advertise and promote their products. A doctor or group of doctors cannot be given favors and entertainment continuously without in some way being affected and perhaps even corrupted. However, in its memorandum the Council expresses the belief that "groups within the profession may, as in the past, accept the hospitality, services, or contributions of Commercial Houses without any obligation, tacit or implied, to further the advertisements of any individual products"—to which statement the PROs of the drug houses can only respond with a delighted horse laugh. "In accepting such contributions," the Council continues, "the body accepting them may acknowledge them openly, naming the particular House which has made the contribution, in a manner that is dignified and appropriate."

One notes here, as elsewhere in the memorandum, that the B.M.A. Council seems more concerned with the dignity of the medical profession than with basic principles. However it is our health that is being indirectly bartered. Why, the same issue of the *British Medical Journal* that contains the memorandum (April 30, 1966) also presents a pertinent paper by Dr. G. M. Wilson of Sheffield University entitled "Ill-Health Due to Drugs." The B.M.A. appears to be speaking with two voices. Something is rotten in the state of Medicine. And not only in Britain. In some of the U.S. medical journals even "scientific" articles are inspired by the pharmaceutical companies. Dr. H. J. Weinstein, formerly with the medical staff of the American drug firm Pfizer, told a committee set up in America under the chairmanship of Senator Estes Kefauver to inquire into the drug industry and the pricing of drugs: "A substantial number of the so-called medical scientific papers that are published on behalf of these drugs are. written within the confines of the pharmaceutical houses concerned."

It seems such papers are sent out to those medical journals in which the pharmaceutical company advertises its products regularly. Dependent on advertising revenue, the journal rarely refuses the article. Dr. Weinstein said: "I was involved in a situation which will, I believe, describe the relations between the pharmaceutical house and the publisher quite adequately. I was assigned the task of writing a paper on a new formulation of a broad spectrum antibiotic. I was informed that this paper had been accepted for publication and the 100,000-plus reprints were ordered before I finished the writing assignment. The paper, of course, was published exactly on schedule, which incidentally was within a few days of the introduction of the product on the market."

Doctors cannot rely on the objectivity of advertisements in magazines—nor even, on occasions it would seem, on the impartiality of "learned" papers in the medical press. If the doctor is bombarded with biased information from all quarters, and is impressionable, as many are, he will become a puppet with a syringe manipulated by pharmaceutical firms for their own profits. Meanwhile, trusting patients will roll up their sleeves and the needle will be plunged in.

Despite, or because of, massive promotional activities the drug firms make enormous profits. The annual sales of drugs in the U.S.A. alone amount to $2500 million. Some American pensioners spend as much as one third of their income on the different medicaments they need. The Association of the British Pharmaceutical Industry has admitted that the average profit of eight American companies based in Britain is 72.83 per cent—and even allowing for money siphoned off for research and administrative costs at their U.S. headquarters, the average profit is still over 33 per cent. The Socialist Medical Association states that the profits made by the pharmaceutical industry as a whole in Britain are at the rate of some 15 per cent compared with the 13.8 per cent earned by other industries. There are many who feel that the drug houses are entitled to earn as much as they legitimately can under a free enterprise capitalist system—whether they operate in the U.S.A., Britain, West Germany, Italy, France, or wherever. On the other hand, in countries like France, Italy, Spain, and America, where no National Health Service exists, many are desperately in need of medicines they cannot afford. And even where the state does foot the bill for drugs there is no reason why it should be fleeced, for then the people as a whole are indirectly deprived of much-needed hospitals that could otherwise be paid for. Ultimately, perhaps, the issue depends on whether or not the profits made are reasonable.

The Kefauver committee revealed some hair-raising facts about the profits of American drug companies. It calculated that a cortisone-type drug, prednisolone, manufactured by the American company Upjohn, cost but 1.57 cents a tablet to produce, bottle, label, pack, etc. Another drug company, Schering, bought the drug at 2.37 cents and sold it to the chemist at 17.90 cents a tablet. The patient finally had to pay 29.8 cents per tablet. In short, Schering's markup was over 650 per cent. On another occasion this same company bought a drug from a French pharmaceutical firm at $3.5 per gram, then bottled and sold 11.7 cents worth of the drug for $8.40. Of this latter transaction Senator Kefauver said to the Schering president: "All you did was put it in a tablet, put it out under your name, and sell it at a mark-up of 7,079 per cent." As Brian Inglis has pointed out in *Drugs, Doctors and Diseases*: "It was hardly surprising, then, that in the five and a half years since it [Schering] had been converted into a corporation its net total profits had exceeded the purchase price of the firm by about three million dollars."

The Kefauver committee also had a great deal to say about the profits made on the extremely popular and much prescribed antibiotic, tetracycline. The patentees of this antibiotic were Pfizer and American Cyanamid, which means that royalties had to be paid to them when the drug was made by another pharmaceutical company. Both Bristol and Upjohn produced the drug—Bristol for 5.03 cents (including 40 per cent royalties paid to the patentees) and Upjohn for 9.3 cents. Both firms sold it to the retail chemist at 31 cents. The patient had to pay 51 cents a capsule. Obviously fantastic profits were being made.

"In 1961," writes Brian Inglis, "a new British company, DDSA Pharmaceuticals, began to market tetracycline. Ordinarily there would have been nothing remarkable about such an event, but in this

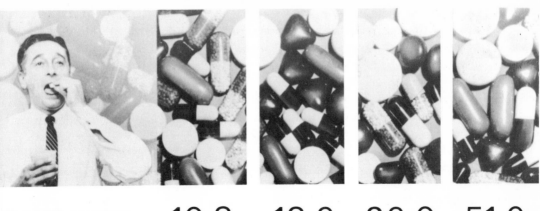

| CONSUMER | 10.8 | 13.9 | 29.0 | 51.0 |

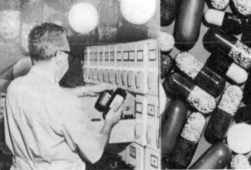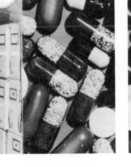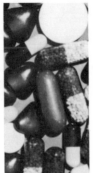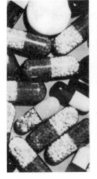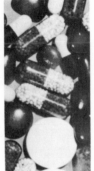

| DRUGGIST | 6.5 | 8.3 | 17.9 | 30.6 |

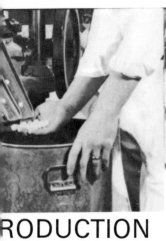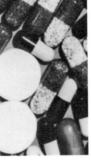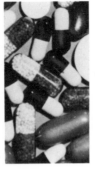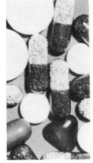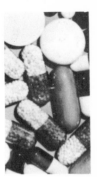

| | 0.7 cents | 1.6 cents | 1.6 cents | 2.9 cents |
| PRODUCTION | MILTOWN TRANQUILIZER | ORINASE ANTIDIABETIC | PREDNISOLONE ARTHRITIS TREATMENT | TETRACYCLINE ANTIBIOTIC |

A chart, published in America at the time of the Kefauver hearings, shows the ratios between the production and selling costs of four major drugs.

279

case there was: the price they were asking for the antibiotic. When tetracycline had been introduced into Britain in the mid-1950s the patentees, Pfizer, and the other companies they had licensed to sell it, charged over £90 [about $250] per 1,000 tablets; expensive, but, thought doctors who prescribed it, well worth the cost because it was an effective "broad spectrum" antibiotic, useful in the treatment of a much wider range of infectious disorders than, say, penicillin. In due course, it could be assumed, the price would come down, as drug prices ordinarily do. In due course, it did; by the early 1960s it had fallen by a third, to a little over £60 [about $170] per 1,000 tablets, which suggested that the firms concerned were keeping keen competitive prices. It came as a shock, therefore, to hear that DDSA were charging a mere £6 10s. 0d. [about $18] per thousand for their tetracycline: little more than one tenth of the—till then—ruling price. DDSA's supplies, it transpired, came from the Continent; either from countries which, like Italy, did not allow patents on drugs, or from behind the Iron Curtain, where Western patents were not recognised anyway."

Communist countries such as Czechoslovakia, Poland, and Hungary are able to supply some antibiotics produced in their state factories

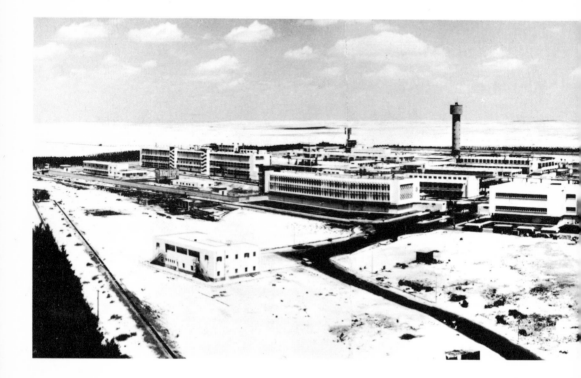

at extremely low prices partly because their governments pay no royalties to the patentees. When in 1961 tetracycline was imported into Britain by the large Carlo Erba company of Milan the Poles were able to offer the antibiotic at an even cheaper price. (Italy does not recognize drug patents. For the equivalent of 1s. 6d.—about 20 cents— the Italians can buy from the Patent Office a copy of any drug patent complete with production details.)

The Pfizer group have been forthright in condemning Western purchases of "cheap communist material." Yet Pfizer, themselves, have bought Hungarian antibiotics for years. They had a contract with Medimpex, the Hungarian state drug firm, which allowed them to acquire oxytetracycline. According to Dr. Andreas Vincze, a Pfizer agent, and Laszlo Hamburger of Medimpex, the basic charge to Pfizer for oxytetracycline was £16 ($44.5) per kilo; but the British retail chemists had to pay £220 ($615) per kilo for the drug marketed by Pfizer under the name of "Terramycin." If these figures are correct Pfizer were making well over 1000 per cent profit on the Hungarian drug. Pfizer have maintained that they had an oversupply of hydrocortisone and wished to market it in Eastern Europe. B. J. G. Page, one of Pfizer's top men in Britain, has said: "The Hungarians hadn't

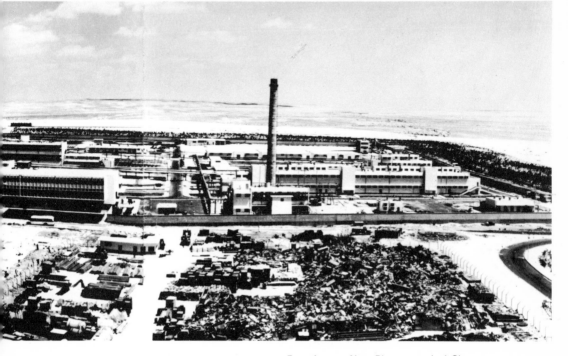

Egypt's new Nasr Pharmaceutical City, 25 miles northwest of Cairo—a vast enterprise backed to a very large extent by Russian money and technical know-how.

any currency to pay us in." So Pfizer took oxytetracycline instead. "We just wanted to keep our hydro-cortisone plant working," said Mr. Page. "We didn't want the oxytetracycline; it was a pain in the neck to us." With the profits that Pfizer seem to have made, most manufacturers would gratefully endure such a pain.

One British expert who has been giving evidence to the Sainsbury committee on the astronomical profit margins made by the pharmaceutical companies is Dr. M. A. Phillips, for 20 years a research chemist with May and Baker. Dr. Phillips is also a Fellow of the Royal Society of Medicine and of the Royal Institute of Chemistry, as well as a director of several drug manufacturing companies. In other words, his experience allows him to speak with authority about such matters. Already he has ventilated certain facts in the national press. On January 2, 1966, he wrote in *The People*: "I must bring into the open a scandal that has remained cloaked in secrecy and repectability for more years that I care to remember. It is the scandal of the outrageous prices that you and I—the ordinary taxpayers—are having to pay for the life-saving and healing drugs which are prescribed for us by our family doctors. . . ." He lists the profits on such drugs as Chloromycetin, Furadantin, Nydrazid, Ceporin, and Synalar. According to Dr. Phillips the lowest profit made on these drugs is 320 per cent and the highest 5000 per cent.

But the British spend less per head on drugs than any other Western community with the exception of the Danes. Based on figures published in 1962, Britain spends an average of 16 shillings (about $2.20) per head of population each year. Holland, however, spends 22s. 2d. (just over $3); Sweden 25s. 8d. (about $3.50); West Germany 26s. 1d. (about $3.66); Italy 47s. 5d. (about $6.60); and Belgium 55s. 4d. (about $7.75).

All over the world, governments, including those of South Africa, the Philippines, and Australia, have inquired, or are inquiring, into the high profits made on drugs by the pharmaceutical industries. The Egyptian government has actively controlled the means of pharmaceutical distribution, and calls for nationalization have been made in several South American countries, notably Brazil and Peru. Argentina, too, has brought in new drug legislation, and in 1963 the government of Colombia proclaimed a generic drug program.

The term "generic" here means simply that drugs are given their real, often difficult, chemical name rather than the pharmaceutical house's easy-to-remember, branded, patented name. Once branded, drugs become infinitely more expensive. The Colombian government, aware that so many people could not afford to pay for patented, branded drugs and as a result had to suffer and even die, called in the biggest drug wholesalers in the U.S.A.—McKesson and Robbins—to market 32 generic drugs. Thus one antibiotic, which sold at 29 cents per capsule under its brand name, was distributed by McKesson and Robbins (without its glamorous name) at 3.6 cents. Vitamin $B_{12}$, sold under its trade name at \$12, fell to \$1.20 when sold generically— and needless to say, McKesson and Robbins were still able to take a handsome profit even at this price. No wonder moves to abolish or amend patents in the public interest have taken place, or are now being considered, in several countries—among them India, New Zealand, Canada, and Turkey. No wonder official disquiet is widespread.

Despite the Kefauver report and adverse publicity, the drug industry in the U.S.A. hailed the year 1965 as "the greatest." That is to say, the volume of drug sales broke all previous records. So did the profits. Nearly one thousand million prescriptions were handed in to retail druggists—an increase of 12.3 per cent over 1964. Madeline Oxford Holland reported in *The Pharmaceutical Journal* of February 26, 1966, that: "Prescription volume in December, 1965, broke all records for a continuing survey which has followed the field for the past 14 years. Eighty-nine million prescriptions were dispensed in December; 40 million of them "new" prescriptions. Statistics show that there are 55 million households in the United States; that means that, in December alone, there were dispensed 1.6 prescriptions for every household in the country. The 1965 total for new prescriptions was 427 million; repeat prescriptions showed a 12.1 per cent increase. In 1965, 10 categories of drugs (led by antibiotics, analgesics, cough and cold remedies, hormones and ataraxics) accounted for 70.9 per cent of the volume, or 277.7 million prescriptions. The number of oral contraceptive prescriptions in 1965 rose 54.3 per cent to account, with other hormone products, for 9.0 per cent of that year's total."

The U.S. companies are not only particularly efficient in selling their drugs; they are also particularly avaricious. They claim that their overheads are extremely high because they engage in expensive research projects in the hope of discovering new drugs that will ultimately benefit the health of humankind. Undoubtedly, new drugs discovered in the laboratories of the pharmaceutical houses have made a major contribution to the progress of medical science. People of all nations have much to thank them for. The cry of, "We do research," however, does not in itself explain the inordinate price of drugs. There are many examples of U.S. firms that have bought drugs discovered by European companies and so have not had to lay out money on their earlier research and development. Pfizer's acquisition of oxytetracycline from Medimpex has already been cited. Another instance is the antidiabetic drug tolbutamide (Orinase), which was discovered by the German firm Hoechst. Hoechst charged the German retail chemist $1.85 for their product. Upjohn, who sold the German drug exclusively in the U.S.A., sold the same amount of it for $4.17. Again, a drug used in the treatment of high blood pressure, reserpine, was developed by the Swiss firm of CIBA who marketed it under the name of Serpasil throughout Europe at between $1 and $2. The American subsidiary of CIBA, however, asked $4.5 for the same quantity of Serpasil. To give but one more example: Rhône-Poulenc, the French firm, charged the retail druggists 51 cents for 50 tablets of the tranquilizer chlorpromazine (Thorazine or Largactil). The U.S. licensee, Smith, Kline and French, charged the retailer $3.03 for the very same drug.

At the Kefauver hearings the American pharmaceutical companies tried to explain away such high profits in terms of the higher labor costs that exist in the U.S.A. This conflicts, though, with the conclusions drawn by Estes Kefauver in his book *In a Few Hands*: ". . . the available evidence suggests that American companies have, if anything, lower unit costs than their European confrères because the chemical industry, of which drug operations are a part, is highly mechanized." A Chemical Fund newsletter reported: "It takes only 833,000 American

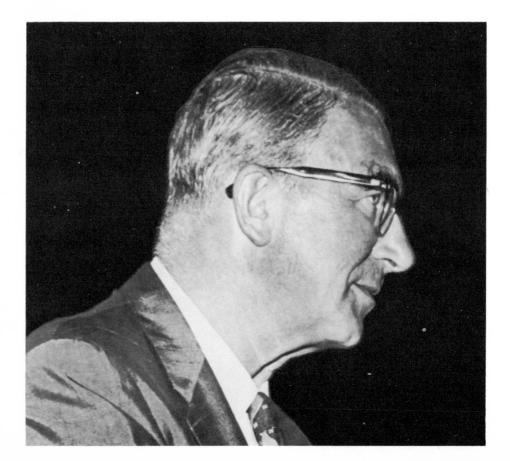

workers to produce 25 billion dollars of chemicals a year; while, in Europe, by comparison, it takes more than 1,400,000 employees to produce only 10 billion of chemicals a year." Hence the argument that drugs have to be priced higher in the U.S.A. than in Europe does not hold.

Perhaps the most inane excuse for the high cost of drugs in the U.S.A. was expounded by Dr. Austin Smith, the president of the Pharmaceutical Manufacturers Association, when he gave evidence before the Kefauver committee. Let me quote Dr. Smith's statement direct from *In a Few Hands*: "Death costs about 900 dollars, and that does not include legal fees or doctor's fees, only the funeral director and the embalming service and the coffins and the monuments and the tombstones and the cemetery services." On the other hand, Dr. Smith suggested that drugs can save a trip to the hospital; and that if hospital costs are stacked against drug costs, any drug—whatever its price—is a bargain. And so for years he has been "speaking of the low cost of drugs." One can imagine the advertising promotion triggered off by Dr. Smith's argument. "This drug is expensive but it is cheaper than death."

How profitable drug selling has been in the U.S.A. can be gauged from the way the shares of certain pharmaceutical companies have rocketed in a relatively short space of time. On February 18, 1959, the *Investor's Reader* reported how a Mr. Harry B. Leeds of Atlantic City, a retail druggist, made his fortune: "He . . . carefully stowed away his 40 shares of Smith, Kline and French common. His original purchase of 10 shares for less than 1,000 dollars early in 1929 had been multiplied by a 4-for-1 split later that bullish year and was already worth $4,800 by 1938. Chances are investor Leeds never realized what a much bigger bonanza lay ahead. At any rate, the stock was still in the safe when his widow Harriet died last year. However, thanks to stock splits in 1947, 1950, and 1954, the holdings had by then expanded into 4,800 shares worth 477,000 dollars. After the usual tax deductions and fees the Atlantic City Court which reviewed the estate approved 390,773.73 dollars for distribution to the Leeds heirs."

There are those who feel that the pharmaceutical companies deserve their excessive profits. In defense of the industry they point out that a number of firms perform a public, disinterested service. For altruistic reasons, they manufacture drugs on which they may make a loss. For example, Crookes-Barnes Laboratories manufacture a preparation intended for use during certain medical emergencies—as when a coma ensues on a liver disfunction. Now this preparation is only called for on some 10,000 occasions a year; yet Crookes-Barnes maintain a stock

United States Senator Estes Kefauver, chairman of the Senate Subcommittee on Antitrust and Monopoly from 1957 until his death in 1963.

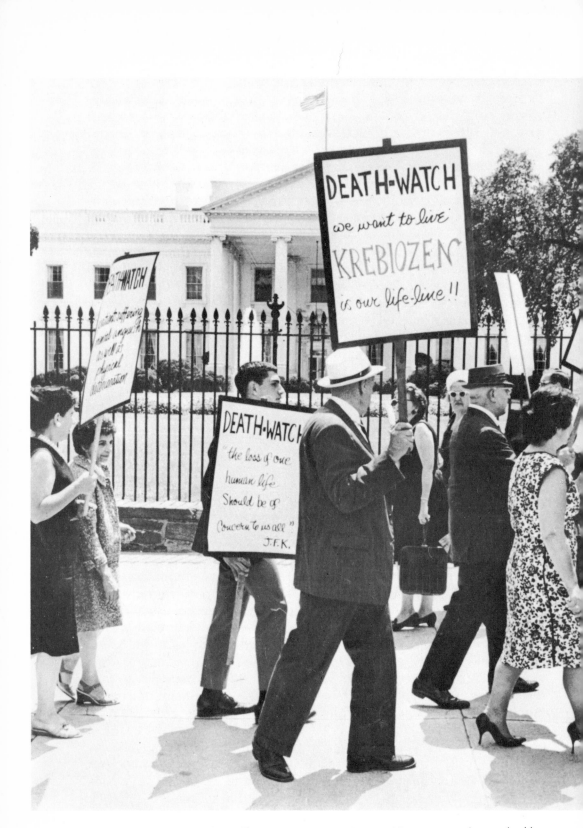

Cancer patients picket the White House in protest against the FDA's ban on the interstate sale of krebiozen in 1963. Although analysis showed that the drug (which cost 10 cents to produce and sold at $9.50) mostly consisted of creatine and mineral oil, these patients remained convinced of its efficacy.

of it in 300 of their wholesale houses. The president of this large firm, Edmund Beckwith, said at the Kefauver hearings: "We maintain 24-hour telephone coverage at our headquarters, maintain prepacked emergency stocks at air freight terminals on both coasts, and routinely absorb all shipping charges right to the hospital door. A few months ago, via our Montreal office and before this particular preparation was available in Canada, we had an emergency call from Winnipeg. A child was dying. Simultaneously we shipped six units from each coast in the U.S. Why both coasts? We couldn't be sure which routing would arrive first. (The East, via Toronto, won by 30 minutes.) Why six units? Because Customs officers sometimes remove samples for analysis and we had to be sure enough got through. Why no charge? Because the risk of even half an hour delay by a Customs officer considering the question of a U.S. firm shipping a drug into Canada for sale would have been intolerable."

There are other firms with other "prestige" drugs on their list. It is admirable that this should be so. For that matter it is admirable that they provide money for charitable organizations, and arrange educational seminars for doctors, and so on. It is admirable, but they can afford it. That they expend large sums of money on research is perhaps a more solid argument for those who defend the drug firms. For example, I.C.I. recently spent £700,000 (about $1,960,000) looking for a new drug to combat a particular virus. They never found what they were looking for. Such an occurrence is a common one. Only one in 3000 chemicals researched and developed becomes marketable. Even so, more money is spent on advertising and promotion than on research. Twenty-two of the biggest companies reported to the Kefauver committee that their combined expenditure on the promotion of drugs during 1958 was $580 million. The companies' research and development costs, though, amounted to only about a quarter of this figure.

Again, much of the research undertaken is directed not toward the discovery of a new drug but rather to finding a modification of one already available but marketed by a competitor. Thus, when the antihistamines were found to counteract certain allergic conditions like hay fever and urticarial skin disorders, the pharmaceutical firms sought slight chemical variants in order to obtain patent rights on antiallergic products. For 15 years, subsequently, they were able to sell their patented, branded, antihistamine-like drugs at much higher prices. More than 300 antihistamine compounds, all with different names, and marketed by different firms, were soon available. All basically had the same properties. All the firms could protest that the high price of their product was due to research.

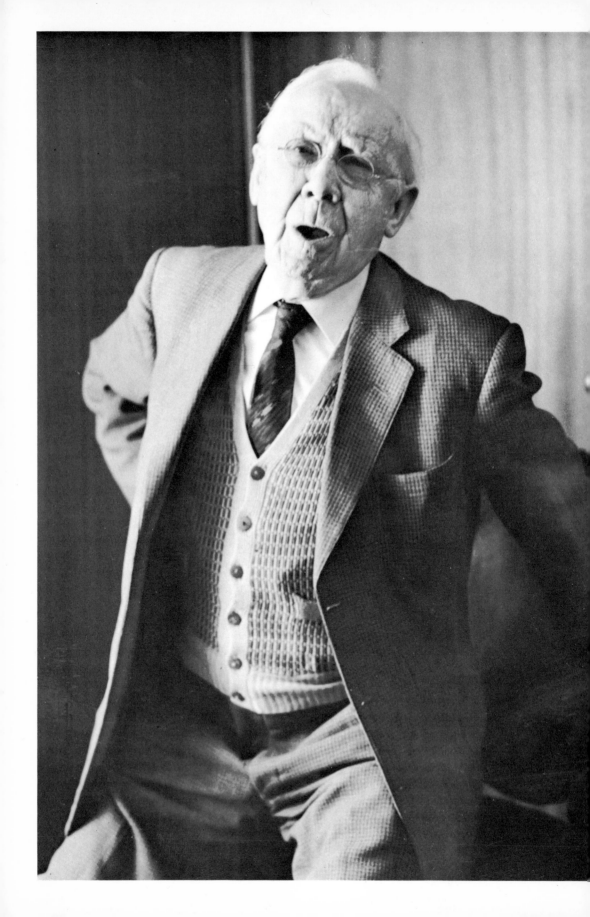

More recently the tranquilizing drugs were researched and branded in the same way. Something like 70 per cent of the money available for research in the U.S. pharmaceutical industry is spent on finding chemical variants that provide only minimal therapeutic benefit to the public at large—though great benefit financially to the individual firms. Real research has been done and is being done. "Miracle drugs" have been and will be discovered as a result; but when the pharmaceutical industry talks about the high cost of drugs arising from the high cost of research, it must be remembered that there are productive and unproductive varieties of research. It is only fair to add here, though, that variants of a drug *may* result in advantages for the patient—where, for instance, the basic drug cannot be given orally and the variant can; or where the latter is longer-lasting in the body and so cuts down the number of injections required; or where the drug, in its varied form, is simply more palatable.

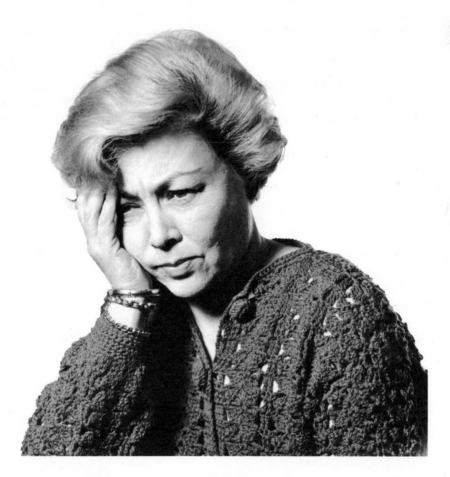

Two of the professional models used—because of their ability to simulate symptoms—in many pharmaceutical adverts aimed at the medical profession. Here they portray a rheumatic (left), and a sufferer from headaches and neuralgia (above).

If patents were done away with or modified, then much of the more wasteful kind of research would diminish. So would the prices of drugs. The companies argue that they need to keep absolute patent rights. They claim that without the protection of such patents competitors might steal their discoveries; that without such a protection they could hardly be expected to spend millions. There would, they say, be stagnation of research. Their arguments are fortified by the fact that no significant new drugs have been discovered in the U.S.S.R. Yet only Belgium, the U.S.A., and Panama allow drugs to be patented without imposing certain limitations to safeguard the public. There is no evidence to suggest that Belgium, the U.S.A., and Panama are more disposed to discover new drugs (as opposed to variants) than other nations.

No important drug has been discovered in Panama. The sub-committee staff at the Kefauver hearings prepared a list of drugs that could be considered to be a real contribution to "the healing art" and gave their country of origin. Only two of the drugs on this list originated in Belgium. This is hardly impressive when set beside Germany's score of 27 significant discoveries. True, the commercial firms in the U.S. have contributed 60 important drugs, but the Kefauver report states: "It may come as something of a surprise to note that the following drugs which are among the most widely used in the world were discovered in countries which have never awarded patents on pharmaceutical products." The report then went on to list the major non-patent drugs.

**Germany:** Acetanilid; Acetophenetidin (Phenacetin); Aspirin; Atabrine (Quinacrine); Diphenylhydantoin; Meperidine (Demerol); Methadone; Pentobarbital (Nembutal); Phenobarbital (Luminal); Phenylephrine; Primaquine; Tolbutamide (Orinase).

**Switzerland:** Androsterone; Desoxycorticosterone; Hydralazine (Apresoline); Phenmetrazine (Preludin); Progesterone; Reserpine; Sulfisomidine (Elkosin); Testosterone.

**France:** Cocaine; Chlorpromazine (Thorazine); Promazine (Sparine); Prochlorperazine (Compazine).

**Sweden:** Lidocaine (Xylocaine); Para-Aminosalicylic acid (PAS); Pentaerythritoltetranitrate (PETN).

**Mexico:** Prednisone; Norethindrone (Norlutin).

Britain has been excluded from the above list because it is unique in that while it did not award product patents during the period 1919–49, it subsequently did, with limitations. I have constructed a table below in which all the most important drugs discovered in Britain during the non-patent period from 1927 are set against those discovered afterwards.

| Type of drug | Non-Patent Period | Patent Period |
|---|---|---|
| HORMONES | Pregnanediol (1927)<br>Dienestrol (1938)<br>Aldosterone (Switzerland and Britain) 1939 | |
| ANTIBIOTICS | Penicillin G 1929<br>Aerosporin (Polymixin B) 1947 | Griseofulvin 1954<br>Phenoxyethyl penicillin 1959 |
| TRANQUILIZERS AND CENTRAL NERVOUS SYSTEM DRUGS | Mephenesin 1946 | Primidone 1954 |
| GENERAL DRUGS | Digitoxin (isolated) 1936<br><br>Magnesium Trisilicate 1936<br><br>Penicillinase 1940<br><br>Pilocarpine 1947<br>Potassium Bromide 1935<br><br>Sulfamethazine 1941<br>Sulfapyridine 1938<br><br>Urethan 1946 | Chlorambucil (Leukeran) 1957<br>Chloroguanide (anti-malarial) 1954<br>Mechlorethamine 1949<br>Myleran 1953<br>Pentolinium Tartrate 1953<br><br>Triiodothyronine (Cytomel) 1952 |

From the above it would appear that no stagnation of research occurred in Britain during the period when no patent was allowed; nor for that matter has there been a significant acceleration in the number of important discoveries since 1949. In short, the argument that patented products are an imperative incentive for researchers to research and for discoveries to be discovered does not seem to be substantiated by fact. Indeed, the Kefauver committee concluded that it would "appear to be warranted that . . . the mere existence of patent protection is not a guarantee of invention, nor is its absence much of a barrier." If a patent is no guarantee of inventiveness it is a guarantee that prices of drugs will leap up, as can be seen from the following table for 1959:

| Product | Average prices (in $) throughout the world | |
| --- | --- | --- |
| | Without Patents | With Patents |
| Prednisone (Meticorten) | 14.75 | 22.36 |
| Chlorpromazine (Thorazine) | 1.24 | 1.89 |
| Prochlorperazine (Compazine) | 0.80 | 2.84 |
| Promazine (Sparine) | 1.57 | 1.98 |
| Meprobamate (Miltown) | 2.53 | 3.31 |
| Reserpine (Serpasil) | 1.73 | 2.79 |
| Tolbutamide (Orinase) | 2.03 | 3.02 |
| Chlorpropamide (Diabinese) | 3.81 | 4.87 |
| Penicillin V | 10.87 | 13.19 |
| Chloramphenicol (Chloromycetin) | 3.17 | 3.77 |
| Chlortetracycline (Aureomycin) | 4.68 | 5.53 |
| Tetracycline (Achromycin) | 4.63 | 5.68 |

In every case the drug price is higher for countries with product patents than without—sometimes considerably. The fact that the U.S. commercial firms often take the public for a financial ride may be deplorable. Worse is the fact that in their hurry to gain quick profits the pharmaceutical companies, on occasions, endanger human lives. When a drug is a commercial success, and it is then discovered that the same drug can cause unpredictable side effects, the manufacturers naturally tend to minimize the drug's dangers. Sometimes they have gone even further and put out misleading information. The story of chloramphenicol, sold by Parke, Davis under the trade name of Chloromycetin, is a case in point. I have touched on the Chloromycetin scandal in the chapter entitled *The Human Guinea Pig*, but I intend to go into further detail here.

As has been said, the commercial success of Chloromycetin was fantastic. It was the second largest selling broad-spectrum antibiotic and was used to combat all kinds of minor infections from earache to tonsillitis, from septic cuts to whooping cough, as well as more serious conditions like typhoid fever for which it is a specific. But in 1950 it was discovered that Chloromycetin could damage the bone marrow and cause serious blood disorders like aplastic anemia—which has a death rate of over 50 per cent. Soon physicians throughout the world began to read reports in their different medical journals of such dangerous Chloromycetin complications. As a result, rightly, an acute decline in the sales of the drug occurred. Parke, Davis apparently did not resign themselves to the financial loss involved. At least they sent out a series of memos containing misleading or false information to their detail men. Thus in their "President's Letter," dated August 12, 1952, the following statement can be read: "Chloromycetin has been officially cleared by the FDA [Food and Drug Administration] and the National Research Council with *no restrictions* on the number or the range of diseases for which Chloromycetin may be administered."

As the Kefauver report indicated: "This statement is false because recommendation No. 2 of the National Research Council states that 'although this complication has thus far been uncommon, it was considered sufficiently important to warrant a warning on the label of the packages of the drugs and the recommendation that chloramphenicol *not be used indiscriminately or for minor infections*.' Obviously when the National Research Council recommended that chloramphenicol 'not be used indiscriminately or for minor infections,' it was proposing a restriction 'on the number' and 'the range of diseases.' This statement is misleading in that it distorts the true nature of the action by FDA and the NRC. What these two bodies did was to permit the continued use and sale of the drug under certain specific conditions, namely, that a warning must be included on the label and the advertisements and that the drug should not be used indiscriminately or for minor ailments. Parke, Davis perverted the permission for continued use under these restrictions into a blanket 'clearance' of the drug."

In fact the Parke, Davis detail men received further memos containing equally distorted information. On November 20, 1952, they received a directive containing the following passages, which they were told to memorize and repeat verbatim to physicians they visited:

"1. . . . intensive investigation by the Food and Drug Administration, carried on with the assistance of a special committee of eminent specialists appointed by the National Research Council, resulted in *unqualified sanction* of continued used of Chloromycetin for all conditions in which it has previously been used." (My italics.)

"2. A sensible caution against indiscriminate use, which we have incorporated into our advertising and labeling, is a *welcome addition* to our literature and to the label on Chloromycetin products, and in our opinion, would be appropriate in those on any potent chemotherapeutic agent. Actually, such caution is an assurance that the full benefits of well-tolerated Chloromycetin will be available and free from misuse." (My italics.)

# "DOCTOR v. CHEMIST."

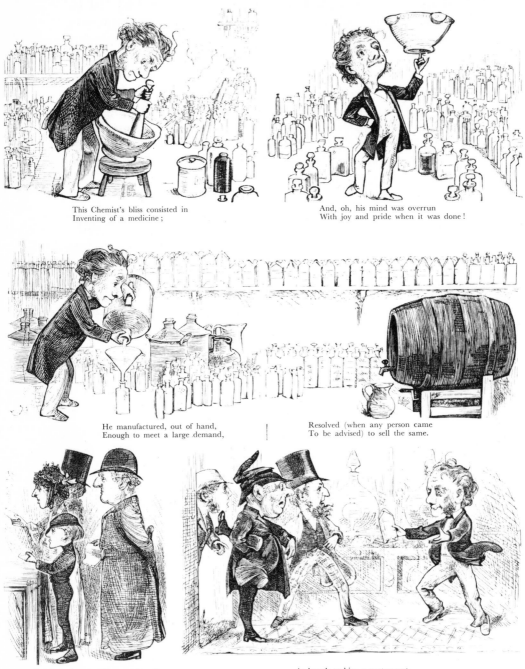

This Chemist's bliss consisted in
Inventing of a medicine;

And, oh, his mind was overrun
With joy and pride when it was done!

He manufactured, out of hand,
Enough to meet a large demand,

Resolved (when any person came
To be advised) to sell the same.

But lo! when people came to call,
They brought prescriptions, one and all;
While no one entered for the sake
Of asking "what he ought to take?"

At length to him a party went
Who'd lost his leg by accident;
The chance had come—it was enough!
That Chemist sold him all the stuff!

294 The popular image of the "chemist" in 19th-century Britain is presented in a contemporary cartoon. He is shown as an unscrupulous rogue, eager to foist his worthless patent cures on any credulous patient who seeks his advice.

So, in the space of a few months, the detail men were told that Chloromycetin had been "officially cleared," that it had passed "intensive investigation," and that these investigations had led to "an unqualified sanction" of the drug. The Kefauver report comments that Parke, Davis "was able to make these incredible assertions because then, as now, the instructions are known only to three parties—the drug companies who concoct them, the detail men who memorize and transmit them, and the Nation's doctors who ultimately receive them." The Kefauver subcommittee had exposed the behavior of Parke, Davis over this matter by securing the highly inflammable copies of the memos sent off to the detail men. According to American author Richard Harris, in his book *The Real Voice*, nothing had made Senator Kefauver so angry as these revelations.

In 1951 Parke, Davis had sold 52 million dollars' worth of Chloromycetin, for doctors were prescribing it indiscriminately. But, by 1955, sales had dropped to 35 million dollars. Before the Kefauver hearings the sales of Chloromycetin had climbed higher than ever to roughly 86 million dollars' worth. Following the hearings the sales of Chloromycetin declined to approximately 68 million dollars. Harry J. Loynd, the president of Parke, Davis, grumbled that Senator Kefauver's hearings had caused "some very unfavorable publicity, I might say unjustified and some of it ridiculous, which cost us a volume loss on Chloromycetin of about fifteen million dollars."

But did all this evidence and the publicity it received irrevocably hold back doctors from prescribing Chloromycetin? It would seem not. As Richard Harris points out: "In 1961, the *Physicians' Desk Reference*, a commercially produced manual of therapeutic agents known as 'the physician's Bible,' carried not the FDA's warning on Chloromycetin but Parke, Davis's amended version, and in 1962 this was dropped in favor of a statement that the doctor could get information on 'dosage, administration, contraindications and precautions' from the package insert, the detail man, or the company. Reports from various parts of the country at the time indicated that many doctors had missed all the furor and were still prescribing Chloromycetin for minor afflictions."

So much for orthodox medical bodies' pious belief that a physician's education allows him to discriminate in his choice of drugs despite the bombardment of advertisements from the pharmaceutical companies. No wonder there are those who take an extremist position and agree with the Victorian physician who said he firmly believed that if all the drugs in the world could be sunk to the bottom of the sea it would be that much better for mankind, and that much worse for the fish. Perhaps extremists of this order would feel differently if the competitive

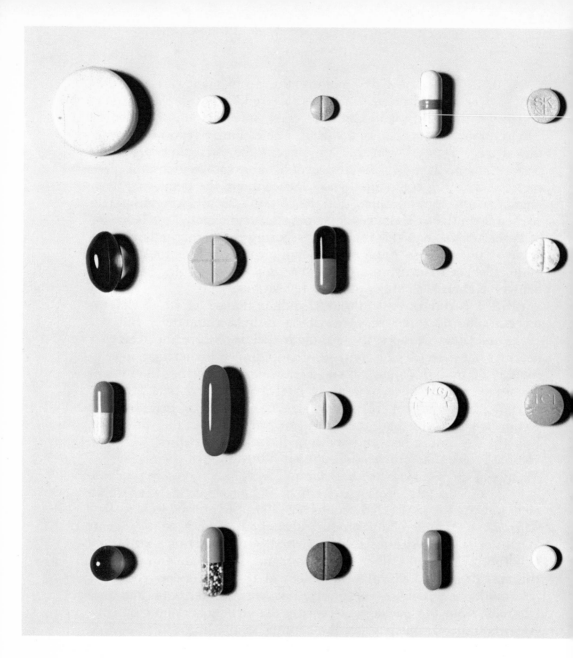

## 40 Major Drugs in International Use Today

*TOP ROW* (left to right)
Pycamisan : for tuberculosis
Enavid-E : for severe dysmenorrhea
Methotrexate : for acute leukemia
Chloromycetin : antibiotic, specific for typhoid
Dexedrine : appetite reducer, antidepressant

*SECOND ROW*
Oblivon : tranquilizer
Lederkyn : against pneumonia
Orbenin : against penicillin-resistant bacteria
Lingraine : for migraine relief
Decadron : pain-reliever for arthritis

*THIRD ROW*
Aventyl : antidepressant
Serensil : nonbarbiturate sedative
Imuran : used in kidney-grafting operations
Flagyl : for genital tract infection in women
Mysoline : anticonvulsant (epilepsy)

*FOURTH ROW*
Atromid-S : preventive for thrombosis
Mebryl : antihistamine for allergies
Camoprima : for malaria
Librium : tranquilizer
Secrodyl : for diagnosis of pregnancy

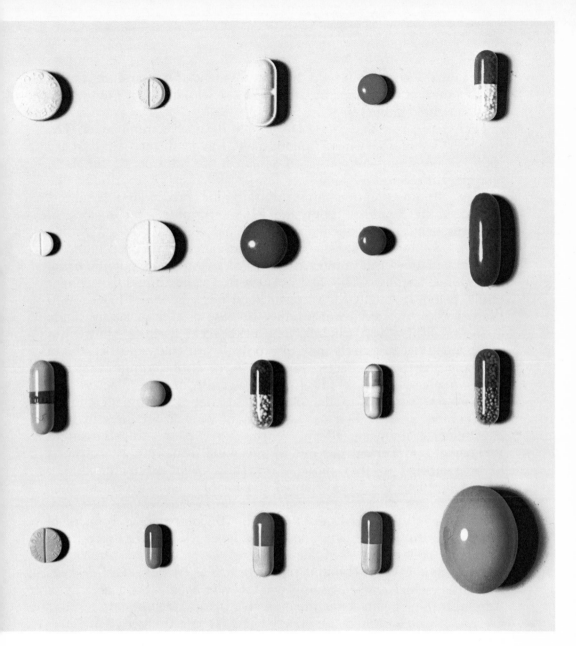

*TOP ROW*
Sulphetrone : for leprosy
Dindevan : anticoagulant
Dimelor : for diabetes
Butazolidin : pain-reliever for arthritis
Drinamyl : for anxiety states

*SECOND ROW*
Nitrong : pain-killer for angina pectoris
Antabuse : alcohol deterrent
Nystatin : for vaginal or intestinal fungi
Telmid : against intestinal worms
Perihemin : for anemias

*THIRD ROW*
Humatin : for intestinal infections
Myleran : relieves chronic myeloid leukemia
Tolnate : tranquilizer
Portyn : for peptic ulcers
Feospan : for iron-deficiency anemias

*FOURTH ROW*
Esbatal : to reduce high blood pressure
Actomol : antidepressant
Vortel : palliative for bronchial asthma
Dytide : for congestive heart diseases
Marboran : for protection against smallpox

297

spirit and the concern for the highest dividends for shareholders did not dictate that new drugs be promoted like washing soap products or new household gadgets.

There are signs that the FDA under its new commissioner, Dr. James L. Goddard (whose appointment was confirmed in January 1965) is becoming altogether tougher in its attitude to the U.S. pharmaceutical industry. Just a few weeks after he took office he ordered an investigation into the migraine prophylactic, Sansert (produced by Sandoz). Then the FDA terminated a clinical trial that was being undertaken on a hormonal contraceptive, MK–665 (Merck). Studies on dogs had shown that cancers had been induced. Within a matter of days later Elipten (CIBA), an antiepileptic drug, was banned because CIBA had not reported some animal experiment results before it sought FDA approval. A week later the FDA seized Warner Chilcott's Peritrate product because of certain claims made in the medical advertisements. The next week, Roche's Madricidin was banned because of its inability to deal with colds and because of the danger of its side effects. Days later some antihistamines that had been widely used as a prophylactic against motion sickness and nausea were ordered to be relabeled so that a warning could be incorporated against their use by pregnant women, for there was the possibility of injurious effects on the fetus. Marezine (Burroughs Wellcome) and Perazil put out by the same firm were also ordered to be relabeled so that more information could be included. On March 8, 1966, the FDA banned the further manufacture of antibiotic lozenges since claims that these were effective against sore throats were ill-founded. As a result, 70 companies' products of tyrothricin, bacitracin, and neomycin lozenges, which represented 25 million dollars' worth of sales per year, were outlawed. On March 18, Madeline Oxford Holland reported in *The Pharmaceutical Journal*: "All drugs which had been approved as safe by the Food and Drug Administration before enactment of the Drug Amendments of 1962 are now to be screened for effectiveness. It is estimated that 3,000 compounds are involved, many of them widely used on both a prescription and non-prescription basis. The drugs to be screened for efficacy are those approved as safe by the drug agency between the start of its screening programme in 1938 and the institution of new procedures in 1962. The latter require that drug makers show not only that their product is safe, but also that it does what they claim. Now it will be up to the manufacturers to show that the earlier drugs are efficacious. In some cases this will be evident from clinical tests already published. For others, new tests, satisfactory to the FDA, will have to be initiated."

And in June 1966 the FDA gave notice that, in the future, all vitamin and mineral pill bottles must be labeled: "Vitamins and minerals are supplied in abundant amounts by the foods we eat. Except for persons with special medical needs there is no scientific basis for recommending routine use of dietary supplements." As a result of this labeling, sales of patent vitamins are likely to tumble.

That the FDA should take such action is commendable; that it is necessary is lamentable.

In this chapter, various aggressive comments have been made on the practices of the pharmaceutical companies, and certain scandalous incidents and facts have been ventilated. There are many eminent doctors, though, some of them Nobel Prize winners, who from time to time defend the drug industry. No doubt many of us become particularly vehement when we discover that a drug is substandard, or can lead to toxic side effects whose nature has been misrepresented by the manufacturers. Perhaps we do tend to be less strict about lapses in the standards of other industries. As the Australian Nobel Prize winner, Lord Florey, said on November 5, 1965, when opening the new Crookes' laboratories in Hampshire, Britain: "There is a great contrast between the attitude of the public to the motor car and to drugs and this is, I consider, a very interesting social phenomenon. We all know that hundreds of people are killed and maimed for life on the roads of this country alone every month; we appear to accept this facet of modern civilization with brutal indifference. But if there should be but one misjudgement with a drug, most searching inquiries are made and severe judgements are pronounced.... It seems to me that the British pharmaceutical industry is doing a good job and it would be a great pity to disturb it on grounds other than those which would be clearly demonstrable to be for the benefit of the country...."

Misjudgments about drugs, though, are not isolated occurrences. They occur too frequently. Very recently tetracycline eyedrops for children, which had been imported into Britain from Italy, were found to be between 57 and 73 per cent lower than the stated strength on the label. Now if a driver of a vehicle is given two gallons of gasoline when he thinks three are going into the tank he is likely to feel outraged at being cheated. Under-strength antibiotics, however, are entirely different, for they can lead to all kinds of dangerous complications. A child, for example, could, under certain circumstances, become blind. So is not vehement indignation at such occurrences a very healthy and natural reaction?

Another Nobel Prize winner who has defended the pharmaceutical industry is Professor E. B. Chain. On December 7, 1965, the Association

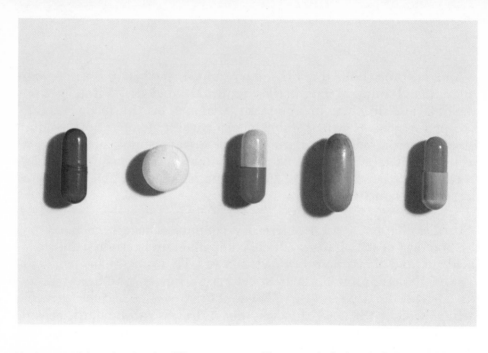

Much research is undertaken by different pharmaceutical companies to produce variations of a basic drug. Above, the antibiotic tetracycline and four of its variants: (from left to right) Tetracyn S.F. (Pfizer), Tetracycline Tablets B.P. (British Pharmaceuticals, London), Tetrex (Bristol Labs.), Achromycin (Lederle), Totomycin (Boots). Right, Professor Ernst Chain speaking in defense of the drug industry during the 1965 teach-in organized at Edinburgh University.

of the British Pharmaceutical Industry arranged a teach-in at Edinburgh University on pharmaceutical profits and the nation's health. On this occasion Professor Chain made three points to his audience of 350 doctors, students, and pharmacists. The three points were that drugs were essential for our health; that the pharmaceutical industry had made innumerable important therapeutic discoveries; and that to control or tamper with the pharmaceutical industry would put a stop to the proved source of new drugs being developed.

Professor Chain was evidently impressed by the way the pharmaceutical companies had made penicillin generally available. "A great deal of original thought and work had to be applied to reach the stage in which penicillin became, as it is now, a cheap and readily available drug." He then continued: "This work was largely carried out in industrial laboratories, and to describe it as a mere 'development' of our fundamental discovery is as far off the mark as to describe our own work at Oxford, namely the discovery of the curative power of penicillin, as a mere 'development' of Fleming's original observations of the antagonistic effect of his mould against various pathogenic bacteria." Professor Chain argued that the same considerations were applicable to Waksman's discovery, streptomycin. "Nearly all other

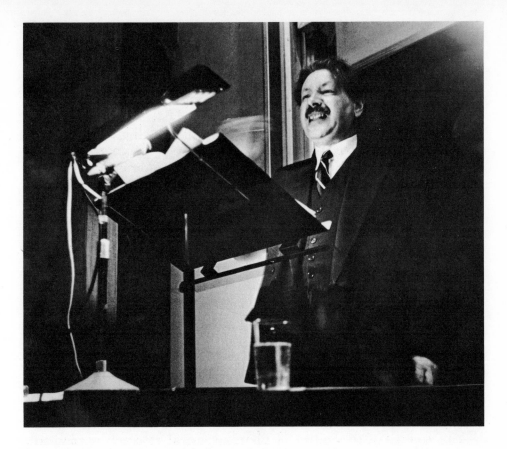

antibiotics of practical importance," he asserted, "have been discovered in industrial laboratories." And he listed: tetracycline,
chloramphenicol, the macrolites—erythromycin, magnamycin, olean-
domycin—the polymixins, griseofulvin, and the semisynthetic penicil-
lins. "I cannot conceive of any other system," said Professor Chain,
"which could replace the pharmaceutical industry in the job which
it has done so successfully."

It is quite true that no one should undervalue the positive contributions of the pharmaceutical companies. But this does not mean that
we should forget the astronomical profits once made on drugs like
tetracycline or the shabby misrepresentations about drugs like
chloramphenicol (Chloromycetin). One can understand the irritation
of Dr. David Kerr, a member of parliament and a general practitioner, when he rose at the same teach-in to say: "As a general
practitioner, I never conceived that I should stand up and tell a Nobel
Prize winner that he was talking out of the back of his test tubes."
Such abuse, however, is no argument. Fact has to be set against fact,
figures against figures. This, Dr. Kerr did later in his speech. He
pointed out that more money is being spent on advertising promotion
than on research, and also that drug companies as a whole make

considerably higher profits than most other industries. When he asked at the same teach-in: "Where is the moral right, for a start, in any shareholder making a profit out of somebody's illness?" he was surely raising a principle that is not applicable to the drug industry alone. He was putting forward a philosophy of economics. Dr. Kerr could just as well have asked: "Where is the moral right in any shareholder making a profit out of the death industry of armaments— guns, tanks, bombs, and so on?" Or for that matter: "Where is the moral right in one man making a profit economically from another man's labor?"

Many may disagree with such an absolutist viewpoint, for its implications are that the pharmaceutical industry should be national-ized. They might say with Professor Chain: "An example of what happens when the state has the monopoly of drug research can be seen in the Soviet Union. During 50 years of state-controlled drug research, not one single new drug in any field of pharmaceuticals has emerged. That is not because of lack of effort: hundreds of people are working in various pharmaceutical research institutes in the Soviet Union but have had no success for financial and many other reasons, of which an incredibly turgid bureaucracy, the unwillingness of anyone to assume responsibility, lack of incentive, lack of competition, and lack of contact with centres of pharmaceutical research abroad are some of the reasons."

Whatever one's view, the danger to world health of a money-grabbing drug industry cannot be underrated, nor for that matter should the pharmaceutical industry's past contributions in terms of new drugs be undervalued. As for myself, I firmly believe that a greater control over the industry is necessary at the very least; an uncontrolled patent system is undesirable; extravagant profits should be curbed; some strict discipline should be enforced to limit the wild promotional activities of the drug industry's advertising managers and PROs; money spent on advertisements should, in my view, be related to the money laid out on *real* research and the present ratios between these activities reversed; firmer action should be taken against those firms guilty of negligence; and not only should the toxicity of drugs be scrutinized with a more formidable aggression, but those proprietary and ethical drugs that have no greater efficacy than placebos should be banned. Finally, doctors need to be educated about new drugs— and not by the pharmaceutical companies. Drastic reforms are required, and since it is the health of nations that is at stake there should be no timidity or favor.

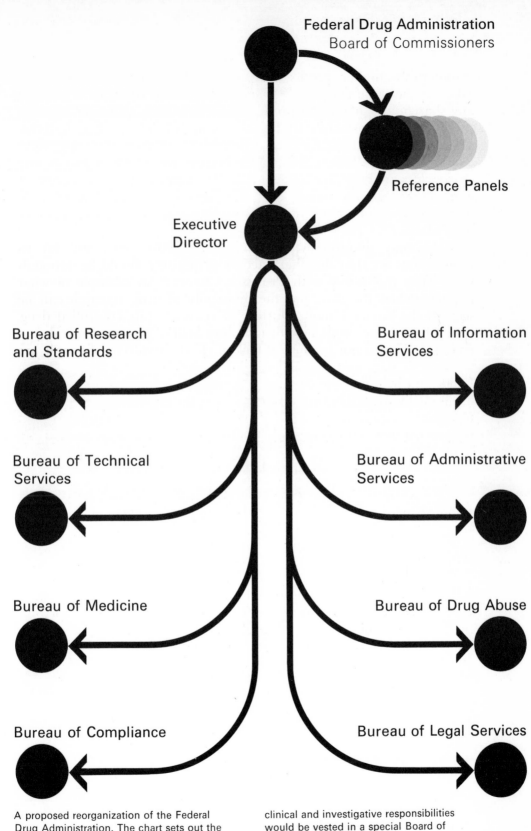

**Federal Drug Administration**
Board of Commissioners

Reference Panels

Executive
Director

Bureau of Research
and Standards

Bureau of Information
Services

Bureau of Technical
Services

Bureau of Administrative
Services

Bureau of Medicine

Bureau of Drug Abuse

Bureau of Compliance

Bureau of Legal Services

A proposed reorganization of the Federal Drug Administration. The chart sets out the structure advocated by Professor Joseph D. Cooper, following his study of drug control problems in America and Britain. Regulatory clinical and investigative responsibilities would be vested in a special Board of Commissioners, with outside reference panels of experts being responsible for studies on drug safety and effect.

303

# 9 Tomorrow and Tomorrow

"That all is not well with medicine and its practice despite the dramatic victories over disease in the past few decades," the president of the Royal Society of Medicine, Lord Cohen of Birkenhead, wrote recently, "will be conceded by even the most superficial observer of the contemporary scene." In the years to come there will undoubtedly be further dramatic discoveries that will relieve much physical suffering and mental devastation. Even so, despite (and, indeed, sometimes because of) such discoveries all will not be perfect in the field of medicine. For victory in any sphere of social activity brings in its wake its own peculiar problems.

It is a truism that medicine does not exist as an isolated entity. It is man-directed. What kind of medical service appertains in future societies will depend on the morals and political organizations of those societies. A writer with a cheerful temperament could easily engage in enthusiastic, utopian hypotheses about the future of medicine; one who is mournful could imagine how new medical discoveries would be employed for nightmarish and evil ends. For the moment, though—leaving aside all differently colored speculations—one can say plainly and concretely that medical research all over the world continues with a bustle and a pace never before witnessed. However, even as one

A ten-week-old human fetus alive in an artificial womb. Control over such human processes as reproduction and birth is now within the grasp of medical science.

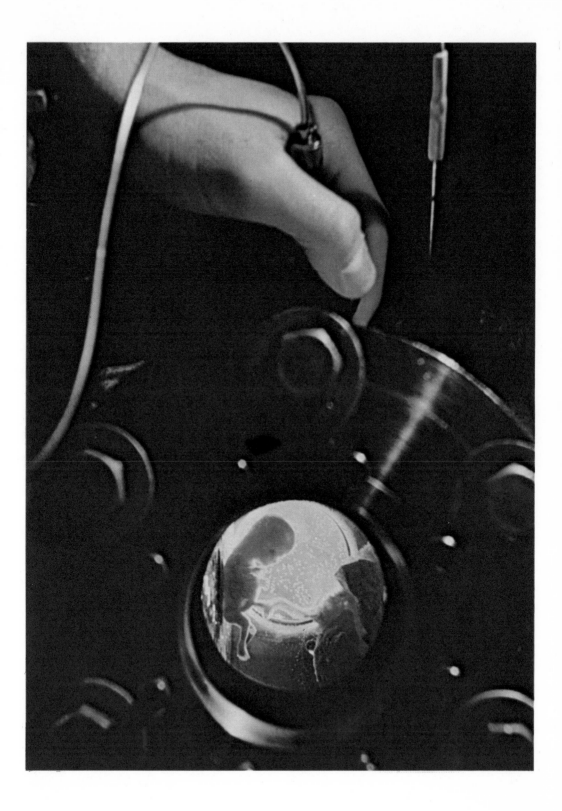

dark door creaks back for the first time, the research doctor with his probing torch comes upon yet another dark, beckoning passageway, to yet another locked door behind which lies yet another dark labyrinth, another mystery.

For example, in 1962 two New York research doctors, A. J. Friedhoff and E. Van Winkle, reported that they had isolated a substance known as DMPE from the urine of 15 schizophrenic patients. (Schizophrenia is a psychosis that can be controlled but not cured; one person in 100 is likely to suffer from a schizophrenic episode during some stage of his life.) Now DMPE is chemically related to the hallucinogenic drug mescaline. Immediately, doctors everywhere began to wonder whether schizophrenia had a specific chemical cause—for schizophrenics do suffer hallucinations. Could DMPE, then, be the chemical agent that induced such waking dreams, such tortured visions?

One method of testing for DMPE in the urine is through "the pink spot test." When this chemical is present a pink spot shows up on an especially prepared strip of paper. In 1965, Professor Cyril Clarke and his colleagues at Liverpool University, who had made use of this pink spot test, published their report. They had previously engaged in a painstaking inquiry into the presence or absence of DMPE in the urine of schizophrenics as compared with controls. They found that 60 per cent of all schizophrenics produced the pink spot on the paper. On the other hand, of 310 people not suffering from that psychosis only one was pink spot positive. Though these results are statistically suggestive, it is thought now that the chemical DMPE is not the direct cause of schizophrenia. This is borne out by the fact that large doses of DMPE given to normal people do not, in fact, induce schizoid symptoms.

Thus a door has been breached, a discovery made, but the labyrinth beyond is as dark as ever. No one knows at present what deep biochemical disorder prevents DMPE from being broken down in the body so that it is excreted in the urine of 60 per cent of schizophrenic patients. It may be that the clue of the pink spot may significantly help solve an age-old mystery: the cause and then the cure of schizophrenia. On the other hand it may be irrelevant: the labyrinth may lead nowhere and the research doctor, unlike Theseus, may discover in the maze no monster but a mouse.

It is the investigation of the mind—the workings of memory and intelligence, the brain's chemical intricacies, normal and disordered— that leads the romantic writer to his most desolate prophecies. Lately, for instance, it has been demonstrated that electric stimulation of a particular part of the brain in man, as well as in animals, can lead to a subjective sensation of happiness. It is even possible to let one half

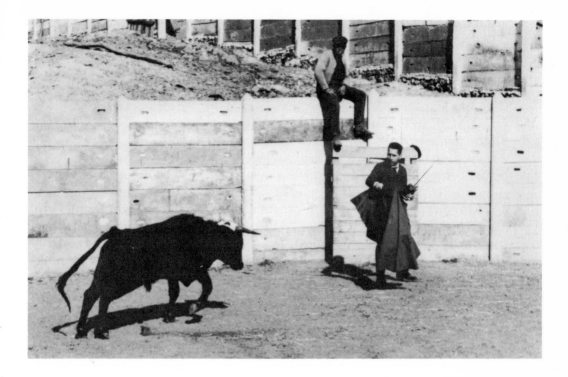

The extent to which an animal's behavior can be controlled by electric stimuli is demonstrated in the bull ring by Dr José Delgado, professor of physiology at Yale University's Medical School. By signaling from a hidden radio transmitter to electrodes in the bull's brain, Dr Delgado halted the animal's charge at will, leaving it docile.

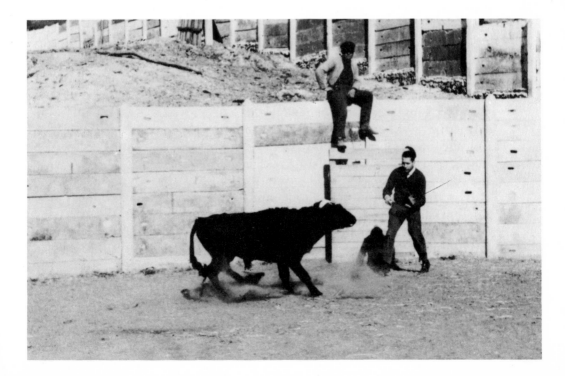

of the organism experience a sense of well-being while the other half continues in its usual state. Where such states of mind can be artificially induced, what fantasies, what sensual and melodramatic imaginings may visit a writer speculating on the world of man tomorrow!

Or consider the prospect of a controlled eugenic policy. There are scientists who advocate active social measures to improve the human genetic quality. Sir Julian Huxley has written in a symposium organized by CIBA called *Man and his Future* that such an improvement in quality by eugenic methods "would take a great load of suffering and frustration off the shoulders of evolving humanity, and would much increase both enjoyment and efficiency. . . . The general level of genetic intelligence could theoretically be raised by eugenic selection; and even a slight rise in its average level would give a marked increase in the number of the outstandingly intelligent and capable people needed to run our increasingly complex societies. Thus a 1·5 per cent increase in mean genetic intelligence quotient (I.Q.), from 100 to 101·5, would increase the production of those with an I.Q. of 160 and over by about 50 per cent. . . . Eugenics will eventually have to have recourse to methods like multiple artificial insemination by preferred donors of high genetic quality. . . . Such a policy will not be easy to execute. However, I confidently look forward to a time when eugenic improvement will become one of the major aims of mankind."

If the imagination boggles at the thought of a world where such eugenic policies are commonplace, how much more may we be astounded by the possible application of recent discoveries concerning a drug that can speed up learning and improve the memory. In the late 1950s Holger Hyden, director of the Institute of Neurobiology at the University of Gothenburg, Sweden, surgically separated single cells from animal brain tissue. To do this he used a dissecting needle less than one tenth of the diameter of a human hair and of course a powerful microscope. As a result of such microscopic surgery Professor Hyden was able to observe minute chemical changes in isolated brain cells. He discovered that the key to memory and learning lay in a chemical component of the brain cell—ribonucleic acid, or RNA. When, over a period of four days, he taught rats to balance on a wire, the efforts of the animals to remember this learning procedure caused the RNA in a certain number of their brain cells to increase by 12 per cent. Professor Hyden estimated that a molecule of RNA could encode 1,000,000,000,000,000 pieces of information in a lifetime.

Following Professor Hyden's work, a psychologist at Michigan University, James V. McConnell, experimented with flatworms. When he subjected these worms to a light and an electric shock the latter caused the worms to contract their bodies. By repeating these experiments he conditioned the worms, in the Pavlovian manner, to contract their bodies whenever the light was shone on them—that is, even without the electric shock. These conditioned worms were then cut up and fed to other worms that had not been subjected to such experiments. It was discovered that the cannibal worms now learned to respond to the light-shock stimulus faster than worms fed on a normal diet. McConnell and his colleagues believed that it was the RNA in the minced worms that was responsible for the increased learning and memory ability of the cannibal worms. Indeed, when they destroyed the RNA content of the minced worm diet—they added an RNA-destroying enzyme to it—the cannibals' rate of learning decreased to the normal pace.

A drug, Cylert, has now been synthesized in the Abbott Laboratories at Chicago. Dr. N. Plotnikoff and Dr. A. J. Glasky, who with others have developed Cylert, say that it speeds up learning and improves memory in animals because it increases brain RNA production by 30–40 per cent. Rats given this drug have learned to perform tricks four to five times faster than untreated rats. As was inevitable, laboratory animal experiments were followed by human trials. At present, 18 male students at the University of Michigan are taking Cylert and undergoing tests. The results of this experiment will probably become available shortly. If it proves to be successful it is likely that old people with failing memories, along with retarded children, will be given the drug. Already RNA is being called "the memory molecule." To put it mildly, this is an oversimplification. All the same, enough experimental evidence has been published for different scientists to talk sardonically about apes in business suits with capsules of RNA in their briefcases and of malevolent powers controlling the memory of vast populations with pills. To paraphrase Mark Twain, one can be worried not by what one cannot understand but by what one can.

Since I seem to be on the frontiers of a world imagined by an Aldous Huxley or a George Orwell, perhaps I should also mention, at least briefly, some of the fantastic propositions made by those who see in suspended animation by deep freezing the possibility of a cure to all our mortal ills. It has been suggested that if a person suffering from an incurable cancer could be put into a state of suspended animation, he could then be resuscitated at some future date when doctors have discovered a means of dealing with such a cancer. Some primitive types of animal life can be frozen so that their internal activity is interrupted, and when they are thawed they appear to resume their normal function again. In 1959 Louis Rey, a prominent French biologist, wrote in *Conservation de la vie par le froid*: "There are some very convincing reasons to think that, thanks to future research, the solution will . . . be found to the problem of suspending the vital life force perhaps indefinitely."

Dr. D. K. C. MacDonald of Ottawa University remarked (after considering how embryo chicken hearts had been cooled to $-190°c$ following treatment with a glycerol solution, and how they had resumed beating after thawing) that maybe "the day will come when, if you want it, you can arrange 'to hibernate' for a thousand years or so in liquid air, and then be 'wakened up' again to see how the world has changed in the meantime." In his book *The Prospect of Immortality* Robert C. W. Ettinger proposes that one day not only those suffering from incurable diseases should be put into a state of suspended animation but the new dead also. For he looks forward to a medical science that can reverse the apparently irreversible and advocates that the dead should not be cremated or buried but frozen and preserved for an indefinite period at a temperature near absolute zero to prevent further deterioration. Many of us may mock such imaginings. But when we, skeptics all, are but dust and colored chemicals, Mr. Ettinger may yet leap out of his refrigerator 100 years hence shouting, "I told you so" to the wind.

The concept of deep freeze preservation for human beings was satirized by Mayakovsky in 1929, in his play *The Bedbug.* In the scene below, a peasant—frozen alive in an earlier age—is revived by doctors.

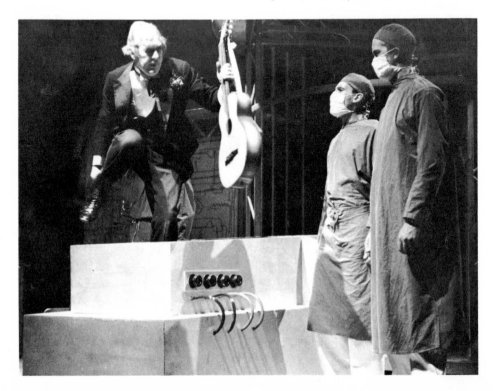

The preservation of human beings in a deep freeze is not a new idea. As long ago as 1776, John Hunter admitted in a lecture that he had taken two living carp and frozen them in a vessel containing river water. When he thawed them out he unhappily saw that the fish were dead. "Till this time," he continued, "I had imagined that it might be possible to prolong life to any period by freezing a person in the frigid zone as I thought all action and waste would cease until the body was thawed. I thought that if a man would give up the last years of his life to this kind of alternate oblivion and action, it might be prolonged to a thousand years; and by getting himself thawed every hundred years he might learn what had happened during his frozen condition. Like other schemes, I thought I should make my fortune by it, but this experiment undeceived me."

Robert Ettinger, however, takes encouragement from more up-to-date experiments in freezing, such as those directed at the problem of cold-storing human tissues for transplantation purposes and from recent surgical procedures for open heart surgery. For over the last decade and a half, hypothermy has been used more and more in such operations. Profound hypothermia, by resting the heart, allows the thoracic surgeon—as one of them has put it—"to operate in a quiet

Below, a clinically "dead" dog, photographed during a deep freeze experiment at the Russian Academy of Medical Sciences. The dog was revived after respiratory and cardiac arrest had been prolonged for two hours.

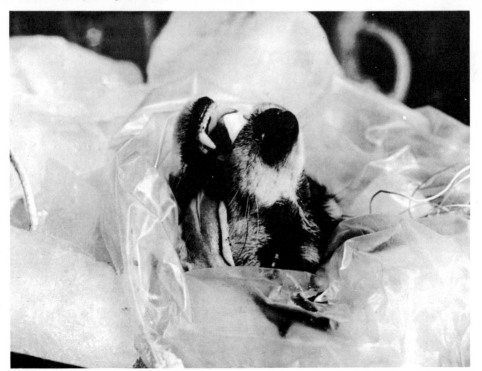

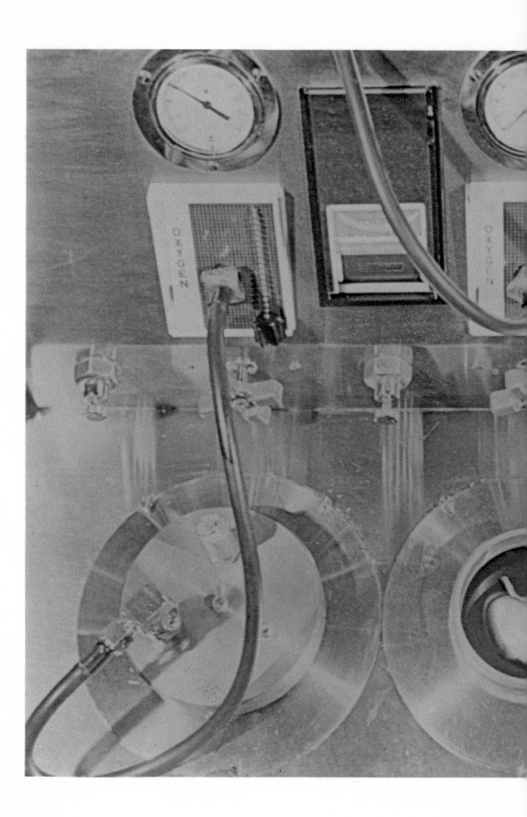

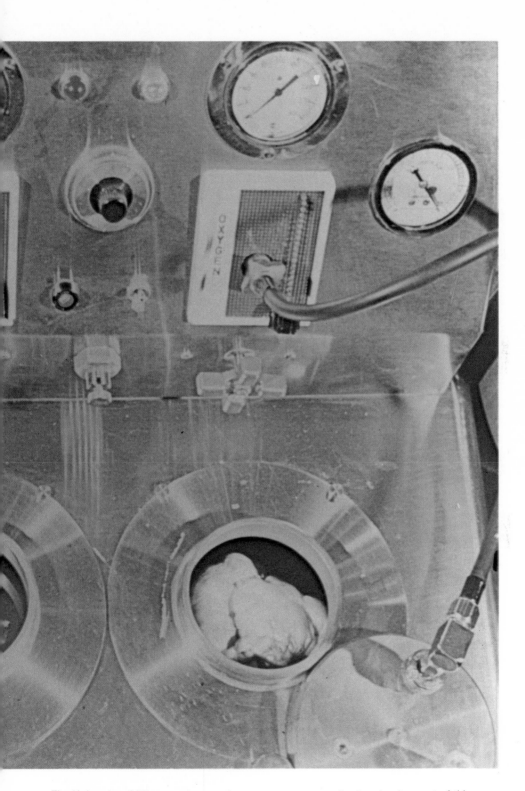

The University of Minnesota's recently completed organ bank in which animal organs can be preserved under optimum conditions—at 1.11 °C, in oxygen, under pressure. Further development of this machine may soon make it possible to preserve banks of human kidneys for transplant purposes.

field." Low temperature surgery has been successful, and through hypothermia, operations have even been carried out on previously inaccessible blood vessels in the brain by arresting the circulation for a prolonged period. Profound hypothermia has been induced through the use of a heart-lung machine, though some surgeons have aimed only at local cooling of the heart by introducing cold blood through the coronary arteries.

Perhaps closer to Ettinger's preoccupations with immortality are the experiments of Dr. Audrey U. Smith of the National Institute for Medical Research at Mill Hill, London. With her colleague J. Farrant she writes in the *Penguin Science Survey B*, 1966:

"The desire to cheat death and to enjoy immortality seems to be universal. People have frequently asked us how soon we shall be able to store whole animals and whole human beings at low temperatures in a state of suspended animation to be resurrected in the future. Until 1952 we had to tell them that, in warm-blooded animals including men, heart beats and breathing stopped and could not be restarted if the body was cooled by more than 10 degrees c. below normal. Then we heard that a young Yugoslav physiologist, Dr. R. Andjus, had succeeded in reviving rats cooled to internal body temperatures just above the freezing point of water and after one hour of respiratory and cardiac arrest. When Dr. Andjus came to work at the National Institute for Medical Research techniques of resuscitation were improved until ninety per cent of ice-cold rats could be brought to life after one hour of apparent death. After recovery they had not lost their memory, judging by their ability to solve problems which they had previously mastered. Golden hamsters were sturdier than rats and some survived three hours' arrested heart beat and breathing after cooling to 0 degrees c.

"The next question was what was the lowest body temperature compatible with revival. Ice-cold and apparently inanimate hamsters were plunged into baths at −5 degrees c. with the result that their body temperatures fell to −0·55 degrees c., the freezing point of plasma. During the course of the next hour the hamsters froze progressively, becoming stiffer and stiffer due to the spread of ice from the skin to the deeper tissues and organs. At the end of the hour they were as hard as a piece of wood and quite lifeless. Nevertheless, after thawing with diathermy and puffing air into the lungs the heart started to beat again, and within about forty-five minutes the animals came to life. Most of them showed no serious ill-effects afterwards and survived till the end of their normal lifespan, and when given the opportunity to mate had large numbers of offspring. If the ears or paws were bent while they were frozen stiff they showed the typical signs of frost-bite

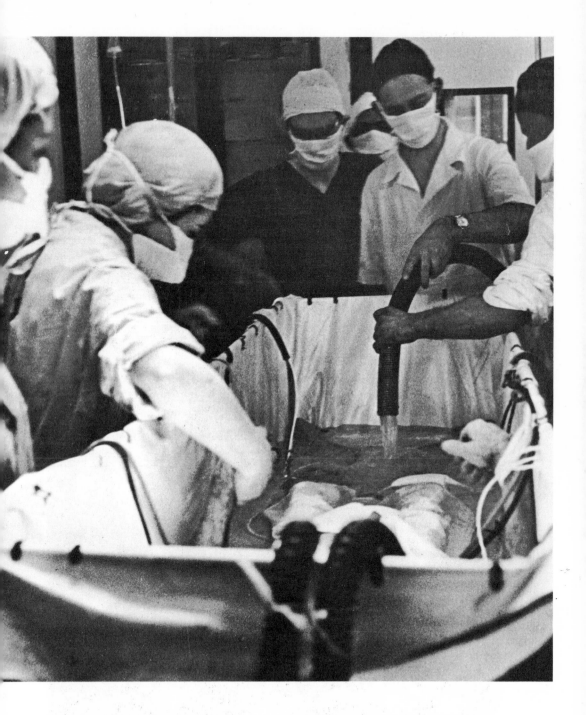

The intra-arterial injection of cytoxic drugs
during whole-body hypothermia is one
of the most advanced techniques of treating
cancer tumors of the head and neck. The

operation is performed after the patient's
body has been reduced to about 29°C. Above,
nurses fill a hypothermic bath—the simple
part of a complex operation.

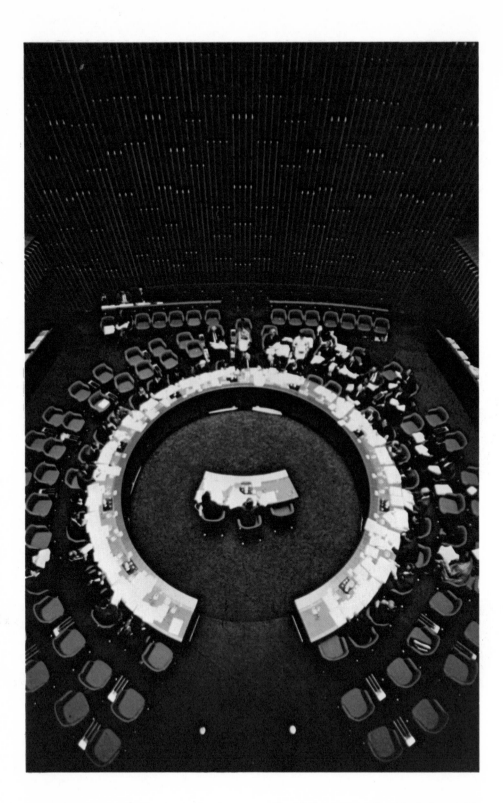

The WHO's executive meets for the first time in the organization's new Geneva headquarters, inaugurated in May 1966.

The WHO, an international body founded in 1948, aims to achieve "the highest possible level of health" for all peoples.

after thawing. If the extremities were not bent or handled roughly there was no frost-bite in spite of the fact that ninety per cent of the water in the skin had been converted to ice at about −4 degrees c. The internal organs of the body still contained some fluid blood although there were ice crystals inside the heart, stomach and even in the brain. The results showed that the hamsters never survived freezing for more than one hour or at a lower external temperature than −5 degrees c. or a lower internal temperature than −1 degree c. Calculations indicated that they did not recover if more than fifty per cent of the total water in the blood and tissues had frozen.

"It was remarkable that animals frozen to this extent could be revived at all and made us revise our previous ideas about death."

How hard it is then to imagine the future practice of medicine when man himself could be eugenically upgraded, his brain affected by subtle chemicals, and his body refrigerated when dead; a world, in short, where we shall all be healthy and intelligent, own prodigious memories, and become immortal. More easy to consider the immediate future of medicine; to turn to those facts that are being uncovered about such major killing diseases as cancer; to some of the extra-ordinary surgical procedures that are tentatively being tried out; to other current research projects whose conclusion would seem likely to belong to the world of tomorrow and not to some far distant utopia or hell.

Undeniably, this century has seen a general improvement in the health of man in most countries of the world: but before we become too complacent it should be recalled that in Africa alone there are more than 14 countries with populations in excess of three million that do not have even one medical school between them. Transmissible diseases in some parts of the world remain a tragic scourge. In our affluent societies we can too easily forget that what millions look forward to is not immortality or the improvement of memory but the eradication of ravaging diseases like leprosy and cholera. (A form of cholera has spread since 1961 throughout most of the countries in the Western Pacific and in South-East Asia. It has traveled westward also, to reach the borders of Europe as well as Africa.) The future task of international medicine is not only to make the healthy nations healthier, but to advocate that medical resources and proven drugs be made available in massive quantities to those countries desperately in need of them. This, of course, is not only a medical problem; it is also an economic one. Nor is it a question of the availability of such sophisticated matters as drugs. It is often a question of basic sanitation and simple hygiene.

Not all the money in the world can at present solve the problem of virus diseases—whether in the advanced countries or in the tropics, where so many virus illnesses are transmitted by insects. Yet more and more knowledge is becoming available. Sooner or later a drug will surely be found to combat virus infections just as antibiotics such as penicillin can now attack the bacterial diseases.

In 1964 the American Professor Byron E. Leach and his colleagues reported in *Nature* that when a substance they called viractin was evaporated into room air, it reduced the incidence of minor upper respiratory diseases of virus origin and of influenza: their conclusion was that it prevented the viruses attaching themselves to and multiplying in cells. Viractin is a distillate of the fermentation products of *Streptomyces griseus*. In laboratory tests, however, there was no evidence to show that viractin inactivated viruses, though it did seem to act on mice after very large doses were given intranasally.

Other scientists have studied the activity of viractin since then and found that even small doses of the common cold virus could multiply in cultures exposed to intense concentrations of viractin. Moreover, when mice infected with influenza A were kept in a room where the air was treated with viractin, they lived no longer than other infected mice exposed only to a normal atmosphere. Leach still feels that it is justifiable to carry out extended clinical trials with viractin on man. Others are more dubious and, at present, the debate continues.

Meanwhile much research is going on with interferon, a substance that inhibits the multiplication of a wide variety of viruses. Interferon was discovered in 1957, at the National Institute for Medical Research, by A. Isaacs and J. Lindenmann. The precise structure of interferon is still not known, though its purification has very recently been accomplished. But it is known that interferon is a very small and simple protein and that it is sometimes produced in the body cells when the latter are invaded by viruses. Invasion by all kinds of viruses seems to stimulate the cells to manufacture interferon and this is evidently one major means whereby the body eventually overcomes a viral infection. Interferon does not seem to be present in the cells when they are unaffected by viruses. Lately, too, large amounts of interferon have been discovered not only in the cells of animals and humans suffering from a virus infection but also in the bloodstream. It would appear that there is some element in a virus that calls forth an interferon reaction from the body cells when it invades them. Viruses contain, within a protein covering, either ribonucleic acid (RNA) or deoxyribonucleic acid (DNA) and it is conjectured that interferon interferes with the synthesis of these components. Thus viral RNA loses its protein covering when subjected to interferon.

More and more is being learned about how interferon actually works. It may be that one day interferon will be used clinically against virus infections, or that a means will be discovered whereby the body will be stimulated to produce protective amounts of interferon naturally. At present, the technical problem of producing adequate quantities of interferon has not been overcome; but here is a research area full of promise, and one that, if successfully concluded, will lead to spectacular advances in medicine.

Intensive work has also been carried out on the relationship between viruses and cancer. As long ago as 1908 cancer of viral origin had been experimentally induced in laboratory animals, and since then many other viruses have proved to be carcinogenic. Still, there was no evidence until lately that such viruses could be implicated in the causation of neoplasms in man. One serious difficulty has been that research doctors could hardly attempt to induce a viral cancer in human beings. Nowadays, though, they have other research "tools." The French scientist Alexis Carrel (1873–1944) once kept alive cells of an embryo chicken heart in the laboratory for 40 years. Today, the human, live cancer HeLa-cell cultures are available in practically every virus research laboratory in the world. These HeLa-cells originate from a cancer of an American lady whose names began He . . . La. . . . With such human tissue-cell cultures, along with electron microscopy (which allows a virus in a cancer cell to be visualized) and other technical advances, cancer virus research has accelerated.

In 1964, Dr. G. Negroni, at the Mill Hill laboratories, London, isolated a microorganism from human tissue-cell cultures that had been inoculated with bone marrow from patients suffering from leukemia. Leukemia has long intrigued cancer virologists, for while, on the one hand, it is a malignant disease, it also has many features characteristic of an infective process. In April 1966, the Imperial Cancer Research Fund's annual report confirmed that this microorganism had been identified as a mycoplasma related to *Mycoplasma pulmonis*. More evidence that infected microorganisms are implicated in the formation of some human malignant tumors has come from the East African Virus Research Institute. In 1958 the British surgeon D. P. Burkitt recognized that a number of apparently unrelated children's cancers in Africa had the same basic properties. These cancers were then named Burkitt's lymphoma, and it has been conjectured in America that this disease is a modified form of leukemia. Recently viruses have been recovered from 10 cases of this particular type of cancer.

Various other interesting facts have emerged. For example, in 1962 John J. Trentin and his American colleagues described how they had inoculated newborn hamsters with a virus and how tumors were produced as a result. The viruses that Trentin used were adenoviruses, types 12 and 18, which in man cause upper respiratory tract infections. Now these viruses contain DNA, which has a close chemical correspondence to the whole DNA of the hamster cell genes that were affected. Two lines of thought followed from this experiment: first, that a virus causing an infection in one species may be implicated in the etiology of a malignant tumor in another species; second, that the virus DNA and the animal genetic cell DNA correspondence may be significant—it may be the key to the change that takes place in a gene (which is composed of DNA), and this mutation may then be copied and reproduced in successive generations of cells. Certainly this correspondence leads research workers to think of interesting theoretical postulates, with practical possibilities. As a leading cancer research doctor, R. J. C. Harris, writes in his book *Cancer*: "Some of those engaged in research with cancer-producing viruses have been much intrigued by the possibility of interpreting carcinogenesis in this way [i.e. in terms of DNA homologues]. Does the normal cell have the 'malignant DNA'—whatever this may be—already present in its nucleus like a fused time-bomb? Can this 'bomb' be set off in the cell by a variety of agencies—chemicals, hormones, radiation, super-infecting viruses—all of which are known to be carcinogenic . . . ?"

The word "cancer" is a generic term covering many different varieties of the disease. Kidney cancers, for example, behave differently from breast cancers or from bone marrow malignancies. Equally, there are different factors involved in the etiology of cancer. The miracle is perhaps not that cancerous growths do occur but that they occur, relatively, so seldom. Each day we lose some two per cent of our total body cells through death; each day billions of new cells are born to replace those lost. It is more remarkable that cells so constantly and frequently obey the limiting laws of health than that occasionally they go wild and multiply continuously and at random—especially when they are so often insulted by carcinogenic agencies such as endocrinal imbalances, chemical irritants like tobacco smoke, natural and man-made radiation, and probably also viral invasion.

It is likely that man has always been subject to neoplastic disease, though its fatal prognosis was only recognized in 300 B.C.—when the tumor would either be treated by arsenical ointments or excised. But experimental cancer research is intrinsically a concern of the 20th century. It is apposite that this should be so, for with aging populations an increase in the incidence of cancer has occurred, and a further increase can be expected in the future. Nor can the radiation following H-bomb testing be altogether discounted. (The Atomic Bomb Casualty

Commission recently indicated that there had been a general increase in cancer among the irradiated survivors of the Hiroshima and Nagasaki explosions.) True, the prognosis of cancer in the popular mind is still as gloomy as the forebodings of those making the diagnosis in 300 B.C. And there are those who point out that despite the colossal amount of research carried out since German pathologists, a century ago, noted the important and seemingly significant resemblance between a cancer cell and an embryonic cell, few fundamental advances have been made. Surgery, though, has become more and more refined, and in certain kinds of cancer—prostate neoplasms and breast cancer, for example—promising results have followed hormone treatment. Then the so-called cytotoxic drugs, like nitrogen mustard and its variants, have been used to poison the cancer cells with some partial success. Professor L. F. Larionov, along with his Russian colleagues, has claimed good results in treating testicular and liver cancers with the cytotoxic drug sarcolysine. The Japanese, using one variant of nitrogen mustard called "nitromin," also claim to have obtained temporary improvements in treating forms of disseminated cancer such as chronic leukemia and malignant varieties of Hodgkin's disease.

It must be admitted, though, that cancer chemotherapy is still in its infancy and, as yet, no drug is known that specifically kills the cancer cells without harming the normal tissues. Nevertheless, the present discoveries about carcinogenesis made by those studying cell function at the molecular level and by those working on cancer virology lead scientists everywhere to be more optimistic about the future therapy of cancer. Thus, the Hungarian Nobel Prize winner Dr. Albert Szent-Györgyi looks forward to "a far-advanced refinement of our present knowledge which will then open the way to the understanding of the deepest problems, the nature of life, how it originated and perfected itself." From the broadening of biology's foundations, Dr. Szent-Györgyi says, "You may wish for anything: a cure-all for cancer, a mastery of mutation, an understanding of hormone action, or a cure for any of the diseases you have especially in mind. None of your wishes need remain unfulfilled, once we have penetrated deep enough into the foundations of life. This is the real promise of medicine."

Such optimism is not confined to scientists working in the field of virology, genetics, and chemistry. For workers in immunology, too, feel they are on the threshhold of advances that will be relevant therapeutically to the cancer problem. In France, Professor Bernard Halpern, who in 1942 discovered the synthetic antihistamines—the first effective medication against allergic conditions—is now working at the Hôpital Broussais in Paris on immunological mechanisms. He has written in the French journal *Réalités* (June 1966): "Immunology also offers a new approach to the problem of cancer. This recent development is based on the following observation: in nearly all cases the structure of tumors is not immunologically identical to the organism's normal structures. Consequently, it should be theoretically possible to vaccinate a cancer sufferer against his own cancer. . . . We can say that the new path of immunology gives us new reasons for hope in the problems of both transplants and cancer."

Since everyone now acknowledges a multifactorial etiology in cancer, perhaps it is not surprising that in recent years even psychiatrists have become interested in this organic disease. If anxiety and depression can lower the resistance of an individual to invading infective pathogens— as has been indicated elsewhere in this book—then it is surely possible that fundamental psychological imbalances could play a role in the production of malignancies. It can even be conjectured that psychological processes may be involved in gene mutation. Such a hypothesis may seem farfetched to some, but there is an impressive amount of data to suggest that the crucial emotion of severe depression that follows the loss of a loved one, for example, can be operative in the formation of some cancers. It has been noted, too, how frequently apparently healed malignancies have recurred soon after the patient has experienced a personal bereavement. Not only psychiatrists recognize the relationship of tumor formation and grief—other kinds of specialists acknowledge it also.

Thus the British surgeon D. Lang Stevenson has commented in his paper *Evolution and the Neurobiogenesis of Neoplasia*: "There is, in fact, evidence strongly to suggest that brain states signifying profound alarm or despondency, particularly in a medium of ageing hormones, are connected with tumor formation and that this indeed may be one of the common causes of human cancers. The time measurement between the event, bereavement of a close contemporary for instance, and the appearance of the tumor has been found constant enough to be statistically significant." Professor J. S. Mitchell, too, in the opening address to the 1963 Conference of the International Psychosomatic Cancer Study Group said: "As a radiotherapist and physician I get to know our patients very well. . . . Not infrequently, one observes the recurrence of a malignant tumor which has been healed for many years, perhaps ten years, sometimes much longer, after surgery or radiotherapy or both methods of treatment. It appears as if tumor cells had lain dormant . . . and then after many years started to grow. Such a recurrence often seems to have been precipitated by an emotional upheaval such as follows the death of a husband, wife or child. . . ." From studies of breast cancer, pathologists have learned that microscopic clusters of malignant cells do remain dormant for years. Why this should be so is no more understood than why 1 in 10,000 malignant tumors should spontaneously regress. Could it be that in the latter cases the patients rediscovered profoundly their "will to live" while in the opposite condition, where recurrences of tumors occur, the severely depressed patients have lost this same unconscious urge to live? Certainly cancer has been described by one psychiatrist as "a passive and unconscious suicide," and from the Department of Psychiatry at Jefferson Medical College, Philadelphia, comes the startling theory that a patient (one perhaps overcome with grief?) may suffer cancer as an alternative to a psychosis.

The relationship between cancer and emotion has also been described by Grant Newton of the Upstate Medical Center, Syracuse, who subjected rats to stress. He described how such stress affected the rats' resistance to implanted tumors. Other evidence to support the role of the psyche in tumor control comes from reports of how patients, dying of cancer, were referred to analysts "for psychological treatment," and sometimes lived much longer than the surgeons or anyone else expected. H. F. Baltrusch of Oldenburg, West Germany, has reported not only significant psychological differences in patients suffering from leukemia as compared with controls, but also his belief that psychotherapeutic guidance of a leukemia patient will lead to a better adjustment to his disease as well as, perhaps, to "an increased survival time." Laurence Le Shan, the American psychologist, is another who advocates that doctors should mobilize the will to live of patients dying from cancer. "If we believe in the value of the individual and the sacred character of human life," he writes, "our concern [the psychotherapists'] does not stop as death approaches. . . . Further, one discovers something that is rarely mentioned in the textbooks of psychology and psychiatry. One sees clearly the strength and dignity of human beings, the deep altruism, the positive qualities that exist at all levels of personality. Working with people who are under the hammer of fate greatly increases one's respect for them and makes one proud of being a human being."

If the problem of cancer is to be solved, if its many causes are to be wholly understood, if more harmless, sophisticated, and specific methods of treatment are to become available, it is obvious that those working in different medical disciplines—surgeons, physicians, psychiatrists, biochemists, geneticists, and immunologists—will all have to play their part together in uncovering that which is, at present, arcane. As medical knowledge advances, specialists in all areas of medicine will have to know more and more about other specialities—

and it will be one important function of postgraduate education in the future to see that they do. This fact is underlined, too, in the field of organ transplantation, where cooperation between different teams of specialists will be required before such surgical procedures become an everyday occurrence. For in this field, despite recent progress, much still remains insoluble. As has already been mentioned (by Professor Bernard Halpern) the solution of some of the immunological problems of transplantation might also have a direct bearing on cancer. Such a hypothesis could well prove true. For the moment, at any rate, we can at least agree with the British philosopher, Alfred North Whitehead, who wrote in 1929: ". . . in the real world it is more important that a proposition be interesting than that it be true. The importance of truth is, that it adds to interest."

The conception of transplantation—of the exchange of a new heart for an old one, a new liver or kidney for a diseased one—is not new. A century and a half ago old organs for new might have sounded like the Aladdin fairy story. Nevertheless, John Hunter "took a sound tooth from a person's head, then made a pretty deep wound with a lancet into the thick part of a cock's comb and pressed the fang of the tooth into this wound, fastening it with threads passed through other parts of the comb."

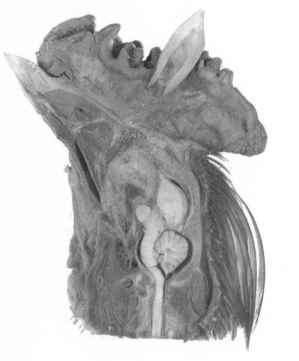

Left, the original cock's head used by John Hunter for his early grafting experiment (preserved in cross section at the Royal College of Surgeons, London). The grafted tooth is clearly visible at the top.

In a pioneer operation at Boston City Hospital, Harvard surgeons fight for the life of a 34-year-old woman dying from a diseased liver. The operation involved the circulation of the patient's blood for two hours through a healthy pig's liver.

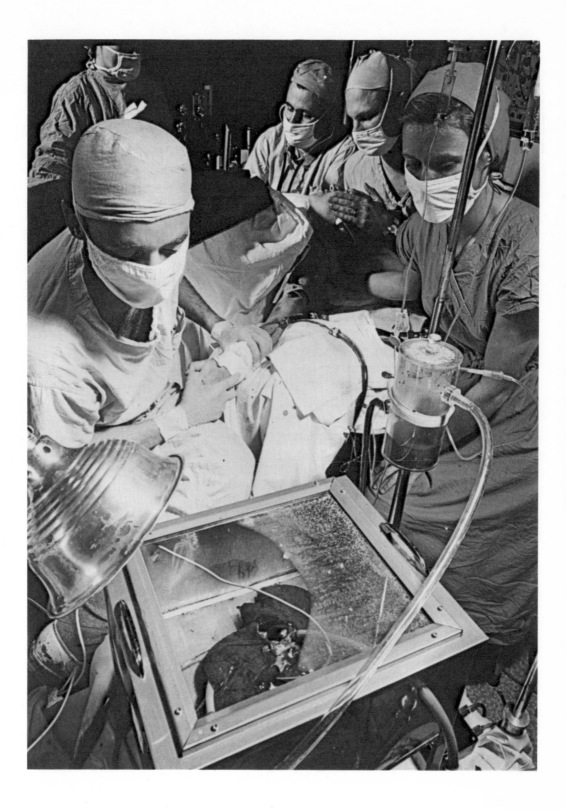

Hunter's early contribution to the problem of transplantation brought forth some derision from his contemporaries. The anatomist Thomas Bell mocked: "Nothing but sanguine expectations created in an ardent mind could account for a man of sound judgement continuing the practice." Hunter was attempting heterotransplantation— that is to say, transplantations of living tissues from one species to another. Today such transplantations are carried out in an attempt to save life. For example, chimpanzee kidneys have been transplanted into human beings with partial success.

That random transplantation operations are not generally a success is due to the fact that the body will, ordinarily, reject the alien cells of the transplanted tissue. The body's defense mechanisms, through its immunological processes, will destroy alien tissue as it would invading bacteria. So the survival of a transplant will depend on the degree of biological compatibility of the donor and the recipient. That the grafting of chimpanzee kidneys into humans has met with partial success has led certain scientists to assume that there is a closer biological affinity between some chimpanzees and some humans than between some humans and others. This is an assumption that will not surprise most of us as we look around at our more dubious friends.

Identical twins have an identical or virtually identical genetic constitution, so—in theory—one organ of one twin could be transplanted into the other. Indeed there have been cases where one twin dying of renal failure (consequent on two damaged kidneys) has survived for years following such a surgical procedure. A remarkable operation on identical twins—Richard and Ronald Herrick—took place at the Peter Bent Brigham Hospital in Boston, U.S.A., on December 23, 1954. It had been decided that Ronald's normal left kidney would be removed and transplanted into Richard's right lower abdomen. Later, after this successful surgery, Richard's own useless left kidney was taken out, and in June 1955 the remaining irrevocably damaged right kidney was also removed. Before December 23, 1954, Richard was dying. In July 1955 the twins had two kidneys between them and were fit. Once, both these kidneys were in Ronald's body. Now they had one each. This was the mathematics of an extraordinarily successful surgical adventure. For, as a result, Richard continued to live actively for a further eight and a half years. The success of this kidney transplantation operation in identical twins led to further transplantation work being done at the Peter Bent Brigham Hospital, as well as the Hôpital Necker in Paris, and at other European centers. By 1963, 20 further transplants between identical twins had been performed at the Peter Bent Brigham Hospital alone—and only 5 of these had failed.

Since most people in need of transplants do not have an identical twin who could be called upon to sacrifice an organ, attempts are being made to neutralize the immunological rejection processes of the recipient to foreign transplants. Since 1948 it has been known that total body irradiation diminishes the activity of these immunological mechanisms. But it was not until 1959 that a human body was irradiated prior to a grafting operation. Dr. Jean Hamburger and his colleagues in Paris achieved some successes with high irradiation doses. Alas, such high radiation leads, in itself, to serious blood disease complications.

Lately, radiomimetic drugs—that is, drugs that act similarly to radiation—have been introduced. The best drug of this kind is probably azathioprine, but it, too, tends to damage bone marrow and to encourage infection. It seems reasonable to prophesy, though, that in the near future better and more refined ways will be found to neutralize the immunological reactions of the body. Then, and then only, will transplantation operations become an altogether more common occurrence.

It could also happen that healthy living people will not be called upon to sacrifice an organ. Already kidneys from fresh cadavers have been used and recent results have been promising. Thus Doctors J. F. Mowbray, S. Cohen, and colleagues at St. Mary's Hospital, London, have reported that of 20 patients in terminal renal failure 8 were still alive with functioning cadaver transplants 3–20 months after their operations, and W. J. Kolff and his colleagues have had similar results in the U.S.A.

The kidneys of most patients dying in hospital, however, are not suitable for transplantation purposes. It is now known, for instance, that patients who have died from disseminated cancer often have undetectable cancer cells in their kidneys. After a successful cadaver kidney transplant these previously undetectable cancer cells can grow, multiply, and spread to kill the new host. Nevertheless cadaver kidney transplantation has a very real future and though further research is clearly needed it will become an increasingly acceptable operation for those patients dying of renal disease.

When the immunological barriers are broken, cadaver transplants other than kidney ones are likely to be performed. Already lung transplantations have been attempted. The first of these was carried out at the University of Mississippi Medical Center on June 12, 1963, by Dr. James D. Hardy, who prior to the operation had, over a period of seven years, performed some 500 lung transplantations in animals. The patient died after 18 days but the transplanted lung functioned

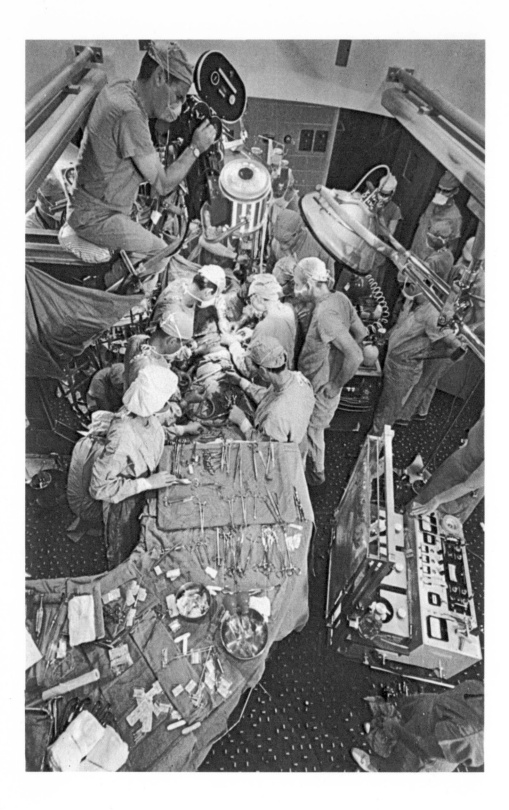

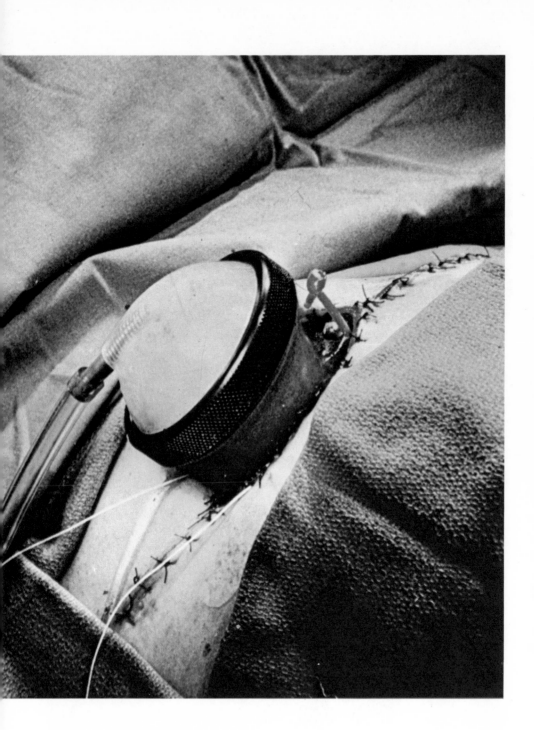

The historic DeBakey operation—an attempt
to relieve a patient's failing heart by
inserting a plastic "bypass" pump powered
by compressed carbon dioxide. Above, the
bypass pump, stitched in position.

during that time. Subsequently, Dr. Hardy commented: "This case demonstrated that human lung transplantation is technically feasible and that the homograft functioned. The way is open to permanent lung transplants between identical twins." At present, doctors have to say regrettably to patients fighting for breath, "Alas we can't give you a new pair of lungs." The day may well come when the patient replies, "Why not, doctor?" And others may well be demanding new livers and even new hearts. Such a hypothesis no longer belongs merely to the pages of fabulous science fiction.

Nor is "spare part surgery" a question of transplantation of organs only. Artificial devices have been invented that may partially or totally replace the body's organs. Recently Russian surgeons reported that they had implanted an artificial urinary bladder into a 24-year-old girl. The patient had apparently suffered from tuberculosis of the bladder so that a large part of the bladder wall had to be removed. The Soviet surgeons from Kiev stated that their patient had made a good recovery. In the U.S.A. millions of dollars are being spent on

Below, the "minicoil" artificial kidney, developed in Britain in 1962. Machines of this kind can help cases of chronic renal failure to lead relatively normal lives.

Right, two types of pacemaker—used to administer regular electric impulses to faulty hearts. The background X ray shows a pacemaker positioned in the body.

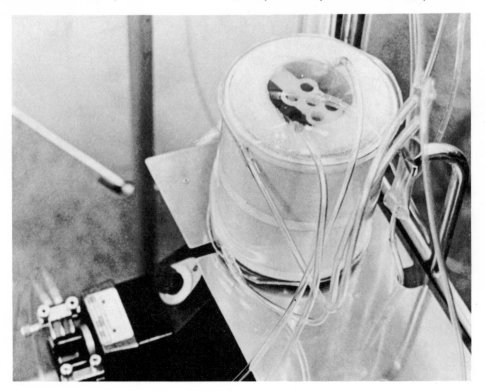

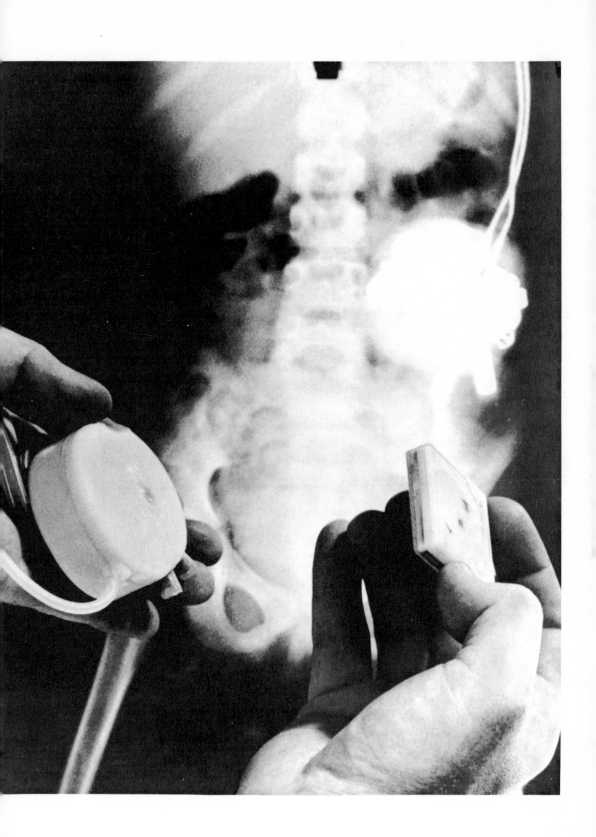

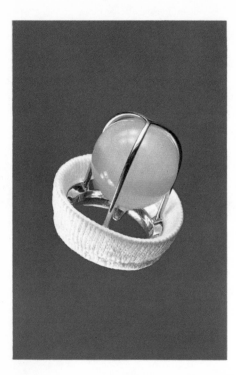

Left, an aortic prosthesis, developed during the 1960s to replace damaged or worn-out valves in the human heart. Below, an aortic valve is inserted into a human heart and its padded ring stitched to the human tissues. Right, another heart valve—a mitral prosthesis—is stitched into position.

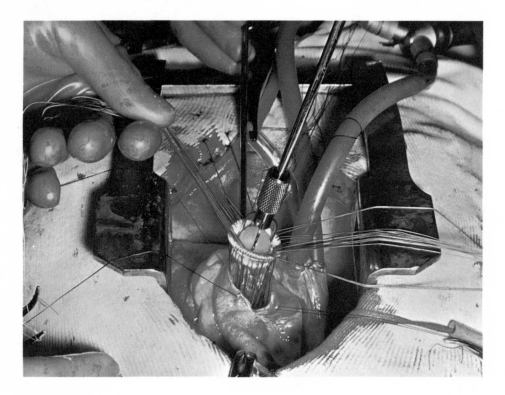

developing an artificial heart or an artificial supplement to the human heart. In April 1966, Dr. Michael DeBakey, at Houston, Texas, inserted a cardiac device that he hoped would temporarily relieve his patient's failing heart and so give it a chance to recover fully. On this occasion the patient died, but undoubtedly there will be many other pioneering operations of this kind in the very near future.

With the development of spare part surgery, doctors and society as a whole will be confronted with unexpected ethical problems. Already some surgeons want permission to remove the healthy kidney of persons who are fatally injured but still living, in order to use it as a graft. Dr. Belding H. Scribner, in his presidential address at the annual meeting of the American Society for Artificial Internal Organs in April 1964, discussed some of these problems—and indeed took up the problem of donor selection for organ transplantation. "On this subject," he said, "I speak to you as a patient as well as a physician because I am looking at you through donated corneas and therefore feel a very personal debt to a society which permitted the evolution of eye banks and willed eyes which makes the donation of corneas possible. As we all know, the problem of donating organs other than the cornea which can be stored in a bank is greatly complicated by the fact that storage for

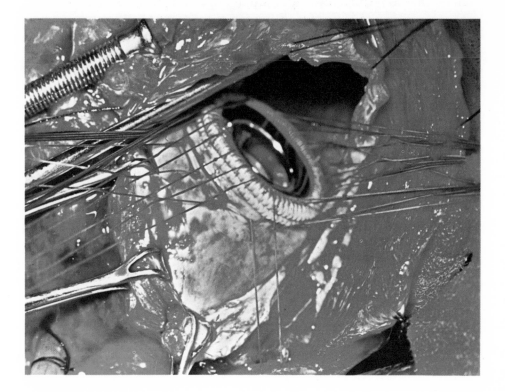

most organs is difficult, if not impossible. Hence, donation prior to or at the moment of death becomes a real consideration and this fact introduces all sorts of ethical, legal and religious complications. For example, in the state of Washington, it is illegal to obtain an autopsy permit prior to death. As a result, our first kidney donor's husband and minister were forced to stand by her bed for eleven long hours watching in horror as the last spark of life ebbed away, and when death finally came, the kidney to be donated had been severely damaged by the terminal agonal events. . . . If I knew that I had a fatal disease I would seriously consider volunteering to donate one of my kidneys while I was still well, and as far as death is concerned, I would like to be able to put into my will a paragraph urging that when my physician felt that the end was near, I be put to sleep and any useful organs taken prior to death. I wonder how many people feel as I do? I think the ethical and legal guidelines should be devised to permit me and others to volunteer in these ways."

Elsewhere is his address, Dr. Scribner raised the problem of "death control." He pointed out that many patients dying from uremia (a toxic condition caused by insufficient secretion of waste products) could be humanely relieved of their slow suffering by the weekly use of an artificial kidney machine (hemodialysis). The dying patient "could live a normal life right up to the end and die quickly and without prolonged suffering. But such a maneuver to provide hemodialysis for a limited period which would avoid all of the suffering and much of the expense that characterizes natural death from uremia is utterly impossible under existing moral, ethical and religious guidelines." At the moment there are not enough artificial kidney machines to rehabilitate people who, given this treatment, would survive. No doubt, though, the question of death with dignity and death control will become an ethical problem that future generations will have to redefine and solve.

At present it is birth control rather than death control that occupies the attention of research doctors. Though the oral contraceptive pills and the new IUCDs (intrauterine contraceptive devices) have only been introduced comparatively recently, even newer refinements in contraception are likely to be introduced in the near future. On

The most advanced form of operating theatre (a hyperbaric oxygen chamber), recently installed at Glasgow's Western Infirmary— the hospital where Joseph Lister introduced antiseptic surgery in the 1860s.

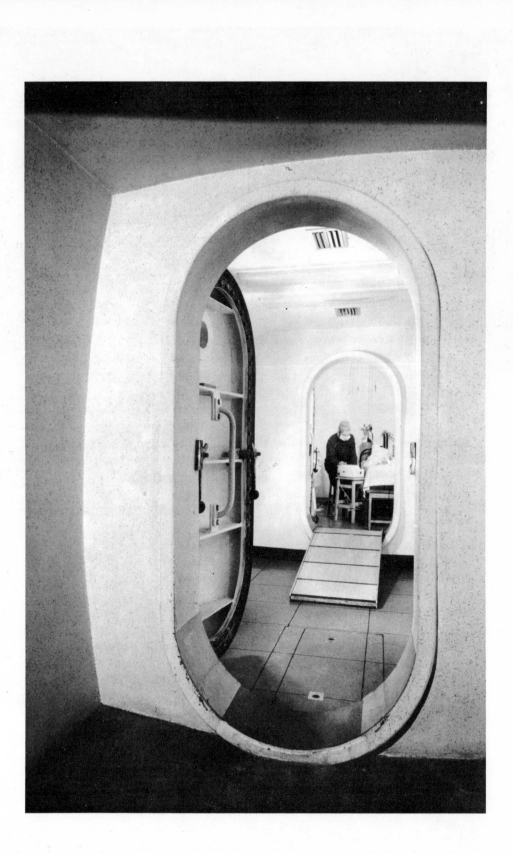

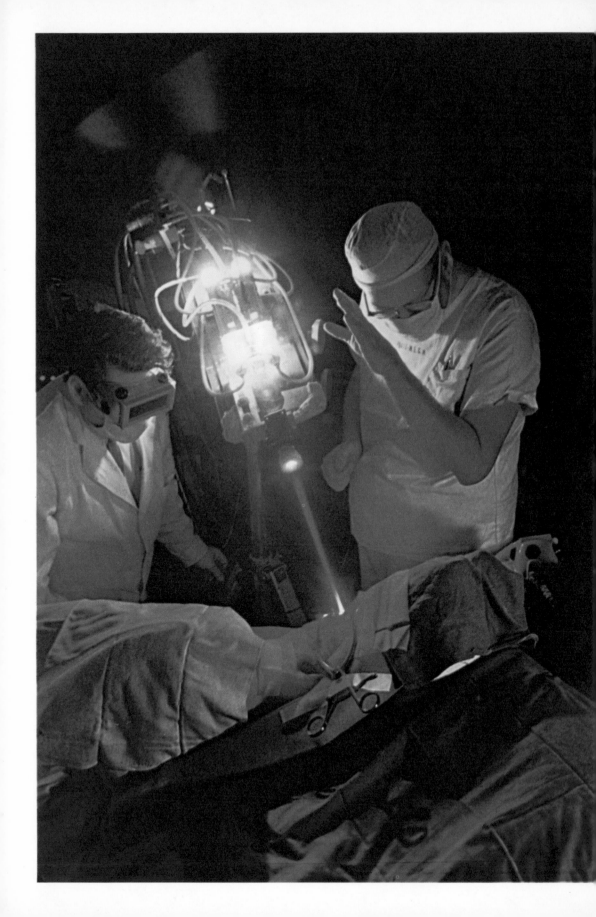

January 19, 1965, Dr. Edward T. Tyler of the University of California reported on the promising results he had obtained among Los Angeles women who had been given long-action contraceptive hormones by once-a-month injections. A year later (in January 1966), Dr. Gregory Pincus of the Worcester Foundation for Experimental Biology in Shrewsbury, Massachusetts, maintained that once-a-year anti-pregnancy vaccination is possible. Animals had already been prevented from conceiving by such annual injections. And in April 1966 Dr. Merrit Callantine, of Parke, Davis research laboratories, reported that success-ful trials had been concluded with animals on a morning-after pill—that is, a pill taken after intercourse. This pill, an analogue of stilboestrol, is at present called CN–5518.

Apart from contraceptive pills, new developments with fertility drugs continue. One of these drugs is clomiphene, a hormone that acts as an anti-fecundity agent in the rabbit and the rat but produces the opposite action in certain childless women. Dr. Peter Bishop at Chelsea Hospital for Women, London, gave the drug to 120 apparently sterile married women. Sixteen of them subsequently became fertile enough to conceive. Infertile men, too, as a result of a new hormone that causes primitive sex cells to develop into mature ones, may soon be able to father children. Dr. Alfred Byrne reported in *The Sunday Times* of April 10, 1966, on work done by Dr. Carl Heller of Washington State and Dr. Yves Clermont of Quebec with convict volunteers from an Oregon jail. "After injecting the convicts with a radio-active 'tracer' they punched out portions of the men's testes and from them made an intensive microscopic study of the reproductive cells at various stages of their development. This revealed that it takes about 74 days for a sperm to mature. Hence the reason that the new hormone therapy must be conducted for 80 to 100 days." This new hormone, known as the human menopausal gonadotrophin, was given for 80 days to 100 men with a low sperm count that had made them infertile. Subsequently 38 of them increased their mature sperm ratios and several later fathered children.

Meanwhile the debate continues about the advantages and dis-advantages of the present oral contraceptive pill. For example, Hilda O'Hare wrote from Cornwall to the *New Statesman* of June 17, 1966: "Many of our clinic patients whom we thought happily settled on the pill have changed to our more recent IUCD method, and still more would do so if only it were 100 per cent effective, as is claimed for the pill. Inquiries as to why they wish to change bring floods of confidences: e.g. 'What is the use of a perfectly safe contraceptive if you lose interest in sex?' . . . 'I just feel different' . . . 'I feel apathetic about the whole thing.' More disturbing are the women who notice no differences

A laser beam replaces the surgeon's knife in a skin cancer operation in America. This intense wave front of light has immense potential in surgery.

themselves but whose husbands ask 'Have you stopped loving me?' or who suffer such a drying of the vaginal tissues that they have to buy a lubricant. Whilst no ordinary man can expect the privileges of a sheikh with a very large harem—a female on heat always available—he surely deserves a better fate than intercourse with a permanently pregnant (physiologically speaking) wife."

That the changing endocrine status of the human female may affect her sexual attractiveness for the male is not a matter raised generally when the pros and cons of the pill are discussed. Lately, though, an 18-month investigation of the sexual behavior of six pairs of adult male and female rhesus monkeys has been concluded, and the findings seem most pertinent. *The Lancet* of May 7, 1966, reports that the female monkeys were regularly introduced into the cages of males for one hour, and experienced observers watched their sexual behavior from behind a one-way mirror. "The most notable finding is that dramatic changes in the sexual behaviour of males result when hormones are administered to their female partners: oestradiol stimulates male copulatory activity and progesterone depresses it. . . . In particular, the mounting activity and ejaculatory capacity of the males is notably diminished by the administration of progesterone. . . . These findings may have implications for the human situation where women are taking progestational substances orally for contraceptive purposes over prolonged periods." Of course what may be relevant for a female rhesus monkey may not be so for a woman. As Max Beerbohm once said, "Women are a sex by themselves, so to speak."

While some scientists are trying to discover ever more effective and safer methods of contraception, others seek means whereby human eggs can be fertilized outside the mother's body. In 1965 it was announced that the Cambridge physiologist Dr. R. G. Edwards had succeeded in culturing human ova up to that point where they were capable of being fertilized by spermatozoa. From this the once bizarre idea that human embryos might be reared in a test tube enters the realms of possibility. Dr. Edwards foresees that cultured human embryos could be used to avoid certain transmissible genetic diseases. For example, hemophilia is a blood disease that results from a genetic defect carried by the chromosomes of the affected female. Hemophilia, however, only affects, clinically, the male of the species. Thus a woman with a familial history of hemophilia could supply ova that could be fertilized in a test tube. Subsequently a female embryo could be selected from the culture and implanted into her womb to ensure that she gave birth to a daughter and not a son. It is possible to imagine other medical uses of human embryos reared in the laboratory; but to some the whole idea will seem repugnant and somewhat crazy.

In the field of molecular biology, too, Brave New World experiments must frighten some who wonder whether there are certain things that man should not try to do. In January 1966, the Australian biologist and Nobel Prize winner Sir Macfarlane Burnet, went as far as to write (in *The Lancet*): "It seems almost indecent to hint that, so far as the advance of medicine is concerned, molecular biology may be an evil thing." Molecular biologists can alter the genetic makeup of viruses and Sir Macfarlane Burnet fears that a new deadly virus might be brought into being that could infect humankind.

Visions of white-coated, heartless men breeding lethal viruses or rearing embryos in the laboratory and bringing forth genetic monsters are all too easy to come by. If one believes with the British writer Malcolm Muggeridge, for example, that, "The way of life in urbanised rich countries, as it exists today and is likely to go on developing, is probably the most degraded and unillumined ever to come to pass on earth," then future medical practice can only be visualized in nightmare terms. Those who believe, however, that today we are more concerned with the dignity and rights of the individual than we have ever been before will look forward to tomorrow's medical discoveries with an altogether different expectancy.

Of course the attitude of the scientist should be utterly objective; but like everyone else he is endowed with subjective feelings of optimism and pessimism that, in any case, vary with his own varying personal life-situations. Speculative crystal gazing, however informed, is not a scientific exercise. Yet it is vital that scientists of all nations should speculate on the practical application of imminent or possible future medical discoveries. Scientific optimism on the one hand can lead to a rich creativity, while pessimism, on the other, can warn us of those dangers we might prefer to ignore. A certain courage is required if we are to think of things we are not accustomed to, and it seems to me that those who are knowledgeable must not only proceed with their scientific enquiries but also, from time to time, take up responsible admonitory stances. The scientist nowadays must look into the abyss even though, as Neitzsche has warned, the abyss may start looking back at him.

# Index

Page numbers in *italics* refer to illustrations.

343

347

Transplantation, 324–7, *324,* 332–4; of
bladder, 330; of heart 332; in identical
twins, 326–7; and irradiation, 327; of
kidney, 327; of lung, 327–30; of organs,
*312,* 321–2, 324; rejection of alien tissue,
326; testicular, *248*ff., *253*; *see also*
surgery
Trentin, John J., 319–20
Trocchi, Alexander, 207
Truman, Harry S., 67
Truth drug, *see* scopolamine
Trypan red, 27
Tuberculosis, 34ff., *34,* 36, 55, 66, 76, 156,
168, 176, 268, *296*; and antibiotics, 37ff.;
bacillus, 36, 78; of bladder, 330;
chemotherapy, 36ff.; history of, 34;
military, 175; quiescent, 67
Tuke, Samuel, 99–102
Tuke, William 99–102
Twain, Mark, 300
Typhoid fever, 139, 144, 292, *296*
Typhus, 128
Tyrothricin, 299

Ulcers, 174, 223; duodenal, 74, 174, *176,*
182; gastrointestinal, 75; peptic, 67, *297*
Unconscious mind, 108, 121; collective, 107;
*see also* Freud, Jung, psychoanalysis,
psychology
University: of Birmingham (England), 230;
of California (U.S.A.), 219, 334; of
Edinburgh (Scotland), 300, *300*; of
Geneva, 255; of Gothenburg (Sweden),
308; of Göttingen (West Germany), 110,
248; Johns Hopkins (U.S.A.), 31, 59, 90;
of Manchester (England), 90; of Michigan
(U.S.A.), 308, 309; of Minnesota (U.S.A.),
*312*; of Mississippi, Medical Center
(U.S.A.), 327; of Montreal (Canada), 73;
of Ottawa (Canada), 310; Queen's, Belfast,
275; of Toronto (Canada), 61; of Virginia
(U.S.A.), 185; of Washington (U.S.A.),
140; Yale (U.S.A.), 141, *307*
Upjohn (pharmaceutical company), 278, 284
Upstate Medical Center (U.S.A.), 323
Urine, 196, 239, 306; in diabetes, 58–9, *60,*
U.S.A., 33, 48, *51, 53,* 54, *56,* 66, *69,* 83, 102,
106, 113, 126, 135, 137, 139, 141, *143,*
146, 154, *155,* 160, *165,* 169, *170,* 172,
180, 182, 183, *186,* 194, 195, 198, 219,
227, 228, 239, *243,* 246, 266, 277ff., *283–4,*
*286,* 290, 318, 319, 326, 327; alcoholism
in, 220–3; drug addiction in, 195, *197,*
198–206, *208,* 211, *214*; use of H3, *259,*
260; infant mortality in, 236; and
longevity 232, *236*; and LSD, 110, 219;
lung cancer in, 231; mental illness in, 88,
98ff., oral contraceptive, 63; poliomyelitis
in, 51; suicide rate, 262
U.S. Army Chemical Center, 135
U.S. Defense Department, 135
U.S. Department of Health, 261
U.S. Public Health Service, 142
U.S.S.R., 46, 108, 135, 139, 141, 250, 290,
302, *311*; alcoholism in, 228; cancer
research in, 321; transplantations, 330

Vaccination, *34, 45,* 48, 232; encephalitis
danger, 46; Jenner, 44ff.; poliomyelitis
vaccine, 50ff., 53ff., 55, 146; against
pregnancy, 337; rabies, 47–8; Salk, 53ff.,
146; smallpox, 44ff., *45,* 55; typhus, 128;
yellow fever, 50ff., *51*; *see also*
immunization, inoculation
Van Winkle, Dr. E., 306
Vienna, 103, 165, 248, 249
Vinaze, Dr. Andreas, 281
Viractin, 318
Virchow, Rudolf, 76
Virology, 41, 143, 320–1; *see also* viruses
Viruses, 41ff., *43,* 54ff., 128, 286, 317–8; and
antibodies, 54ff.; common cold, 41ff., 146;
composition, 41; enterovirus, 53; herpes,
41; poliomyelitis, 50ff., *53*; rabies, 47ff.,
6; rhinoviruses, 41; size of, 41; smallpox,
44ff.; viractin, 318; yellow fever, 50;
*see also* infection
Vitamins, 41, 58, *85,* 97, 156, 174; A, 82;
advertisements 83, 299; antineuritic,
56; B12, 79, 82, 159, 283; C, 57, 82; D,
82; growth-stimulating, 56; K, 58, 82; and
malnutrition, 82–5; supplements, 83
Voronoff, Serge, 248–54, *253,* 261
Vortel, *297*

Wade, Prof. O. L., 275
Wagner, Robert F., 199
Wakefield, Edward, *100*
Waksman, Prof. Selman A., 36ff., 56, 78, 301
Walker, Kenneth, 80
Warfare, 135ff.; biological, 139–40;
chemical, *136,* 140; germ, 137, 139, *139*;
psychochemical, 135–7; radiological, 140;
research on, 136
Warner, William R., & Co., 270
Warner Chilcott (pharmaceutical company),
298
Waugh, Evelyn, 270
Weber, Max, 185
Weinstein, Dr. H. J., 277
Weiss, B., 90
Weiss, Edward, 182
Wells, H. G., 62
Weyer, Johann, *95*
Weygandt, Prof. Wilhelm, 79
Whipple, George H., 56–7, 80–1
White, Edward, *155*
White, William C., 37
Whitehead, Alfred North, 324
Whitehead, Ted, 273
Wikler, Dr. Abraham, 210
Williams, L. Norman, 130
Wilson, Dr. G. M., 277
Wirths, Edward, 134
Witchcraft, 94, *95*
World Health Organization, *34, 43,* 50, 65,
85, 263, 316; on drug addiction, 188–90;
on mental illness, 88

Yellow fever, 43, 48ff., 50, *51*; vaccine, 48
Yellowlees, Dr., 179
Young, James Harvey, 160
Yugoslavia, 26, 255, 314

# Acknowledgments

Key to picture positions: (T) top (C) center (B) bottom; and combinations, e.g. (TL) top left (BR) bottom right.

Photos Paul Almasy: 202–3, 212 225(B)

Photos Warren Andrew, Ph.D., M.D., Indiana University, Indianapolis: 237

The Arthritis and Rheumatism Council, London: 68

Associated Press: 129(TR), 139, 279, 284

Courtesy of Farbenfabriken Bayer, Leverkusen: 32(T)

Courtesy Bayerischen Staatsgemalde-sammlungen, München: 105

The Bettmann Archive Inc.: 95(TL), 97

Reproduced from Sir Robert W. Boyce, *Mosquito or Man?*, John Murray (Publishers) Ltd., London, 1909: 51(TL)

British Museum (photographs reproduced by courtesy of the Trustees): 161(B), 162–6; photos John Freeman: 34, 49(T), 60, 100, 101(T), 157, 221(T), 234(B), 244

Brown Brothers, New York: 28(B)

Photos Bucharest Institute of Geriatrics: 258–259

Photos Mike Busselle: 177, 181(BR), 216–7, 264–5, 269, 271–2, 288–9

Romano Cagnoni, London: 208(B), 209

Camera Press Ltd., London: 129(TL)

J. Allan Cash: 25

Photos Ciba Ltd., Basle: 32(B)

Ciba Pharmaceutical Company, Summit, New Jersey, 1950: 96

Photo Cleveland Clinic: 70

Photo Gerry Cranham: 57

Culver Pictures: 104

Photos José M. R. Delgado, *Evolution of Physical Control of the Brain* (James Arthur Lecture on the Evolution of the Human Brain, American Museum of Natural History, New York, 1965): 307

Edwards Laboratories Inc., photos Studio Briggs: 332

Photo Max Ehlert: 256(T)

*Electronic Medical Digest*, 1924, 1946: 170–1

Epinal Museum, photo Ciba Ltd., Basle: 64

Epoque Limited, London: 234(T)

Photo Jack Esten: 256(B)

European Picture Service, New York: 127

Photo Free Chinese Centre, London: 241

Photo John Freeman: 229

Photo Collection Ernst L. Freud, London: 92

Photos Mario Giacomelli, Ancona: 175, 240(T)

Glaxo Research Limited, photos Behram Kapadia: 21, 29(T)

Courtesy Billy Graham Evangelistic Association Ltd., London: 186

Courtesy Board of Governors, Guy's Hospital, London: 121

Imperial War Museum, London: 136

Photo Behram Kapadia: 184(B)

Laboratoire d'Histophysiologie, Collège de France, Paris: 247

Photo courtesy Lederle Laboratories, Division American Cynamid Co.: 39(T)

Photo The Library of Congress, Washington, D.C.: 161(TR)

*Life* © 1967, Time Inc.: 274, 305, 312–3, 325, 328–9

Magnum. Photos Werner Bischof: 84; Henri Cartier-Bresson: 150; George Rodger: 167; Ian Berry, 192–3; Bob Henriques: 221(B)

Felix Mann, *Atlas of Acupuncture*, Heinemann Medical Books Ltd., London: 176(L); courtesy Felix Mann: 176(R)

Mansell Collection: 77

Mead Johnson Laboratories: 151

Photo Adolf Morath: 181(BL)

*Münchener Medizinische Wochenschrift* (Galerie Hervorragender Ärzte und Naturforscher) J. F. Lehmanns Verlag, München: 80

Musée d'Oswiencim, Poland: 125, 132–3

Courtesy Bureau of Narcotics, Treasury Department, Washington, D.C.: 213

The National Association for Mental Health, photo John Brooke: 120

Courtesy Director of the Art Department, Netherne & Fairdene Hospitals, Coulsdon, photos Mike Busselle: 89, 116–7, 189

Photo Morris Newcomb: 310

Novosti Press Agency: 311

*On the Bowery*, Prod. & Dir. Lionel Rogosin and Mark Sufrin, U.S.A., 1955: 225(T)

Photo PAF International: 240(B)

Photo courtesy the Parke-Bernet Galleries, Inc., and Mrs. A. Varick Stout, the owner: 69

Photos Lynn Pelham, courtesy Camera Press Ltd., and the Curtis Publishing Company: 191, 198–9

Chas. Pfizer & Co. Inc., New York: 28(T), 39(B)

Photopress, Zürich: 250

Paul Popper Ltd.: 51(TR), 208(T)

Powick Hospital, LSD Unit, Worcester, photos John Brooke: 112–3

Radio Times Hulton Picture Library: 95(TR), 226

Photo Rapho, Paris: 101(B)

Courtesy Rediffusion Television, London: 119; photo Maurice Hatton: 118

*Report*, London, photo Robert E. Wilson: 152–3

Photos C. F. Robinow: 24(TL & TR); photo-micrograph C. F. Robinow, Woutera van Iterson, and RCA laboratories: 24(BL)

Courtesy A. H. Robins Company, Inc.: 72

Reproduced by kind permission of the President and Council of the Royal College of Surgeons of England: 324

*Saturday Evening Post*, © 1967 The Curtis Publishing Company: 214

© 1962, *Scientific American*. All rights reserved: 236, 238

Courtesy *The Scotsman*: 138

Prof. Selye, *Second Annual Report on Stress*, Acta Inc., Medical Publishers, Montreal; Courtesy the author: 73

Photos Senior Citizens Village Inc., sponsored

by California League of Senior Citizens:
242–3

Photos Kurt Severin, South Miami: 197, 215

Photo courtesy the Smithsonian Institution,
161(TL)

Photo Staatliche Museen, Berlin-Dahlem: 233

Photo Studio Briggs: 301

Photos *The Sunday Times*, London: 296–7

By courtesy of the Trustees of the Tate
Gallery, London: 109

United Nations photo: 49(B)

United Press International (U.K.) Ltd.: 65,
143, 286

Courtesy Prof. Pasteur Vallery-Radot: 48(B)

*Weekend Telegraph*. Photos Anthony
Howarth: 147; Alexander Low: 200–1,
204–5

Wellcome Historical Medical Museum: 44(B),
184(T), 245, 253

WHO photos: 29(B), 35, 42–3, 45,
52(T & B), 71, 85, 93, 224, 316, 331

Photomicrograph Wild Heerbrugg Ltd.:
24(CT)

*World Medicine*: 280–1, 300, 315, 330, 335–6

**Text Credits**

*How the Poor Die* by George Orwell,
reprinted by permission of Miss Sonia
Brownell and Secker and Warburg Ltd.

*The Story of Puerperal Fever—1800-1950*
by Leonard Colebrook, published by the
British Medical Journal.

*The Conquest of Tuberculosis* by Selman A.
Waksman, published in Great Britain by
Robert Hale Ltd; published in the U.S.A.
by the University of California Press.

*Man, Nature and Disease* by Richard
Fiennes, published by George Weidenfeld
and Nicolson Ltd; reprinted in the U.S.A.
by permission of the New American
Library, Inc.

*The Stress of Life* by Hans Selye, Copyright
© 1956 by McGraw-Hill, Inc. Used by
permission of McGraw-Hill Book Company;
published in Great Britain by
Longmans, Green & Co. Ltd.

*Medizin von Morgen* (*Frontiers of
Medicine*) edited by Rudolph Friedrich,
reprinted by permission of Liveright
Publishers. New York. Copyright © 1961,
by Liveright Publishers. "Frontiers of
Medicine" (*Sunday Times* Magazine
special issue, December 6, 1964). Article by
Ludovic Kennedy.

"Madness, Badness, Sadness" in *Collected
Essays* by Aldous Huxley; published in
Great Britain by Chatto and Windus Ltd;
published in the U.S.A. by Harper and Row.
Reprinted by permission of Mrs. Laura
Huxley.

*The Life and Work of Sigmund Freud* by
Ernest Jones, published in Great Britain
by the Hogarth Press; published in the
U.S.A. by Basic Books, Inc., New York.
Reprinted by permission of Mrs. Katherine
Jones.

*Drugs of Hallucination* by Sidney Cohen,
published in Great Britain by Martin Secker
and Warburg Ltd; proprietors, Atheneum
Publishers.

*Auschwitz in England* by M. M. Hill and
L. N. Williams, published in Great Britain by
MacGibbon and Kee Ltd.; reprinted in the
U.S.A. by permission of Stein and Day.

*Perspectives in Biology and Medicine*.
Volume VI, No. 4—"Medical Ethics and
Biological Warfare" by Dr. Theodor
Rosebury, reprinted by permission of
The University of Chicago Press.

*Social Pathology* by L. Guy Brown,
published by F. S. Crofts in 1942; reprinted
by permission of Appleton-Century-Crofts,
U.S.A.

*Narcotics, Delinquency & Social Policy* by
Chein *et al.*, published in Great Britain by
Tavistock Publications Ltd; published in
the U.S.A. as *The Road to H* by Basic
Books, Inc., 1964.

*Cain's Book* by Alexander Trocchi,
published by Grove Press, Copyright ©
1960 by Grove Press Inc.; published in
Great Britain by Calder and Boyars Ltd.

*A Journey to Paradise* by Robert Graves;
reprinted by permission of Mr. Graves, and
Collins-Knowlton-Wing, Inc. (U.S.A.).

*The Life of Dylan Thomas* by Constantine
FitzGibbon, published by J. M. Dent &
Sons Ltd; reprinted by permission of the
Trustees for the Copyrights of the late
Dylan Thomas.

*Rejuvenation by Grafting* by Serge
Voronoff, published by George Allen &
Unwin Ltd.

*The Image of A Remedy; its power and
manipulation* by Professor O. L. Wade,
published by the Pergamon Press Ltd.,
1963.

*Drugs, Doctors and Diseases* by Brian
Inglis, published by André Deutsch Ltd;
reprinted in the U.S.A. by permission of
Curtis Brown Ltd.

*Man and His Future* edited by
G. Wolstenholme; published by J. & A.
Churchill Ltd. for the Ciba Foundation.
"Progress in Low Temperature Biology" by
J. Farrant and Audrey Smith." Penguin
Science Survey B—1966", published by
Penguin Books.

*The Semi-Artificial Man* by Harold M.
Schmeck, copyright © 1965 by Harold M.
Schmeck, Jr.; published in Great Britain by
George G. Harrap & Co. Ltd; published in
the U.S.A. by Walker and Co.

If the publishers have unwittingly infringed
copyright in any picture or photograph
reproduced in this book, they offer their
apologies and will—upon being satisfied
as to the owner's title—pay an
appropriate fee.